Clinical Skills for Healthcare Assistants

Paula Ingram
*RGN, Dip(Nursing), BN(Hons), Dip(Management), FETC
Senior Practitioner, Clinical Skills, NHS Lothian, Edinburgh*

and

Irene Lavery
*RGN, SCM, BSc Nursing Studies, PG Cert in Professional
Education, Continuing Professional and Practice Development
Practitioner, CPPD Unit, NHS Lothian, Edinburgh*

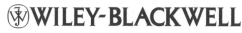**WILEY-BLACKWELL**

A John Wiley & Sons, Ltd., Publication

This edition first published 2009
© 2009 Paula Ingram and Irene Lavery

Wiley-Blackwell is an imprint of John Wiley & Sons, formed by the merger of Wiley's global Scientific, Technical and Medical business with Blackwell Publishing.

Registered office
John Wiley & Sons Ltd, The Atrium, Southern Gate, Chichester, West Sussex, PO19 8SQ, United Kingdom

Editorial office
John Wiley & Sons Ltd, The Atrium, Southern Gate, Chichester, West Sussex, PO19 8SQ, United Kingdom

For details of our global editorial offices, for customer services and for information about how to apply for permission to reuse the copyright material in this book please see our website at www.wiley.com/wiley-blackwell.

Library of Congress Cataloging-in-Publication Data

Clinical skills for healthcare assistants / Paula Ingram and Irene Lavery.
     p. ; cm.
   Includes bibliographical references and index.
   ISBN 978-0-470-51071-1 (pbk. : alk. paper)   1. Nurses' aides.   2. Clinical medicine.
I. Ingram, Paula, 1969-   II. Lavery, Irene, 1956-
   [DNLM: 1. Nurses' Aides–Great Britain–Handbooks.   2. Nursing   Care–methods–Great Britain–Handbooks. WY 49 C6418 2009]
   RT84.C65 2009
   610.7306'98–dc22
                                                                        2008036190

A catalogue record for this book is available from the British Library.

Set in 10/12 pt Sabon by Aptara® Inc., New Delhi, India
Printed and bound in Singapore by Ho Printing Singapore Pte Ltd

Contents

Section 1: Fundamental skills

Section 2: Core clinical skills

Section 3: Complex clinical skills

Preface

This book is aimed at giving readers a comprehensive, easy-to-read resource that will guide them through the clinical skills that they wish to master. It is not a definitive list, but offers a range of what we have termed fundamental skills integral to all clinical practice, core clinical skills, and more advanced skills that require complex practice and so may be less commonly used.

Paula Ingram has taught many clinical skills in a variety of roles namely research nurse, nurse practitioner, ward manager, clinical skills coordinator and, currently, senior practitioner: clinical skills. Irene Lavery has wide experience of clinical skills both in her past role as a charge nurse in respiratory care and in her current role in continuing professional and practice development. Both authors have also collaborated on writing several clinical skills articles.

These previous roles have given both authors experience of the potential barriers and problems with regard to learning clinical skills and help to make the book easy to understand with learning points, case studies and checklists.

We intend that the book be used as a resource for anyone involved in practising or teaching clinical skills. The book can be used for individual skills or in its entirety, and aims to support consistent standards in clinical skills in healthcare practice. However, we do not intend this book to be used as the sole resource to teach a skill, but as a support to existing learning or teaching.

The target audience are healthcare assistants, with the term 'healthcare assistant' encompassing a range of roles with diverse titles, e.g. nursing assistant, clinical support worker. However, we anticipate that it will be a useful resource for newly qualified practitioners and students in health and social care.

Paula Ingram and Irene Lavery

Acknowledgements

We would like to thank our family, friends and colleagues for their moral support, and sincere thanks to the following people in NHS Lothian for their guidance and support; Carol Crowther, Mary Parkhouse, Fiona Cook and Ansley McGibbon.

Thanks also go to Pat Holdsworth, Michelle Caie, Emma J Smith, Lesley MacLean, Catherine Thomson, Maria Pilcher, Jenny Lee, Susan Morrow, David Dewar, Steve Kesterton, Lynsey Dey and Sandy Fleming for their support, proof reading and suggestions. Sincere thanks also to the Illustrator, Barry J. Kirk.

Finally thanks to the following for proof reading and/or giving permission for materials; Suzanne Delaney and Geraldine Brady, and Maggie Byers for her team's competency framework.

We couldn't have written this without them all.

Introduction

The book has been split into three sections:

1. **Section 1** covers fundamental skills applicable to all staff, and is essential as a prerequisite before performing all clinical skills.

2. **Section 2** contains core clinical skills, which includes most of the clinical skills required for clinical practice, and are often taught at a local level.

3. **Section 3** outlines complex clinical skills that require more in-depth training and may be restricted to specialist areas of practice and often require the direct supervision of registered nurses.

Each chapter has the same structure, starting with the aims and objectives of the chapter, followed by the explanation of why the skill is performed, relevant anatomy and physiology, related aspects and terminology, how to perform the skill and common problems. Throughout each chapter case studies and reflection points relating to the topic will be included, encouraging the reader to apply to their own practice. The final section addresses both self and formal assessment where required.

The use of checklists, pictures and clear, concise theory is aimed at making the book a comprehensive yet easy to read resource for all.

Section 1
Fundamental skills

Chapter 1

Accountability

Learning objectives

- Identify the current plans regarding regulation of healthcare assistants
- Define accountability
- Relate accountability to the healthcare assistants role
- Describe the duty of care and how it relates to negligence
- Discuss the process of obtaining consent
- List the key elements of the Mental Capacity Bill

Aim of this chapter

The aim of this chapter is for healthcare assistants to understand the issues and concept of accountability relating both to their role and to others around them.

This chapter covers accountability and issues surrounding accountability in relation to clinical skills. The role of the healthcare assistant has changed dramatically over the past decade, with healthcare assistants taking on roles traditionally associated with registered nurses, including clinical skills (Hancock and Campbell 2006). The introduction of healthcare assistants has been seen as both a necessary and a vital response to previous resource constraints, and to the declining availability of enrolled, student and registered nursing staff on the wards or in the community, with healthcare assistants providing a valuable alternative (Thornley 2000; McKenna et al. 2004).

Healthcare assistants are employed in a variety of clinical settings and carry out a range of tasks and procedures which has led to the distinction between a nurse and a healthcare assistant becoming blurred (McKenna et al. 2004). However, tasks and procedures are being undertaken without regulation, clear boundaries, or systematic education or training (McKenna et al. 2004). Growth in the number of healthcare assistants has increased dramatically and this group is now the fastest growing occupational group in the NHS (Storey 2007). This provides a valuable contribution in healthcare in relation to clinical skills provision for patients.

Regulatory body

Healthcare assistants can join the Royal College of Nursing (RCN) if their routine health or social care work is delegated to them by a registered nurse or midwife, or they have a qualification in health and care level one of the National Qualifications Framework in England, Wales and Northern Ireland or level three of the Scottish Credit and Qualifications framework in Scotland (RCN 2009). The need to regulate healthcare assistants was first raised in *The NHS Plan* (Department of Health [DH] 2000a) and in March 2004 a consultation document was published examining the proposal for extending regulation of healthcare staff (DH 2004). A benefit to regulation would be closing a current loophole that poses a threat to patient safety. This loophole allows previously registered nurses who have been struck off the Nursing and Midwifery Council (NMC) register (see later) to work as healthcare assistants (Nazarko 1999). This could mean that, in practice, patients could be cared for by a healthcare assistant who has previously been sacked for reasons that could include poor quality patient care. Duffin (2006) reports on a convicted rapist who was struck off the NMC register taking up a post as a care assistant at a nursing home for people with mental illness, and how this brought two main issues to the fore: the fact that there was no register for support workers, and that no one oversaw their conduct.

For registered nurses the NMC is the main focus for regulatory accountability. Other professional groups also have professional bodies, e.g. doctors are accountable to the General Medical Council (GMC).

Reflection point

Identify other professional groups within your clinical area and find out the professional bodies to which they report.

Storey (2007) identifies the following reasons for healthcare assistant role regulation to occur:

- To protect the public
- To protect the individual healthcare assistant
- To provide clarity in defining roles of healthcare assistants and healthcare professionals.

Regulation of healthcare assistants is currently being debated but is likely to happen in the future with the general consensus that they should be regulated, the problem being who should do the regulating (Storey 2007).

In Scotland a short working group looked at regulation of healthcare assistants, and the outcome indicated a model of service-led regulation with the addition of a centralised, mandatory, occupational register (Scottish Executive 2006). This led to a project led by the Scottish Executive (2006) with the aim of securing an appropriate form of regulation for healthcare assistants on the grounds of public protection. A supported pilot has been set up with proposed national standards that link to the strand of Agenda for Change concerning knowledge and skills, which will allow the transfer of knowledge and skills for healthcare assistants across the UK. This would ensure that areas such as the recruitment process and conduct and practice would all have a set standard and therefore promote public safety (Scottish Executive 2006). It would also stop healthcare assistants being recruited into posts without any induction or formal training (Parish 2006). The DH (2006a) are looking to adopt this UK-wide employer-led approach to the regulation of this group based on the outcomes of the project. However, the RCN has concerns that, if the central regulation does not encompass all staff who are responsible, or report to nurses, it will not be comprehensive enough (RCN 2006). The NMC is also anxious that they are involved in both developing and implementing an appropriate model (NMC 2006).

What is evident is that current practices will not remain the same, and the current situation with no healthcare assistant register and no professional body to reside over conduct issues will not continue. Proposals in the future for a single code for any health professional in the UK have been suggested, although arguments about whether this can or should be combined in a single body are currently being debated (Caulfield 2005). In the interim healthcare assistants can voice their opinions to unions and their employers while waiting on policy-makers to decide on how registration will be implemented (McKenna et al. 2004).

What do we mean by accountability?

Accountability can be defined as being responsible for the outcome of actions and, as a consequence, taking the blame when something goes wrong (Caulfield 2005). Jacobs (2004) reports that accountability is difficult to describe and that nobody is really sure what it means except that the concept is intrinsically linked to professionalism. For qualified nurses, it is being able to justify actions that require a knowledge base on which decisions are made.

The NMC (2008) states that individual nurses, as professionals, must be accountable for their actions and any omissions in practice. Furthermore, they must also be able to justify decisions that are made. The Code (2008) also states that nurses must:

- Make the care of people their first concern, treating them as individuals and respecting their dignity
- Work with others to protect and promote the health and wellbeing of those in their care, their families and carers, and the wider community
- Provide a high standard of practice and care at all times
- Be open and honest, act with integrity and uphold the reputation of their profession.

Areas of accountability and developing roles

Dimond (2004) reports four areas of responsibility relating to registered nurses as shown in Figure 1.1. As mentioned above, healthcare assistants do not have a professional body, and are therefore not accountable to a profession, but they are accountable in the other areas that are shown and discussed.

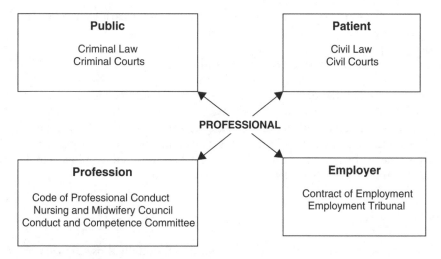

Figure 1.1   Accountability for the registered nurse. (Reproduced from Dimond [2004], with the permission of Pearson.)

Public

Accountability to the public would involve a breach of criminal law and prosecution through the criminal courts (Dimond 2004). An example of this would be if a healthcare assistant caused the death of a patient through their practice. The individual would be prosecuted through the criminal courts for that crime.

Patients

Civil law is actionable in the civil courts and may or may not be a crime (Dimond 2004). Individuals can take out legal proceedings against any healthcare professional, including healthcare assistants. The organisation will take responsibility for this under a concept known as vicarious liability (see later), providing the worker has followed policies and procedures. The law imposes a duty of care (see later) on a practitioner, including healthcare assistants, in circumstances where it is reasonably foreseeable that the practitioner could harm a patient through their action or failure to act (Cox 2006). Healthcare assistants are legally accountable to the patient for any errors that they may make through civil law (RCN 2007). An example here could be if, during cannulation, a healthcare assistant hit a nerve and caused pain, and the patient wished to take legal proceedings.

Employer

The healthcare assistant is accountable to their employer as the contract of employment forms a contractual arrangement and details the employment duties (Caulfield 2005; RCN 2007). It is considered good practice that all employees are given a job description and personal specifications detailing their role and responsibilities (RCN 2007). In relation to healthcare assistants, where the role can be poorly defined and duties therefore misunderstood, the RCN (2007) have suggested that the following guidelines be put in place for primary health care, but the principles are important, and can be related to all areas of practice:

- A clear list of appropriate tasks, with adequate training to enable them to undertake the tasks as necessary
- Clear guidance on role boundaries
- Agreed protocols for the delivery of care
- Clarification of the issues around delegation, accountability, vicarious liability and indemnity insurance (see later)
- Supervision, support and guidance in the role
- Opportunity to develop new roles as practice and patients' needs allow.

It is also recommended that clear lines of responsibility should be identified so it is clear what healthcare assistants are responsible for and to whom. This can be problematic, as Workman (1996) reported, because, if qualified nurses lack clarity in their own role, it has an effect on the role of the healthcare assistant. In addition this can be further complicated in the community setting, because the healthcare assistant and nurse may have different employers making the lines of accountability unclear (Nazarko 1999).

Delegation

Where healthcare assistants who take on tasks that are traditionally those carried out by qualified professionals and are directly given these tasks by qualified staff; these staff remain accountable for the appropriateness of the delegation and for ensuring that adequate supervision or support is provided (Tilley and Watson 2004). A failure to supervise can lead to the nurse who delegates being sued for negligence (discussed later) by the worker to whom she has caused harm, or the patient who has suffered harm (Young 1994). Therefore, delegation of duties to healthcare assistants should be delegated in the knowledge that they will be carried out to the quality standard expected by a nurse who would normally undertake the task (Dimond 2004). This requires an understanding of the role of both the qualified nurse and the healthcare assistant (McKenna et al. 2004).

Reflection point

A registered nurse (RN) delegates the task of taking a patient's temperature using a tympanic thermometer (this measures the temperature in the tympanic membrane in the ear). You have never seen the piece of equipment before. What would your response be? Do you think that this is an appropriate task to delegate?

In the document *Supervision, Accountability and Delegation of Activities to Support Workers: A guide for registered practitioners and support workers*, developed by the RCN, together with The Royal College of Speech and Language Therapists, the British Dietetic Association and the Chartered Society of Physiotherapy (RCN et al. 2006), the following guidance is given about delegation:

Delegation is the process by which a registered practitioner can allocate work to a healthcare assistant who is deemed competent to undertake that task, and the worker then carries the responsibility for that task. Registered practitioners have a legal responsibility to have determined the knowledge and skill level required to perform the delegated task and therefore they are accountable for delegating the task. The healthcare assistant is accountable for accepting the delegated task, as well as being responsible for their actions in carrying it out. There is also a distinction between delegation and assignment. In relation to delegation, the support worker is responsible while the registered practitioner retains accountability whereas with assignment, both the responsibility and accountability for an activity passes from one individual to the other.

It is essential that delegation is appropriate and the principles of delegation adapted from the RCN document (RCN et al. 2006) are shown in Box 1.1.

Reflection point

In relation to these principles, identify and reflect on the tasks that are delegated to you within your own organisation. Seek out any local policies and procedures that are in place to define the tasks that can be undertaken following competency-based training.

Choosing tasks or roles to be undertaken by a healthcare assistant is actually a complex professional activity; it depends on the registered practitioner's professional opinion and, for any

---

Box 1.1 Principles of delegation

- The primary motivation for delegation is to serve the interests of the patient/client, which in turn protects the public.
- The registered practitioner undertakes appropriate assessment, planning, implementation and evaluation of the delegated role.
- The person to whom the task is delegated must have the appropriate role, level of experience and competence to carry it out. This will ensure that the task is appropriate to the individual.
- Registered practitioners must not delegate tasks and responsibilities to colleagues who are outside their level of skill and experience. This will ensure that inappropriate tasks are not delegated.
- The healthcare assistant should undertake training to ensure competency in carrying out any tasks required. This training should be provided by the employer and in some instances will involve supervised practice of the skill before competence is achieved.
- The task to be delegated is discussed and, if both the practitioner and support worker feel confident, the healthcare assistant can then carry out the delegated work/task. This ensures parties are consulted and in agreement.
- The level of supervision and feedback provided is appropriate to the task being delegated. This will be based on the recorded knowledge and competence of the healthcare assistant, the needs of the patient/client, the service setting and the tasks assigned.
- Regular supervision time is agreed and adhered to. This ensures that ongoing support is available.
- In a multiprofessional setting, supervision arrangements will vary and depend on the number of disciplines in the team and the line management structures of the registered practitioners. This is a matter that should be checked locally.
- The organisational structure has well-defined lines of accountability and healthcare assistants are clear about their own accountability. This should be fully discussed and agreed.
- The healthcare assistant shares responsibility for raising any issues in supervision and may initiate discussion or request additional information and/or support. This allows areas of concern to be raised and rectified.
- The healthcare assistant will be expected to make decisions within the context of a set of goals/care plan, which have been negotiated with the patient/client and the healthcare team.
- The healthcare assistant must be aware of the extent of their expertise at all times and seek support from available sources, when appropriate. Where possible, sources of support should be clearly identified with line managers when commencing the role and/or taking on new tasks.
- Documentation is completed by the appropriate person and within employers' protocols and professional standards. This will be different for all organisations and should be checked locally.

---

particular task, there are no general rules (RCN 2007). The NMC (2008) state that for a registered nurse to delegate effectively they must:

- Establish that anyone who is delegated a task can carry out those instructions
- Confirm that the outcome of the delegated tasks meets the required standards
- Ensure that everyone to whom they are responsible is supervised and supported.

In addition it is important to consider the competence of the healthcare assistant in relation to the activity to be delegated and this is discussed next.

The established view is that the public are not concerned about what qualifications individuals possess, only that they are properly trained to carry out the tasks that they perform, and therefore they are unlikely to challenge any change in the role of the healthcare assistant (Hancock and Campbell 2006). In the interest of patient safety, absence of a nationally recognised standard for healthcare assistants linked to an educational programme is overdue (DH 2000b; Field and Smith 2003). Where possible this training should be part of a nationally recognised qualification, e.g. National Vocational Qualification (NVQ) or, in Scotland, Scottish Vocational Qualification

(SVQ). Advantages to this training programme are the potential for a formal recognition of experiential learning, which accredits learning 'on the job' and which many staff may achieve outwith a classroom setting (Thornley 2000). Robertson (2006) suggests that, in theory at least, the potential for training and development for healthcare assistants has never been greater. Local policies and procedures will dictate how clinical skills training and competencies are obtained, and these can be supplementary to those achieved within the NVQ/SVQ framework.

For high-quality educational programmes to function well, it is essential that individuals participating in the delivery of this training should be competent in the skills that they are teaching, and also able to compile accurate records (RCN 2007). The advantages of these qualifications are shown in Box 1.2 (RCN 2007).

Box 1.2 Advantages of qualifications

- Encourages close working relationships between registered and support staff
- Ensures a formal assessment of practical competence across the whole range of support activity undertaken in the workplace
- Provides encouragement for support workers to develop knowledge that underpins the practical aspects of their work
- Allows development of transferable and recognisable knowledge and skills

---

If defined standards of practice were in place, the RCN (2007) would suggest that this would ensure optimum, safe patient care. However, it is also essential that qualified nurses understand these qualifications and the underpinning principles, to ensure that the limitations of the healthcare assistants role are understood (Workman 1996). In specialities such as critical care, there is a feeling that a specialised critical care competency framework would also be beneficial (Ormandy et al. 2004).

Related aspects and terminology

Vicarious liability

This is defined as the liability of an employer for the wrongful acts of an employee committed while in the course of employment. This principle operates to make an employer liable, along with the employee, for any negligence caused by the employee provided that they are operating within the organisation's policies and procedures (Tingle 2004). For example, you have performed venepuncture (the taking or drawing of blood) from a patient, having completed all the appropriate education and competency required by your employer. Unfortunately, the next day the patient has bruising at the site. As you had followed all policies and procedures, should the patient sue, the organisation would take responsibility for your actions.

Indemnity insurance

If a patient sues the employing hospital for negligence due to a nurse or healthcare assistant causing injury, the organisation would cover the nurse under vicarious liability (see above). However, the patient can also decide to sue the nurse or a healthcare assistant as a separate case and, in this instance, indemnity insurance would pay for the nurse's legal costs and the compensation paid to the patient (Caulfield 2005).

The NMC (2008) recommends that professionals in their role for advising, treating and caring for patients take out indemnity insurance. If there are instances where vicarious liability is not accepted, it is pertinent that adequate indemnity insurance is in place. Where indemnity insurance is not secured, patients will need to be fully informed about this, and how this would impact in the event of a professional negligence claim.

If nurses are part of a trade union indemnity cover is usually part of the membership. In cases where registered nurses are not required to have this in place then nor are healthcare assistants. In most instances healthcare assistants will be covered by vicarious liability but this is an area that may change over the next few years. If healthcare assistants work outside their organisation, then care should be taken over establishing whether the other employer, e.g. nursing agency, provides vicarious liability, or if indemnity insurance is required.

Duty of care and negligence

Where a patient or relative is dissatisfied with the care received from either an organisation or an individual, they can sue for clinical negligence. For this to be successful the claimants (patient/relative) must prove the four elements shown in Box 1.3.

Box 1.3 The four elements required to prove clinical negligence

1. The nurse had a duty to provide care to the patient and to follow an acceptable standard of care
It must be established that a legal duty of care is owed to our neighbours, who can be identified as people who are around us (Tingle 2004). Only those who are directly responsible for giving care owe the patient a duty of care, and the concept of duty of care is central to any case of negligence. Once the responsibility for the care of a patient is assumed, it is also assumed that they are owed a legal duty of care (Cox 2006).

An example would be that you are delegated the task of taking a patient's blood pressure; the patient is then owed a duty of care by the healthcare assistant who has been delegated the task.

2. The nurse failed to adhere to the standard of care and there was a breach in the duty
It is generally accepted that every patient should be entitled to a similar standard of care in relation to a particular healthcare intervention, irrespective of where, when or by whom that care is delivered (Cox 2006).

An example would be knowingly not cleansing the skin (as per local policy) before an invasive procedure, e.g. cannulation.

3. The nurse's failure to adhere to the standard of care caused the patient's injuries
The patient was injured due to a substandard of care. An example would be harming a patient by not adhering to the organisation's policy regarding reuse of lancets for blood glucose measurement.

4. The claimant suffered damages as a result of the negligent actions. The damages may be physical, psychological or financial (Showers 1999)
The final part has to prove that the patient was harmed, and the law defines negligence as failure to exercise the degree of care that a reasonable nurse would exercise under the same or similar circumstances (Showers 1999).

An example of this would be a patient developing nerve damage after a healthcare assistant performed venepuncture (taking blood) due to the lack of knowledge of the healthcare assistant, who had not completed competency-based assessment with regard to this skill.

With the role of the healthcare assistant continually changing, often both the individuals performing the job and their managers can be uncertain or confused about the extent of this duty (Cox 2006). The Department of Health published a document *Modernising Nursing Careers: Setting the direction* (DH 2006b), which talks of specialist and advancing roles for registered nurses. As registered nurses take on these roles, it may well widen the role of the healthcare assistant in response to this change.

Reasonable care

In the UK, judges, without input from a jury, consider cases of negligence (Martin 2005). To successfully defend a negligence claim, the standard of care required derives from the case of *Bolam v Friern Hospital Management Committee* 1957. This case of negligence was brought against a hospital by a psychiatric patient called John Bolam who was undergoing electrical convulsive therapy (ECT). During treatment, when the patient convulsed, he sustained several pelvic fractures. The patient then sued for negligence as he did not receive a muscle relaxant or did not have any means of restraint in place during the convulsive period, factors that would have reduced the risk of fracture. The fact that these risks had not been explained to the patient was also cited. The judge then stated the following definition of what is reasonable:

> ...the test is the standard of the ordinary skilled man exercising and professing to have that special skill. A man need not possess the highest expert skill at the risk of being found negligent ... it is sufficient if he exercises the skill of an ordinary man exercising that particular art.
>
> McNair J in *Bolam v Friern Hospital Management Committee* 1957

The doctor was not then found guilty of negligence because he acted in accordance with the practice accepted at the time. This case became the leading reference in medical negligence cases and allowed the courts to accept, without question, a body of professional opinion, as long as that opinion is accepted. Indeed, the court will always take the final decision in negligence cases and, although unusual, this can result in the decision not to apply the Bolam test (Corcoran 2000).

To be successful in proving negligence the claimant must prove a direct link between the breach of the duty of care and the harm that occurred (known as causation); if there is no direct link the action for negligence will not succeed (Martin 2005).

Despite the Bolam test involving medical staff, it is still used in relation to nurses to decide if a professional's actions are reasonable (Ford et al. 2000). A registered nurse professing to have nursing skills must use those skills at an ordinary competent level when exercising the art of nursing. This does not apply to individuals such as healthcare assistants, who do not possess nursing registration and the competent level of skills, and therefore healthcare assistants are not in a position to assess nursing needs, because they have no 'special nursing skills' for this task (Ford et al. 2000).

Consent

When undertaking clinical skills, obtaining valid consent is essential in safeguarding both the healthcare assistant and the patient. Valid consent comprises three main elements (Gates et al. 2004):

1. It is given by a competent person (or their representative)
2. It is given voluntarily
3. It is informed.

Obtaining consent is an opportunity to discuss the procedure fully with the patient and this may involve reassurance and support, especially if the procedure is new to the patient or they have had a previous bad experience. Where possible, choose a quiet environment where you will not be interrupted and give the patient plenty of time to be able to ask questions. Once you are happy that the patient fully understands the procedure and any possible complications, this should be documented.

As mentioned above valid consent must be given voluntarily and freely but it must also be without influence or undue pressure to accept or refuse treatment (Lavery 2003). Care should also be taken to ensure that the elements of voluntariness, appropriate information and capacity have been fulfilled, because otherwise even written consent becomes invalid (GMC 2001). Sometimes patients can infer consent, e.g. rolling up a sleeve ready to have blood taken; however, information and consent must still be obtained. In relation to clinical skills, where the procedure is minor, it is acknowledged that verbal consent is usually acceptable (Lavery and Ingram 2005).

The NMC (2008) state that, in gaining consent:

- It must be given before any treatment or care commences.
- If individuals accept or decline treatment and care, their wishes must be respected and supported.
- People have a right to be fully involved in decisions about their care.

Capacity

The role of the qualified nurse in relation to mental capacity is that they must be aware of the current legislation and ensure that people who lack capacity remain at the centre of decision-making and are fully safeguarded (NMC 2008).

In the speciality of learning disability, capacity and competence are viewed as the ability of the person to understand the information given to them and make an informed decision about their care (Gates et al. 2004). For this particular speciality the DH has issued specific guidance entitled *Seeking Consent: Working with people with learning disabilities* (DH 2001), and it is recommended that this should be accessed where necessary.

In Scotland there is an Adults with Incapacity Act (Scotland) 2000 (Scottish Executive 2000) and incapacity can be defined as an adult over the age of 16 incapable of:

- acting or
- making decisions or
- communicating decisions or
- understanding decisions or
- retaining the memory of decisions.

Lack of capacity may occur, with only one of the above applying, with particular reference to mental illness or inability to communicate because of physical disability. It may be the case that you are the first person to notice a loss of capacity in a patient and, in these instances, further advice and help should be sought.

Reflection point

Identify patients in your care with possible disabilities that would reduce their capacity.

If the patient is deemed incapable of giving consent then treatment will be strictly undertaken in relation to the Incapacity Act or the Mental Health (Care and Treatment) (Scotland) Act 2003.

Part 5 of the Adults with Incapacity Act (relating to medical treatment and research) allowing treatment to be given to safeguard or promote the physical and mental health of an adult who is unable to consent.

In England, the Department for Constitutional Affairs published a factsheet in April 2004 that summarises the key principles of the then Mental Incapacity Bill (now renamed the Mental Capacity Bill). The key principles from this are adapted in Box 1.4.

Box 1.4 Key principles of incapacity (adapted from Department for Constitutional Affairs 2004)

- An assumption of capacity: every adult has the right to make their own decisions and must be assumed to have capacity to do so unless it is proved otherwise.
- Capacity is decision specific: a new assessment must be taken each time that a decision is to be made and no blanket label of incapacity is allowed.
- Participation in decision-making: everyone should be encouraged and enabled to make decisions with help and support given to allow an expression of choice.
- Individuals must retain the right to make what might be seen as eccentric or unwise decisions.
- All decisions must be in the person's bests interests, giving consideration to what the person would have wanted.
- Decisions made on behalf of someone else should be those that are least restrictive of their basic rights and freedoms.

www.dca.gov.uk/menincap/mcbfactsheet.htm

Summary

In summary, accountability of healthcare assistants is currently evolving with impending registration. This will impact on and control the activity of healthcare assistants, something that would be in keeping with the trend for all other healthcare staff (Johnson et al. 2002). In the interim, and following registration, healthcare assistants should ensure that tasks are clearly defined in their job description. In addition a recognised qualification should be sought such as an NVQ/SVQ to ensure safe practice by competent practitioners.

Case study 1.1

A patient requires blood to be taken. You are asked to perform this task. You have had training and done a couple of supervised practice, but have not yet had your final assessment. You take the blood with no injury to the patient. Would this be acceptable, stating your rationale?

Case study 1.2

Mrs Phillips, a 58 year old, requires an indwelling urinary catheter inserted, but has refused before. Discuss how you proceed to try to gain her consent. Are there issues about her capacity that you should consider?

✔ Self-assessment

Assessment	Aspects	
Accountability	*Have you considered all aspects of this section?*	**Achieved ✔**
	To whom are you accountable?	
	The different areas of accountability	
	The healthcare assistant role and delegation	
	Vicarious liability	
Patient	*Have you considered all aspects of this section?*	**Achieved ✔**
	Duty of care and negligence	
	Reasonable care	
	Consent	
	Capacity	

Table of cases

Bolam v Friern Hospital Management Committee [1957] 2 All ER 118–28.

References

Caulfield H (2005) *Accountability*. Oxford: Blackwell Publishing.

Corcoran M (2000) What is negligence? *British Journal of Urology* **86**: 280–285

Cox C (2006) Bound to care. *Nursing Standard* **21**(2): 16–18

Department for Constitutional Affairs (2004) Mental Incapacity Bill (now renamed the Mental Capacity Bill). Factsheet April 2004. Available at: www.dca.gov.uk/menincap/mcbfactsheet.htm (last accessed 1 March 2008).

Department of Health (DH) (2000a) *Meeting the Challenge*. London: The Stationery Office.

Department of Health (2000b) *Recruiting and Retaining Nurses, Midwives and Health Visitors in the NHS: A progress report*. London: DH.

Department of Health (2001) *Seeking Consent: Working with people with learning disabilities*. London: HMSO.

Department of Health (2004) *Improvement, Expansion and Reform: the next 3 years. Priorities and Planning Framework 2003–2006*. London: DH. Available at: www.dh.gov.uk/assetRoot/04/07/02/02/04070202.pdf (last accessed 1 March 2008).

Department of Health (2006a) *The NHS Plan*. London: HMSO.

Department of Health (2006b) *Modernising Nursing Careers*. London: HMSO.

Dimond B (2004) *Legal Aspects of Nursing*, 4th edn. London: Prentice Hall.

Duffin C (2006) Registered post. *Nursing Standard* **21**(3): 18–21.

Field L, Smith B (2003) An essential course for healthcare assistants. *Nursing Standard* **17**(44): 33–35.

Ford P, McCormack B, Wills T, Dewing J (2000) Defining the boundaries: nursing and personal care. *Nursing Standard* **15**(3): 43–45.

Gates B, Wolverson M, Wray J (2004) Accountability and clinical governance in learning disability nursing. In: Tilley S, Watson R (eds), *Accountability in Nursing and Midwifery*, 2nd edn. Oxford: Blackwell, pp. 117–122.

General Medical Council (2001) *Good Medical Practice*. London: GMC.

Hancock H, Campbell S (2006) Developing the role of the healthcare assistant. *Nursing Standard* 20(49): 35–41.

Jacobs K (2004) Accountability and clinical governance in nursing: a critical overview of the topic. In: Tilley S, Watson R (eds), *Accountability in Nursing and Midwifery*, 2nd edn. Oxford: Blackwell, pp. 21–36.

Johnson MRD, Allsop J, Clark M, et al. (2002) *Regulation of Health Care Assistants. The future health worker*. London: Institute of Public Policy Research. Available at: www.Ippr.org.uk (accessed 1 March 2008).

Lavery I (2003) Peripheral intravenous therapy and patient consent. *Nursing Standard* 17(28): 40–2.

Lavery I, Ingram P (2005) Venepuncture: best practice. *Nursing Standard* 19(49): 55–65.

McKenna H, Hasson, Keeney, S (2004) Patient safety and quality of care: the role of the health care assistant. *Journal of Nursing Management* 12: 452–459.

Martin J (2005) Clinical negligence and patient compensation. *Nursing Standard* 19(25): 35–39.

Nazarko L (1999) Delegation dilemmas. *Nursing Standard* 14(13–15): 59–61.

Nursing and Midwifery Council (NMC) (2006) *Review of the Regulation of the Non-medical Healthcare Professions*. London: Royal College of Nursing.

Nursing and Midwifery Council (2008) *The Code. Standards of conduct, performance and ethics for nurses and midwives*. London: NMC.

Ormandy P, Long A, Hulme C, Johnson M (2004) The role of the senior health care worker in critical care. *Nursing in Critical Care* 9(4): 151–158.

Parish C (2006) Healthcare assistants employed on wards 'without any training'. *Nursing Standard* 21 (13): 6.

Robertson, G (2006) Sharing the care. *Nursing Standard* 21(1): 22–25.

Royal College of Nursing (2006) *Review of the Regulation of the Non-medical Healthcare Professions*. London: RCN.

Royal College of Nursing (2007) *Primary Health Care. Health care assistants in general practice delegation and accountability*. London: RCN.

Royal College of Nursing (2009) *Full health care support worker*. London: RCN. Available at https://www.rcn.org.uk/membership/categories/category30 (last accessed 3 June 2009).

Royal College of Nursing, Royal College of Speech and Language Therapists, British Dietetic Association and Chartered Society of Physiotherapy (2006) *Supervision, Accountability and Delegation of Activities to Support Workers: A guide for registered practitioners and support workers*. London: RCN.

Scottish Executive (2006) *National Standards Relating to Healthcare Support Workers in Scotland. Consultation Document*. Edinburgh: Scottish Executive. Available at: http://tinyurl.com/2xedym (accessed 8 September 2007).

Showers J (1999) Protection from negligence law suits. *Nursing Management* 30(9): 23–28.

Storey L (2007) Regulation of healthcare assistants: an ongoing debate. *British Journal of Healthcare Assistants* 1(1): 15–17.

Thornley C (2000) A question of competence? Re-evaluating the roles of the nursing auxiliary and health care assistant in the NHS. *Journal of Clinical Nursing* 9: 451–458.

Tilley S, Watson R, eds (2004) *Accountability in Nursing and Midwifery*, 2nd edn. Oxford: Blackwell.

Tingle J (2004) The legal accountability of the nurse. In: Tilley S, Watson R (eds), *Accountability in Nursing and Midwifery*, 2nd edn. Oxford: Blackwell, pp. 47–69.

Workman B (1996) An investigation into how the health care assistants perceive their role as 'support workers' to the qualified staff. *Journal of Advanced Nursing* 23: 612–619.

Young AP (1994) *Law and Professional Conduct in Nursing*, 2nd edn. London: Scutari Press.

Chapter 2

Communication in healthcare

Learning objectives

- Define effective communication, in relation to healthcare settings
- Identify communication methods and reason for use in practice
- Discuss appropriate communication methods and approaches
- Describe possible communication barriers and ways to overcome

Aim of this chapter

The aim of this chapter is to explore communication methods and challenges related to the healthcare setting, and to enable the reader to maximise their skills in communicating with patients and their family/carers, their colleagues and the wider healthcare team.

Why good communication is important

Communication is a vast and complex topic and so this chapter focuses on the healthcare assistant communicating in a work context with patients, and challenges the reader to look at communication in a different light. *Look at Figure 2.1. What can you see? It might depend on your perspective. Refer to end of the chapter for ideas.*

Definition of communication

> ... imparting or exchange of information, letter, message, etc; social dealings.
>
> (Swannell 1986)

Berglund and Saltman (2002) propose that awareness of different behavioural styles, and therefore varying needs, in an interaction is a good starting point for more effective communication. Although the focus of this chapter is on work settings, consider the difference with respect to a social everyday lifestyle communication and a work-related communication.

Different types of relationships determine the appropriate style of communication, e.g. how we talk with our family will differ from how we talk with our manager, and so some choices of communication are already made for us by the situation or the context.

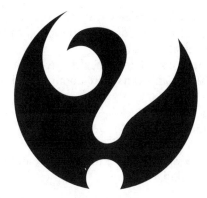

Figure 2.1   Reproduced from Von Oech (1990) with permission.

 Reflection point

This might be a useful point to stop and consider why we need to communicate.

Communication is essential:

- to give instructions
- to ask for information
- to express needs and feelings
- to exchange ideas and thoughts, to entertain
- to give and seek reassurances
- to share experiences.

Swain et al. (2004) noted that it is becoming increasingly accepted that patients need full information to make decisions that are informed and that empower them. To do this they propose the following:

- Check what the patient already knows
- Invite the patient to ask questions
- Make explanations clear and accessible, without the use of unfamiliar jargon
- Avoid a patronising approach
- Support any verbal explanation, where possible, with written information, pictures/diagrams
- Encourage patients to clarify and check out their understanding – ask more questions
- Check that patients have understood, e.g. ask them to repeat instructions: 'I take this pill once in the morning'
- Refer the patient to other sources of information.

So communication is two way, with sender(s) and receiver(s), with the purpose of passing on a message with information; therefore it needs to be to the right person/people, at the right time and in language that is comprehensible to all.

Communication is often the main complaint in healthcare and an Information Services Division (ISD) survey (2005) identified that complaints were about the following:

- 14.5% staff attitudes/behaviours
- 14.5% verbal and oral communication.

These complaints can affect the quality of a patient's care, and is why this book suggests that communication is a fundamental skill.

Communication methods

Let us now review some key aspects of communication in healthcare.

Reflection point

What methods of communication are used in healthcare? Please list below.
Considering this list, write down how most communication is made in healthcare.

Gietzedlt and Jones (2002) proposed that language is made up of two intricately woven parts – verbal and non-verbal cues – and neither can function without the other. They work as a team to produce meaning.

Many people might consider verbal communication as the main method of communicating, but Dickson et al. (1997), Ellis et al. (2003) and Swain et al. (2004) noted that, although the verbal method is important to aid effective communication, the largest aspect of communicating is through non-verbal methods. Ellis et al. (2003) remind us that, in face-to-face communication, a message is received through one or more of the five senses: sight, hearing, smell, taste and touch.

Research by Mehrabian (1972) suggests that:

- 55% of communication is through non-verbal methods
- tone accounts for 38%
- finally, verbal communication is 7% of the total message, so we can see that attention to non-verbal methods is crucial.

So, when communicating, it is important that actions match words because that is what people see, e.g. smiling when saying, 'Hello, pleased to see you', and not frowning, because the receiver might misunderstand the message. In fact the sender may be frowning because it is a very sunny day and they can't see the other's face clearly, but the receiver will see the frown and may think, 'He doesn't really want to talk to me'.

Non-verbal communication

Reflection point

Non-verbal is often classified as body language, so name three ways of communicating using body language:

1

2

3

Dickson et al. (1997) highlighted the six main functions of non-verbal communication:

1. Replacing speech
2. Complementing the verbal message: this is considered the main function of non-verbal communication
3. Regulating and controlling the flow of communication, e.g. nodding, and eye contact to indicate continue speaking
4. Providing feedback, as above
5. Helping define relationships between people, e.g. a white coat to denote role, i.e. doctor
6. Conveying emotional states.

Components of non-verbal communication include: touch, proximity, orientation, posture, body movements, facial expressions, eye contact and appearance.

Touch

In healthcare, touch is one of the most powerful ways that we have of communicating non-verbally. Here culture and gender issues may arise, and so the healthcare assistant should observe the patient for cues as to comfort and acceptance. However, in the scenario in Box 2.1, Sara may have sat down with Annie and held her hand while they had the same conversation, and certainly then Annie would have felt really listened to and cared for.

Proximity

Proximity is about space, and Dickson et al. (1997) suggest that in western cultures we have four zones:

1. Intimate zone of 0–50 cm
2. Personal zone of 50 cm–1.2 m
3. Social/consultative zone 1.2–3.5 m
4. Public zone 3.5 m and above.

Box 2.1 Scenario

It is 07:15 on a busy Saturday shift in an acute hospital ward, when Mrs Annie Wilson, a 54-year-old patient with acute asthma, has rung her bedside buzzer.

Healthcare assistant Sara Smith goes into the single room in response to the buzzer.

Annie: 'Thank goodness, you've come.'

Sara: 'Hello Annie, what's the problem'?

Annie: 'I can't breathe.'

Sara: 'Can't breathe? Oh dear, let me check your oxygen.'

Annie: 'I'm so frightened, I haven't slept a wink.'

Sara: 'Why are you frightened, Annie?'

Annie: 'Because of my asthma, I feel I can't breathe, like I'm choking.'

Sara: 'Now, Annie, you know you are on treatment for your asthma and you are safe in hospital as we are around all the time.'

Annie: 'I still feel like I'm choking, it's terrible . . . .'

Sara: 'I'm sure it must be. What can I do to help make you feel better? Would it help if I put on your fan as it's a bit stuffy in here?'

Annie: 'I was cold and it made too much noise.'

Sara: 'Let's try it, and I'll get you a blanket. How would that be?'

Annie: 'OK, if you think that'll help. Don't leave me please.'

Sara: 'I am only going to get you a blanket.'

They further noted interestingly that, in healthcare, patients' personal space and even intimate space is regularly invaded by staff, often without seeking the patient's permission, and they say that this can increase the vulnerability and loss of control that a patient feels in healthcare. Thus always consider when approaching the patient, particularly if about to undertake a clinical skill, that they should be allowed to give permission, e.g. ask, 'Is it alright if I take your blood pressure?' Then the healthcare assistant can proceed and the patient feels in control of the situation.

Orientation

Orientation is about where and how the communication takes place. Thus, when talking to a patient in a wheelchair, consider the level and where possible make sure that you communicate at eye level, so sit down too. Often in healthcare we talk over objects, e.g. the patient is on one side of a desk or bed and the healthcare assistant is on the other; this artificial barrier can affect the quality of communication too, so consider how to minimise these.

Posture

Posture includes how one stands or sits, looking relaxed and interested, e.g. leaning forward to listen. This links to orientation, and again, in healthcare, if a patient is in bed and we approach them to talk, remember that we are towering above and it can look very dominant or controlling, so sit down.

Body movements

Body movements are a powerful means of conveying non-verbal communication; imagine if Sara (see Box 2.1) had stood with her arms folded during the conversation, what message Annie would have picked up? Probably that Sara does not care or is not interested. However, body language can be misunderstood, as Sara may have had her arms crossed because she was tired and cold after a long night shift.

Be aware also that cultural variances might play a part, e.g. hand gestures in some cultures might offend; Hindle (2003) stated that a gesture that we commonly use in the UK for OK is a circle made with our index finger and thumb; with the other fingers pointing up, this means to a Tunisian, 'I am going to kill you'. Gietzedlt and Jones (2002) noted that Bulgarians and Greeks might signal 'no' by nodding and 'yes' by shaking their head from side to side, unlike most other peoples of the world. So for effective communication be aware of and observe body language during any interaction.

Facial expressions

Think of facial expressions; one example has already been used with frowning, but our faces are often said to tell the story, as we roll our eyes and may not even realise that we are doing so. So, when someone says, 'I see you're unhappy about my idea', it is because of the cue that they have observed, but cues can be misread, so, for communication to be effective, it is about all aspects of communication working together, delivering the same message.

Eye contact

Many suggest that the eyes are a powerful means of communicating non-verbal messages, e.g. the child misbehaving becomes aware of a glare from a parent and swiftly knows that she is in trouble! Eye contact can include or exclude.

Again cultural variances may play a part as some eastern cultures feel that eye contact is rude. This again requires vigilance and observation, and adjusting your eye contact accordingly; however, most cultures would consider avoidance of eye contact as rude. Dickson et al. (1997) identified in western society that the listener usually looks at the speaker about twice as much as the speaker looks at the listener, and that the gaze should be comfortable and appropriate.

Appearance

Finally appearance is a means of communicating non-verbally, e.g. how we dress may reflect our mood or task. In a hospital setting we often ask the patient to get undressed and take away that form of expression (communication). Think of dressing for a night out with friends versus a first date; bet that your wardrobe choice is very different!

So non-verbal cues can be important for the observant healthcare assistant, e.g. while taking blood, the healthcare assistant notices that the patient is looking away and is restless; this body language may tell the healthcare assistant that the patient is nervous or frightened and so they can give reassurance and explanations.

Tone in communication

Now let us briefly think about tone and its importance in effective communication, and again vigilance and self-awareness are necessary. How do we sound to others? If we speak loudly because a person is hard of hearing, will they hear the tone as angry? In healthcare a conversation might be carried out over the phone with a patient's family member so consider how much of the message is lost if they can hear only the tone and words.

Email is another form of communication, and this is where only 7% of the verbal message is left, which is often why people misread a tone in an email, and why people often use pictures to clarify mood, called an 'emoticon'; this one means, I am happy: :>)).

Ellis et al. (2003) say that language can be used to mystify, impress or dominate, and give social position, and not merely inform. This is where tone becomes crucial, as well as the choice of words used, e.g. using jargon that confuses. Imagine that you have been sent a clinic appointment and are a young teenager, so, on arrival at the reception, you ask for Nurse Led, because printed at the top of your appointment card is Nurse Led Clinic. This is an example of jargon and, if the receptionist finds it funny and laughs while explaining, the tone may cause the young teenager to become embarrassed or even angry, resulting in a total breakdown in communication.

Verbal communication

The written word is still classed as verbal communication. There are many advantages with written language, because it allows distribution and uniformity of instruction and information, and so can be re-read and thought over or reflected upon, and is also a permanent record.

Reflection point

However, there may be restrictions on the effectiveness of the written word? Write here what these might be.

People's reading skills need to be considered, so, for instance, can they read, e.g. lost spectacles or font size too small, are they literate (able to read), do they have dyslexia (disorder in reading or writing), is the information too technical, or is English not their first language? All these factors will affect the quality of the written word as a means of communication.

What about the quality of the healthcare assistant's writing if documenting in a care plan? Again this will need consideration; Gietzedlt and Jones (2002) cite a tool to assess the clarity or readability of any piece of work, called the Gunning FOG Index. It simply notes that the lower the score the easier to read, so try comparing a paragraph from a newspaper, e.g. *The Sun* with *The Telegraph*. Refer to the addendum at the end of the chapter for the FOG Index as a guide to this, and writing is explored in more detail in Chapter 4 in relation to writing for record-keeping purposes.

Strategies to improve communication

This section reviews some of the challenges facing effective communication in healthcare.

Reflection point

What might be barriers to effective communication in healthcare?

Let us consider the three aspects related to communication (each of these aspects is reviewed in the scenario in Box 2.1):

- The sender
- The receiver(s)
- The situation: includes environmental factors.

Reflection point

What recommendations might be suggested to enhance the conversation in Box 2.1?

Let us pause here and think over the short conversation:

- Is there evidence of active listening?
- Is there evidence of open questions?
- Is there evidence of any leading questions?
- Is this conversation effective?

Related aspects and terminology

Active listening

Active listening is a process and the most important aspect is to *accept* what is heard, so that the conversation is heard from the sender's (e.g. in Box 2.1, the patient Annie's) point of view (Burnard 1992; Ellis et al. 2003). The receiver is listening for clues – words or phrases – that say what the sender is feeling and expressing. Listening is therefore crucial for effective communication.

In Annie's case she says, 'I'm frightened' and the receiver (Sara) shows that she has heard by acknowledging this; one way is to repeat the word or phrase, so Sara replies, 'Why are you frightened?'. Here Sara has used Annie's word and asked her a question to allow her to expand on this initial statement; this is defined as an 'open' question.

An open question

An open question is phrased in a way that invites the other person to open up and say more, and usually starts with what, why, how, when or where. This encourages a reply, so that there is more in-depth understanding of the situation (Burnard 1997). Closed questions, which usually require a yes or no answer or confirmation of details, e.g. 'Tell me your name', are useful for confirming what is known. In this situation it is more helpful to allow Annie 'space' to tell why she is frightened. 'How' is a useful way of starting a question but take care because this can sometimes lead to one-word answers, e.g. 'How are you feeling?' 'Tired'! Swain et al. (2004) also note that caution should be used for 'why' and suggest limiting its use, otherwise it might feel like an interrogation to the receiver!

Leading questions

This links to leading questions; the risk with these is getting the answer that was wanted and maybe not what was needed, e.g. 'You do want to get up now, don't you?'. There was an example in Box 2.1 with the fan suggestion and, although it may be helpful, Sara has possibly missed the cue about Annie's fear of choking. So care must be taken to use questions that allow the person to expand on and go behind a simple statement.

In one author's experience, a real conversation led to the identification that the patient thought that if she fell asleep her breathing would become poorer and so her oxygen levels would drop, and she would then fall into a coma and die. Only through open questions did we arrive at this fear and so were able to discuss this and allay the fear.

Common problems or communication barriers

Hindle (2003) calls barriers in communication filters. She noted that attitudes and beliefs can influence and act as a filter, and used as an example the situation in which a patient believes that they have cancer and is dying so they may ignore or avoid hearing the message. Assumptions play a large part too as a filter, e.g. how often has a patient overlooked communication with a healthcare assistant because the patient assumes that they do not know? *Maybe you have experienced this.*

Swain et al. (2004) highlighted a number of barriers to developing effective communication as:

- cultural
- organisational
- professional.

We have already explored some cultural aspects within non-verbal and verbal communication.

Organisational barriers can include lack of time, too much work pressure or lack of skills, and staff often fear some situations because they feel that they lack the necessary skills for that communication situation, e.g. speaking with an angry relative.

Swain et al. (2004) also proposed that professional barriers might be linked to professional training, especially if lengthy, because it creates a social distance and could shape their ('professional') perceptions of illness, losing sight of the patient's perspective or position. Effective communication means hearing the message from the sender's perspective and not from our own understanding or assumptions.

Betts (2003) attributed four problems with nursing and communication to:

(1) lack of self-awareness
(2) lack of systematic interpersonal skills training
(3) lack of a conceptual (theory) framework
(4) lack of clarity of purpose: what is the aim of the dialogue in the first place?

Physical barriers

Other barriers to effective communication might relate to a patient's condition, e.g. Annie may find talking difficult due to her asthma and acute breathlessness. Other factors that may affect the patient's ability to communicate or understand communication range from poorly fitting dentures, poor hearing, to poor sight or maybe not wearing their hearing aid or glasses.

Conditions such as cerebral vascular accidents (stroke) may affect a patient's speech (dysphasia) and also a patient may be less able to process a conversation, or the words that they choose may not be appropriate to or 'fit' the conversation. A stutter or other form of speech impediment may cause poor communication. A patient who suffers from dementia or acute confusion may be unable to process a message and so responds less appropriately, as could a patient with a brain or head injury or illness, and the patient in an intensive setting on a ventilator will also have a communication challenge. A learning disability may impede or hinder the ability to understand and process a message.

We also need to consider environmental barriers. These will depend on the environment; however, broadly we might consider noise as a barrier, e.g. machines bleeping, other people talking, trolleys.

Allied to this might be the lack of privacy, especially in a hospital setting. Lighting and room space are other factors and, in the community setting, environmental factors may include other family members or pets!

If it is too cold or hot people can become distracted, blocking effective communication. Talking to someone while you stand in front of a window can create a shadow over your face and poor-sighted or hearing-impaired or deaf people will lose the ability to see your face and your mouth, and so limit their ability to 'see' the conversation.

The case study 2.1 will help in consideration of some environmental aspects.

Case study 2.1

Mr Wang, a Chinese man in his 60s, is being admitted to his bed in the ward. Part of the admission requires asking about his bowel habits; he appears not to understand the question and answers with a 'yes'.

What action might the healthcare assistant admitting him need to consider?

Possible factors might be that the patient is embarrassed in a public place, is hard of hearing or does not understand English. Never assume anything.

What options might be available to the healthcare assistant would again depend on the setting, but there might be a private room where he could be admitted. If hearing were identified as a problem writing the question down could possibly help. If English were not his first language a professional (trained) translator could help. It is recommended not to use family members or friends even when their English is good, because this may breach confidentiality and also cause embarrassment between the family or friends and the patient. McAleer (2006) noted that this factor was also evident in relation to sign language translators.

Some situations might be aided with the use of pre-prepared cards with symbols and words; however, these would have limited application. A drawing instead of words may also assist, but take care not to patronise or use inappropriate pictures.

So, environmental barriers need careful attention, including:

- layout
- lighting
- ventilation
- distractions in the area.

All these are known to affect communication, e.g. if the lighting is poor a patient with a sight problem might not be able to see and so communication may break down.

Summary of good communication

- Is respectful of the person being talked to
- Is clear
- Does not use jargon, technical words or abbreviations
- Is empathic and sensitive to the receiver's (patient) needs
- Takes account of the receiver's abilities/disabilities.

Self-assessment

This simple checklist would aid any communication and ensure it is effective.

Figure 2.1 is either a bird, or a question mark, or if you turn it upside down it's a seal juggling a ball on its nose.

All these aspects can be addressed through a simple self-assessment tool cited by Egan (1990) as **SOLER** in Table 2.1.

Table 2.1 Checklist for effective communication

SOLER	Achieved ✔
Sit **S**quarely in relation to the patient	
Maintain an **O**pen posture	
Lean slightly towards the patient	
Maintain reasonable **E**ye contact with the patient	
Relax (sit comfortably and supported)	

Reproduced with permission from Cengage Learning.

Addendum

Gunning FOG Index (Gunning 1952)

Gunning FOG Index: from http://en.wikipedia.org/wiki/Gunning-Fog_Index, accessed 27/02/08 and permission obtained from wikipedia. Also available at: www.tasc.ac.uk/sdev1/drobis/profcom/fog.htm (accessed 11 January 2006).

Step 1	Count out a 100-word passage. Make sure that the passage ends with a full stop, even if you go slightly above or below exactly 100 words
Step 2	Find the average sentence length by dividing 100 by the number of sentences in the selected passage, e.g. 8 sentences $= 100 \div 8 = 12.5$
Step 3	Count the number of words with three or more syllables (e.g. syllables). This number gives you the percentage of 'hard words' in the passage, e.g. 9
Don't count	Proper nouns, e.g. Irene, Paris Combinations of easy words such as typewriter or newsletter Verb forms with ends: es, ing or ed, e.g. transmitted Jargon familiar to your reader
Step 4	Add the average sentence length (Step 2) to the number of 'hard words' (step 3), e.g. $12.5 + 9 = 21.5$
Step 5	Multiply the total in Step 4 by 0.4 to get the reading level for the passage, e.g. $21.5 \times 0.4 = 8.6$
Note	Easy reading range is 6–10. The average person reads at level 9. Step 5 score was based on a sample from this chapter

Remember, when writing, that the aim is to be understood, so keep to the KIS principle = keep it simple. Aim for a reasonable FOG score, because the last thing we need is the confusion that we often get with fog!

References

Berglund C, Saltman D (2002) *Communication for Health Care*. South Melbourne: Oxford University Press.

Betts A (2003) Improving communication. In: Ellis RB, Gates B, Kenworthy N (eds), *Interpersonal Communication in Nursing*, 2nd edn. Edinburgh: Churchill Livingstone, pp. 73–86.

Burnard P (1992) *A Communication Skills Guide for Health Care Workers*. London: Edward Arnold.

Burnard P (1997) *Effective Communication Skills for Health Professionals*. Cheltenham: N. Thornes.

Dickson D, Hargie O, Morrow N (1997) *Communication Skills Training for Health Professionals*. London: Chapman & Hall.

Egan G, ed. (1990) *The Skilled Helper: A systematic approach to effective helping* 4th edn. Pacific Grove, CA: Brooks Cole.

Ellis RB, Gates B, Kenworthy N, eds (2003) *Interpersonal Communication in Nursing*, 2nd edn. Edinburgh: Churchill Livingstone.

Gietzedlt D, Jones G (2002) What language? In: Berglund C, Saltman D (eds), *Communication for Health Care*. South Melbourne: Oxford University Press, pp. 15–32.

Gunning R (1952) *The Technique of Clear Writing* Oxford: McGraw-Hill.

Hindle SA (2003) Psychological factors affecting communication. In: Ellis RB, Gates B, Kenworthy N (eds), *Interpersonal Communication in Nursing*, 2nd edn. Edinburgh: Churchill Livingstone, pp. 53–72.

Information Services Division (2005) Scottish Health Statistics. Available at: www.isdscotland.org/isd/5113.html (accessed 30 January 2008).

McAleer M (2006) Communicating effectively with deaf patients *Nursing Standard* 20(19): 51–54.

Mehrabian A (1972) *Nonverbal Communication*. Chicago: Aldine-Atherto. Available at: www.kaaj.com/psych (accessed 25 January 2006).

Swannell J, ed. (1986) *The Little Oxford Dictionary of Current English*. Oxford: Clarendon Press.

Swain J, Clark J, Parry K, French S, Reynolds F (2004) *Enabling Relationships in Health and Social Care*. Oxford: Butterworth Heinemann.

Von Oech R (1990) *A Whack on the Side of the Head*. London: HarperCollins Publishers; visit www.creativethink.com.

Chapter 3

Psychological care

Learning objectives

- State the main psychological aspects associated with clinical skills
- Describe the psychological assessment of patients
- Identify specific psychological factors that may affect patients
- Review strategies to optimise psychological wellbeing

Aim of this chapter

The aim of this chapter is to explore psychological aspects of patient care, and its relation to the clinical skills and procedures within this book.

What is meant by psychological care?

Walker et al. (2004) describe psychology as the study of human behaviour, thought processes and emotions, so psychological care is caring for the mind. Mitchell (2007) notes that, currently, little formal psychological nursing intervention is undertaken or, if it is, such care is marginalised (given less attention). This chapter reviews how a psychological assessment can be addressed and how this can aid the healthcare assistant, to ensure that the patient receives a holistic package of care, enhancing the patient experience.

Reflection point

If you were being admitted to hospital, what aspects of care and treatment might make you anxious?

Individuals are unique, so assessment is critical to identify their concerns or fears.

When patients are admitted to hospital or attend a GP surgery, they may be experiencing stress, which could result from their illness, fear of the unknown, fear about painful treatments or concerns over the impact that a potential illness may have on their life, family, work and social community. The skill for the healthcare assistant is to identify and support a patient through this stressful period, and to do that they must first ensure that they have a clear understanding of patients and their concerns.

Psychological assessment in the healthcare setting

Consider, as Mitchell (2007) describes, patients entering a strange and often sterile environment such as a hospital, where they will probably be partially undressed, e.g. for 12-lead ECG, and unsure about what is happening or about to happen. They will be waiting for instructions and procedures (often unpleasant) from a variety of healthcare staff (many strangers to them), all the while trying to retain information and ask questions – no wonder stress and anxiety levels are high!

Thomas (2005) states the importance of identifying 'problem patients' in advance of procedures. It may be possible to identify such patients from their past history, e.g. poor experience during last inpatient stay, a known phobia, e.g. needles, or known learning disability or mental health problem. Also consider the parent of a child, who also needs support and education, because Thomas (2005) suggests that parents can respond unexpectedly, e.g. seen it all on TV's ER, but suddenly can't face a situation and snatch their child and run!

Mitchell (2007) identifies self efficacy – the belief in one's own ability to cope with a stressful situation or challenging demand, often based on past experiences, e.g. coped with an emergency admission with diabetes before, so believe they will manage again. Therefore when assessing the patient pre-procedure, the healthcare assistant should identify this and the ways in which the patient may cope or maintain control, e.g. patients could manage their own blood sugar tests, so therefore they can choose which finger to sample from. *Please check that this is acceptable policy locally.*

Mitchell (2007) also suggests considering environmental factors, noting that the friendliness of staff is crucial, especially in busy, sterile clinical areas, because they often feel impersonal and unfriendly. Comfort is also important, with the use of soft lighting, pictures and flowers helping to 'normalise' the area and helping the patient to relax.

Noise can often increase stress and distract patients (and staff), and although distraction can be a strategy to help patients' cope, here it may be a problem, e.g. when the healthcare assistant explains the preparation for a 12-lead ECG, the patient misses the important information because of distraction.

Doellman (2003) explored psychological aspects in paediatrics and venepuncture, and concluded that preparation for any procedure is a valuable intervention. A child life specialist is cited by Doellman (2003) as an aid for assessment of what support and preparation the child and parents may need; in the UK this may be part of the role of a play specialist. Children younger than 7 years should be prepared as close to the time of the procedure as possible, probably no sooner than 1 hour before the procedure (Doellman 2003). Older children can be prepared in advance, even the day before, and this extra time allows the child to process the information without increasing anxiety levels.

Parents' knowledge of how their children react to stressful situations will help the healthcare assistant determine the appropriate timing of preparation, as well as which coping strategies would be most useful. Doellman (2003) adds further that the developmental and emotional level of the child can be assessed or acknowledged during the preparation period. Thus the healthcare assistant must check the child's records and talk with the parents, to obtain any pertinent information that can aid in undertaking the clinical skill safely and competently.

Fundudis (2003) notes that assessment of children's personality and temperament allows their psychological maturity and competence to be measured, including their language skills, memory and reasoning skills. A child may understand the need for a certain procedure, that it might involve some discomfort and the need to stay in hospital for a few days, but they need to understand any associated risks, e.g. the possible impact on their health if they refuse a procedure.

Thomas (2005) noted the importance of children's psychological preparation before procedures; noting the use of professional clowns has been successful. The individual assessment of each child is necessary to identify the need for specialist intervention, e.g. play therapist, and to clarify the role of the parent, e.g. as chaperone (if suitable and acceptable in the clinical area, because parents may not be able to accompany their child into theatre (Thomas, 2005)).

Before any procedure these aspects must be considered, because they will help the healthcare assistant identify and plan or offer strategies to help the patient cope.

The importance of psychological care in the healthcare setting

Psychological factors

Some factors have already been mentioned, e.g. fear and stress; however, there is a range of factors that the healthcare assistant should consider.

Stress

The symptoms of stress are based on the body's autonomic nervous system response (fight or flight) of arousal. Table 3.1 shows the body's autonomic responses.

Lewith and Horn (1987) note that stress, fear and pain cannot be avoided by running away or conquered by a physical fight, and this state of arousal can actually make things worse – it reduces patients' ability to think and plan logically.

Mitchell (2007) noted that maintaining a positive outlook when experiencing a stressful medical event has a positive influence on postoperative recovery, whereas the negative effects of stress can have a negative influence, e.g. delay wound healing.

Walker et al. (2004) identified a range of symptoms from the stress response, which are discussed in Table 3.2.

Often patients can be unaware of the effects of stress until careful questioning, commonly at admission but also before some procedures, when the healthcare assistant checks that the patient understands the procedure.

Reflection point

Go through the clinical skills listed in the other chapters and list the ways that stress might affect the tests or results.

Table 3.1 Body's autonomic responses

Body organ/system	Effect
Heart and cardiac system	Heart rate and blood pressure increases
Lungs	Respiratory rate and depth of breathing increases
Liver	Glucose is released for muscular activity
Brain	Blood re-routed here to aid decision making
Eyes	Pupils dilate to aid visualisation of threat
Stomach and digestive system	Blood diverted away from, to organs as above
Skin	Blood diverted – leads to pallor and sweating

Adapted from Cannon (1932), cited in Walker et al. (2004), and Lewith and Horn (1987).

Table 3.2 Stress response symptoms

Aspects	Symptoms
Physiological	Altered sleep pattern, e.g. insomnia, waking early or not getting to sleep Indigestion, nausea, diarrhoea Headaches, muscle tension Panic attacks
Cognitive	Feeling a failure, low self-esteem or confidence Worrying a lot, perhaps about things that didn't normally matter Not wanting to be bothered, apathetic about issues Difficulty in making decisions, confusion
Emotional	Feeling upset, crying more than normal Feeling irritable Unreasonable behaviour Fears that are not reasonable Loss of being able to see life in a fun way or loss of sense of humour
Behavioural	Irregular eating habits, e.g. comfort eating, not eating at all or overindulging Taking time off for minor illnesses (which would not normally result in absence) Using stimulants, e.g. drugs, alcohol, tobacco Withdrawing from usual activities, e.g. not seeing friends or going out as much

Adapted from Walker et al. (2004).

Pain

Large (1996) reminds us that pain is an unpleasant sensory and emotional experience, but it is the patient's experience, so if the patient says that there is pain, there is pain – unless the patient is lying about their experience. The psychological effects of acute pain are almost always a cause for anxiety and avoidance, as befits its function as a warning mechanism (Large 1996). Children learn to avoid stimuli (as do adults) that they associate with pain, e.g. matches burn.

Walker et al. (2004) suggest that pain-related fear is often more disabling than the pain itself. Lewith and Horn (1987) described anticipatory pain in children, where they recognise a potentially painful situation and show distress before the procedure begins, e.g. have had bloods taken before and start to cry as the healthcare assistant approaches. This is an equally valid concept for adults, who, although they may not cry, may anticipate pain and become stressed and anxious, which can have an affect on the procedure, e.g. inserting a cannula in a patient who is tense is likely to be more painful, unless this is recognised and managed.

Chronic pain is associated with a range of psychological problems, e.g. helplessness, hopelessness and suicide. Patients often feel isolated, experience loss of self or anger, or feel devalued, because chronic pain can affect lifestyle, employment and relationships (Large 1996). It is not the scope of this book to explore this area in depth, but some aspects are worth reviewing relating to panic and phobia anxiety.

Lewith and Horn (1987) noted that pain is a symptom of a disorder or disease; it serves a useful purpose in that it alerts us to take action or stop what we are doing. They suggest that the essential factors in psychological pain control are understanding, mental calmness and physical relaxation – the ability to focus on something other than the pain; this is explored later.

Finally Large (1996) outlined some psychological processes as a *cause of pain*:

- Muscle tension leading to more pain
- Suppressed anger causing tension, e.g. headaches, migraine
- Sick role, where a patient plays a role of being unwell to gain sympathy.

Phobias

Thomas (2005) indicated that phobias are common in children, e.g. needle or mask phobias; and other factors that influence anxiety are age, gender and temperament, as well as previous hospital experiences. However, many adults can be just as prone to phobias and again needles are commonly a source of anxiety. Walker et al. (2004) describe phobias as the persistent fear of a specific object or situation and they can lead to panic, so careful assessment is essential to identify these factors.

Panic or anxiety

This is described as a consequence of uncertainty and unpredictability. It is often the result of a new situation, e.g. emergency admission to hospital, where the person lacks the appropriate information, or of their inability to make sense of what's happening, e.g. a patient with dementia (Walker et al. 2004).

Confusion

McIlween and Gross (1997) and Walker et al. (2004) mention this because it affects the patient's memory and ability to process information, e.g. in an older patient with dementia, or in younger patients as a result of injury or drugs. In patients with dementia the memory loss can increase the patient's agitation, which in turn makes the memory problem worse (Walker et al. 2004).

Culture

Doellman (2003) suggests that it is useful to understand a patient's culture, e.g. pain may be culture specific, so a child within a culture group learns what people expect and accept about expressing pain. Consider the UK's culture of the 'stiff upper lip' or, as Lewith and Horn (1987) stated, 'big boys don't cry'; we might expect indigenous British people not to show their pain, whereas other cultures may express pain more freely. Cultural beliefs may influence acceptance, or not, of treatments because many consider 'traditional or folk' medicine, e.g. herbal medicine, more acceptable and so may delay decisions about accepting 'conventional' treatment.

Doellman (2003) noted that some cultures view the body as a whole and that invasive procedures can alter this, e.g. shaving hair may be prohibited in some cultures and might be necessary for several clinical procedures, e.g. chest lead placement in a 12-lead ECG procedure or securing a cannula. The concept of space (also discussed in Chapter 2) can be a cultural issue. Doellman (2003) cites Chinese people feeling more comfortable in a side-by-side or right-angle approach and feeling uncomfortable when placed in a face-to-face situation, e.g. when explaining a clinical procedure. Thus consideration of these aspects is necessary when communicating with patients or families, otherwise it may increase their stress and anxiety levels.

Grieving process

This can encompass many different types of behaviour, e.g. anger, guilt, aggression and denial (Walker et al. 2004). McIlween and Gross (1997) describe this as a psychological and bodily reaction to bereavement (could include loss of, for example, fitness, employment, body image, due to illness or treatments). Many stages of this process have been described (McIlween and Gross 1997; Walker et al. 2004); Table 3.3 outlines some aspects.

Table 3.3 Stages of grief and possible outcomes

Stage	Possible outcome examples
Disbelief or shock	'I don't believe I have a heart condition' from 12-lead ECG test
Denial	'I'm not diabetic' when told result of blood sugar test
Depression	'I can't cope with a long-term catheter and its effect on my life'
Guilt	'If only I hadn't smoked,' when told of lung disease from a peak flow test
Anxiety	'How will I cope with taking medication x for the rest of my life?'
Anger/aggression	'It's all your fault, you got bowel test wrong. I don't have bowel cancer.'

McIlween and Gross (1997) note that these vary and some authors describe them as phases or stages. The final stage is often described as acceptance, as the person comes to terms with loss, but timeframes vary considerably and people can 'jump' around stages, and do not necessarily follow any progression. A patient may react to bad news, i.e. told that they have a heart condition after tests, e.g. 12-lead ECG and blood tests, in different ways, so it may be helpful to be aware of these stages. This can help the healthcare assistant to respond in a supportive caring manner, and to suggest or offer coping strategies.

Sick role

Large (1996) mentions this; it is where a patient 'plays' a role to gain sympathy and support. If this role is threatened the patient may respond unexpectedly, and exhibit similar behaviours to those discussed in the grieving process. It may also impact on the patient's ability to participate, e.g. if the healthcare assistant is helping to teach a patient to self-catheterise to achieve some independence, the patient may not wish to do this and so become unwilling to learn or participate.

Conflict

This may occur as part of grieving or anxiety about the loss of a role, e.g. sick role; Walker et al. (2004) note that conflict must be avoided by effective strategies. The healthcare assistant must try to understand the patient's perspective or point of view.

Strategies to optimise psychological wellbeing

Large (1996) noted that, in relation to pain, but relevant to all psychological factors, there are a range of strategies (mental and physical) for coping, the key being the ability to be flexible and adaptable. The first step for the healthcare assistant is to maintain effective communication and identify what may be most effective with the patient.

Communication

Thomas (2005) suggests that the healthcare assistant needs to speak the language of the patient; this does not mean learning Chinese, but does mean listening and getting to know the patient, using words and language that they will understand. A simple, clear explanation can reduce anxiety. However, Thomas (2005) notes that patients who are mentally challenged, e.g. have a learning disability, may require someone close to them to 'interpret' for them, i.e. parent, family member or community nurse specialist.

Mitchell (2007) describes the use of supporting statements in a positive manner, whether verbal or written, e.g. 'This hospital performs many surgical procedures safely'. Doellman (2003) indicated that talking with patients would help identify their preferences for coping strategies, e.g. where suitable and possible a teenager can choose their own music, rather than have a choice imposed.

Finally, Large (1996) states that the key to effective communication is listening, and suggests that this can help break down barriers, e.g. the sick role. Effective communication is central to any healthcare assistant's role and is why this book contains a chapter on this subject.

Information

Doellman (2003) spoke of information in relation to children but it is just as appropriate for patients of any age. Information is necessary to prepare the patient. Doellman (2003) noted parents and children need information about the importance of the procedure to the child's health and diagnosis (why the procedure must be done), e.g. a child with a high fever and cough should be told: 'Taking a blood sample will help identify the specific bacteria (bug) in your lungs so that you get the right antibiotic for the pneumonia (infection in lung) to help you get better quickly.'

In addition, Doellman (2003) indicates the importance of age-appropriate information, such as why and where the procedure will take place, what will be happening and how it will feel. Such information should be presented to the patient, e.g. referring to a tourniquet as a 'tight hug' around the arm, and also being told that this is the tricky part of the procedure. Thus, the child is alerted to the feeling.

Walker et al. (2004) and Mitchell (2007) describe this as information support; the challenge is to pitch information at the right level and suitability for the patient. Getting the balance and timing right is essential, because too much too soon will increase anxiety levels; however, some patients may need more information to help them prepare and manage their anxiety levels (Mitchell 2007). Pre-information can be helpful, to prepare the patient in advance of the procedure, e.g. for catheterisation. Information can allow a patient more control, choice and understanding of what is happening, which is why many of the chapters identify patient education aspects, e.g. peripheral cannulation. A review of Chapter 2 may also be of value.

Thus, the intent of effective communication and appropriate information is to have a patient who is aware and reassured about what is happening or going to happen.

Assessment

Careful assessment includes both communication and information; this is not just to inform, educate and gain consent, but also to ensure that all factors have been assessed, both physical and psychological.

Doellman (2003) outlines this for preparation of the family and the child, suggesting several tactics to help assess their understanding, which can also act as coping strategies:

- Show instructional video (pre-admission is best) followed later by Q&A
- Q&A (questions and answer) session: face-to-face discussion on admission
- Photo album that shows the procedure step by step and pictures of the equipment for the procedure and room, e.g. theatre, peak flow meter
- Procedure kit: this allows a child to play with and touch the equipment used for the procedure, e.g. catheter, tourniquet and play doll. The child's own doll can be used if the child is agreeable but consider this, as they do not want unpleasant associations with their doll later.

- Therapeutic play; using a doll and with a specialist (play therapist), doctor or nurse' the healthcare professional could carry out role play of the procedure with the child
- Story telling: this can also be used during the procedure.

These points all demonstrate the child's, as well as the parents', understanding and acceptance of the procedure, and allows healthcare staff to assess what strategies might be most suited to the child, e.g. a child shows fear of a catheter, so discuss the use of local anaesthetic gel and clinical holding (see Chapter 11).

Dougherty and Lister (2004) noted the use of open questions (discussed in Chapter 2) to assess psychological care needs as:

- How do you feel?
- Do you have any worries or concerns?
- What has helped you cope in the past and what is helping at the moment?

Patient involvement

Mitchell (2007) stated that this allows control over self, and can help a patient cope by reducing anxiety, e.g. choose to self-catheterise at a time suitable for the patient. Choice might also include privacy aspects; rather than have the procedure in a ward behind flimsy screens where everyone can hear, the patient can choose, e.g. toilet to self-catheterise or where a procedure may cause embarrassment, e.g. opening bowels for a bowel test, the patient could opt for the privacy of a toilet too.

Large (1996) called this self-efficacy; it means that the patient is encouraged to take control. A breathless patient may be grateful to be allowed to choose a bed by a window or door, to feel in control of the fresh air, and so may help them manage their breathing and feel more reassured and safe.

Reflection point

You are preparing a 13-year-old boy for a peak flow test. How could you check out his understanding of the procedure?

Timing/pacing

As mentioned earlier, ensuring that the patient has the right information and communication at the right time are important. Mitchell (2007) highlights this and points out that the healthcare assistant must ensure that the patient is not too groggy or sleepy, e.g. under post-procedure sedation, because they may not be able to absorb any information.

Doellman (2003) discussed this in relation to children, and stated judgement is essential, so if a child shows signs of distress, stop. Allow them to calm down and relax, then review the situation, and pace further information giving to suit the child, or indeed any patient.

Emotional support

This was defined by Walker et al. (2004) as offering reassurance and encouragement.

Children specific

Doellman (2003) discusses the use of play and clowns in their practice, and many paediatric settings will employ play specialists and clowns. Their role acts as a support to staff and can offer many strategies suitable for the child and age related too. Interventions suitable for children will also be discussed next.

Pharmacological (drug-related) options

Medicines that may be used might be limited to registered nurses or doctors only; please check your local policies.

Doellman (2003) discusses local anaesthetics, e.g. creams/gels, subdermal injections (under the skin), for use in venepuncture and cannulation, and these must be prescribed and administered by an authorised healthcare professional trained in their use. She also discusses non-invasive needle-free local anaesthesia called iontophoresis, which uses a mild electric current from a small battery-powered unit delivering a water-soluble ionic medication into a selected tissue, e.g. arm (known as Numby). Doellman (2003) notes its use only in children aged over 6 years, because younger children do not apparently tolerate the tingling sensation well. Please check your local policy about this equipment and its use.

Sedation is an option (Doellman 2003); however Mitchell (2007) urges caution as although sedation can be beneficial, it also has side effects, e.g. patient may be too drowsy to respond to questions, and other interventions have less side effects.

One final option may be the use of general anaesthesia, however it would be unlikely for any of the clinical skills listed and discussed within this book.

Both these options would not likely be within the scope of a healthcare assistant.

Non-pharmacological options

These encompass a range of options. Large (1996) lists relaxation, hypnosis and behavioural therapy, e.g. counselling, whereas Doellman (2003) notes distraction, massage, guided imagery, modelling and music, and Mitchell (2007) suggests cognitive coping strategies, e.g. visualisation. Table 3.4 lists the options.

Therapeutic sense of self

Mitchell (2007) describes this as the beneficial effects that the presence of a healthcare worker, e.g. assistant, can have on a patient, especially in the acute care setting. This is due to the support and reassurance that a healthcare assistant can provide, offering supportive positive communications and providing some coping strategies, e.g. a patient with a fear of needles before sampling (venepuncture) is supported by the healthcare assistant using a breathing technique and topical local anaesthetic gel. Having a partner or friend present while waiting can help ease anxiety and, in some cases, e.g. children, patient with a learning disability, being present (if willing and it's suitable) during a procedure may also help. With children, a parent can hold the child while the procedure is carried out, e.g. insertion of a peripheral cannula or blood being sampled from a finger for blood sugar testing. The presence of a friend, parent or family member can often reassure,

Table 3.4 Non-pharmacological options

Option	Action
Massage	Can be helpful for all ages, but only if patient wishes; can reduce pain and anxiety, and increases relaxation
Guided imagery	Most effective with children 8 years and over (or adults); patient imagines a positive place or setting, e.g. playing on a beach, sitting by a gently flowing river
Relaxation	Works well with older children (and adults) because they can be taught to breathe slowly and relax different muscle groups; younger children can be asked to slowly blow out imaginary birthday candles; relaxation can work well with soothing music
Modelling	This is where a play specialist describes the child's role in the procedure, e.g. 'Your job will be to hold your arm as still as you can and to look at the toy/book, and this will help the healthcare assistant with their job'. Reinforcing the positive behaviour during the procedure helps, saying, for example, 'I really like the way that you are holding your arm so still'
	Parents can be taught to model positive behaviour too, so sit with child, offer positive statements and hold their hand
Music	Choice by child (or adult) is preferable; however, sound machines that provide birds chirping, waves rolling or soft heartbeat can be very soothing to small infants
Distraction	Watch a movie (TV); easy and quick, and frees up staff, but Mitchell (2007) notes that might not suit all, as too basic and may not soothe some people
Visualisation	Positive thoughts can dispel false or unfounded fears, and similar to guided imagery, patient thinks of a personal positive situation

Adapted from Large (1996), Doellman (2003) and Mitchell (2007).

and make the person, especially a child, feel safe. Walker et al. (2004) noted the importance of social support, which offers a sense of belonging gained from family and friends.

This aspect should not be overlooked, and it is often the presence of a healthcare assistant, or any other healthcare staff, that is of great benefit to the patient's psychological wellbeing. It is also good practice with many invasive procedures; acting as a chaperone and being able to answer questions, or just *being there*, can be a huge relief to an anxious patient.

Instrumental support

Walker et al. (2004) suggest that this is about offering practical and tangible support, and might include sitting with patients and talking about their fears or offering them comfort, e.g. a cup of tea! Solutions are therefore directed at specific aspects to help reassure and relax the patient.

Related aspects and terminology

Apathetic: withdrawn and quiet, lacking energy, associated with depression.

Common problems

As noted earlier by Mitchell (2007) the risk of ignoring or overlooking psychological aspects – the patient's physical needs are met, but their emotional and psychological ones are not – is serious.

The patient may not respond to treatment or communications in the manner expected (McIlween and Gross 1997). The patient's feeling of loss or anxiety may lead to unexpected behaviours, which could cause problems, e.g. coping with anger can be threatening to the healthcare assistant and others, because this behaviour, if not handled effectively, may escalate into violence. The patient who withdraws due to confusion or fear will also pose a challenge; how to effectively care and communicate when the patient is passive or apathetic?

Staff may lack confidence in assessing psychological needs, but by use of open questions, as suggested by Dougherty and Lister (2004), the healthcare assistant can invite patients to discuss any fears or concerns that they have. From this initial dialogue, the patient, together with the healthcare assistant, can identify what strategies are available and suitable. An associated aspect is recording this information, because many staff may not recognise documentation as an essential part of practice (McGeehan 2006). This is an area where the healthcare assistant must ensure good practice, and so record any communications promptly and clearly, without making subjective statements about a patient, e.g. 'looking worried' (UNISON 2003).

Another aspect to consider is the diversity of staff involved in any one patient's care, because this can lead to problems with maintaining effective communication, while acknowledging confidentiality, and can pose a challenge.

Summary

This chapter has a narrow focus of just clinical skills; we acknowledge this and suggest that the reader explores the wider aspects of psychological care. It is not the scope of this book to explore mental health issues, but, if in doubt about a patient's psychological state, seek advice from a registered colleague.

If you do not know the patient, some mental health symptoms may be 'masked' or hidden by the process of admission and undergoing procedures, particularly invasive ones such as peripheral cannulation (inserting a cannula). Always seek advice, if in doubt ask.

Case study 3.1

Mr Helmut Jung has been admitted as an emergency with chest pain, while on holiday from Germany. He is 66 years old and seems to speak reasonable English. His wife is back at the hotel, calling his family in Hamburg and gathering his medicines and nightclothes. He is in pain and very anxious.

You have been asked to prepare him for a standard 12-lead ECG procedure. What aspects would you need to consider to help prepare him psychologically?

You do not need to understand the actual procedure of recording a standard 12-lead ECG. This asks the healthcare assistant to consider any situation that requires psychological preparation – what the reader would do and why.

✔	Self-assessment

Assessment	Aspects	Achieved ✔
Psychological care	*Have you considered all aspects of this section?*	
	Patient assessment	
	Psychological factors	
	Coping strategies	
	Problems and reporting concerns	

References

Doellman D (2003) Pharmacological versus nonpharmacological techniques in reducing venopuncture psychological trauma in pediatric patients. *Journal of Infusion* **26**: 103–109.

Dougherty L, Lister S, eds (2004) *The Royal Marsden Hospital Manual of Clinical Nursing Procedures*, 7th edn. Oxford: Blackwell Publishing.

Fundudis T (2003) Consent issues in medico-legal procedures: how competent are children to make their own decisions. *Child and Adolescent Mental Health* **8**(1): 18–22.

Large RG (1996) Psychological aspects of pain. *Annals of Rheumatic Diseases* **55**: 340–345.

Lewith G, Horn S (1987) *Drug-free Pain Relief*. Rochester: Thorsons Publisher Inc.

McIlween R, Gross R (1997) *Developmental Psychology*. London: Hodder & Stoughton.

McGeehan R (2006) Best practice in record keeping. *Nursing Standard* **21**(17): 51–55.

Mitchell M (2007) Psychological care of patients undergoing elective surgery *Nursing Standard* **21**(30): 48–55.

Thomas J (2005) Brute force or gentle persuasion? *Pediatric Anesthesia* **15**: 355–357.

UNISON (2003) *The Duty of Care*. London: UNISON.

Walker J, Payne S, Smith P, Jarrett N (2004) *Psychology for Nurses and the Caring Professions*. Milton Keynes: Open University Press.

Chapter 4

Documentation and record keeping

Learning objectives

- Identify why accurate and prompt records are essential
- Outline the standards for good record keeping
- Discuss the types of documentation in relation to clinical skills
- Describe legal requirements in relation to record keeping.

Aim of this chapter

The aim of this chapter is to explore the standards required for patient documentation and record keeping, with the focus on records and documentation relating to clinical skills, e.g. TPR (temperature, pulse and respiration) chart. The importance of recording and maintaining accurate and prompt records along with legal aspects is also discussed.

The importance and purpose of documentation in relation to clinical skills

Birt (1998), Hutchinson and Sharples (2006), and McGeehan (2006) noted that the purpose of records is to provide a complete patient journey and enable the continuity of care across the whole team. Nolan et al. (2005) described these as a formal record of each patient's needs, setting out care goals and plans to deliver that care.

The union UNISON (2003) identified the duty of care of healthcare assistants (also discussed in Chapter 1), and in relation to record keeping they indicated the standard expected of any competent skilled person (healthcare assistant) is:

- to keep accurate and contemporaneous (up to date) records of their work
- to protect confidential information, except where there is a wider duty of care (e.g. if in the public interest).

The Nursing and Midwifery Council (NMC 2005), the ruling body for registered nurses and midwives, state that guidelines for records and record keeping should:

- be written as soon as possible after an event has occurred
- be factual, consistent and accurate

- be accurately timed, dated and signed
- be written clearly and in a manner that cannot be erased
- not include abbreviations, jargon, meaningless phrases, irrelevant speculation or offensive subjective statements
- be written so that any alterations or additions are timed, dated and signed, in order that the original entry can be read clearly
- be readable on any photocopy.

These guidelines are applicable to any healthcare professional and are good practice.

In relation to clinical skills, records are maintained in order that a patient's condition can be observed and monitored, e.g. the record of a patient with diabetes would contain information about blood sugar levels in the urine or blood. These ongoing records, at defined times, e.g. before meals, will allow the patient to receive the correct treatment. In a person with diabetes, this might be to adjust the dose of insulin that the patient receives. Dimond (2002) states that prompt and accurate observations, and recording on the appropriate documentation, are essential for safe and good quality patient care. However, McGeehan (2006) noted that record keeping is often thought of as a chore done at the end of a shift, although in fact clinical skills need recording immediately after the procedure, e.g. blood pressure.

As noted above, records ensure that all the members of the healthcare team are aware of what is happening to that patient, any treatment(s) that they are receiving, and the effects, both positive and negative, e.g. analgesia (pain medication) has reduced pain or not. This is part of effective communication (see Chapter 2).

Therefore the written language has to be clear, with no jargon or abbreviations (unless approved (*check locally what abbreviations, if any, are approved*, e.g. TPR) and written or printed so that they are legible (clear) to the reader (McGeehan 2006). It is also important to remember the need for a permanent record, a requirement in law, so entries must be in black ink; this is required in case documents need to be photocopied, because a pencil entry can be rubbed out or smudged or altered, and so is unclear. Birt (1998) stated that information recorded illegibly or inadequately may have a detrimental effect on a patient's health, because it might lead to errors.

Effective records allow staff to monitor patients over 24-hour periods, for every day that they receive healthcare. If a patient was suffering from chest pain and part of the care was to have the patient's vital signs observed (e.g. temperature, pulse and respiratory rate), and they received an analgesic, monitoring can help develop a picture of the patient's response to the treatment. Thus, if the pain were not responding to the analgesic, the pulse and respiratory rate could remain elevated, showing the potential need for more analgesic. Only through keeping accurate records and reviewing them on an ongoing basis can healthcare staff provide the most effective and responsive care possible. Dougherty and Lister (2004) emphasise that documents help in assessing patients and can hold a baseline (a reading that acts as a reference for future readings) of data, e.g. BP, and allows ongoing monitoring of patient needs. This is crucial as a patient's condition can be unpredictable and complex.

Dougherty and Lister (2004) identified examples of subjective statements in records (Table 4.1).

One of the challenges in healthcare is the variety of staff involved in any one patient's care, and the information that each person needs to carry out because their role varies, so confidentiality must be considered. The Data Protection Act 1998 and the Freedom of Information Act (FOIA) 2005 are important, and healthcare assistants must be aware of the impact that these Acts have on their role. Nolan et al. (2005) describe these and note that the Data Protection Act 1998 restricts the way in which personal information can be used, and limits those who can access information about individuals. Evans (2005) indicated that the Freedom of Information Act 2000

Table 4.1 Examples of records

Poor example	Good example
Upset today	Patient states: 'feeling upset'
Appears depressed	Patient says: 'I am concerned about my treatment and how it will affect me'

Adapted from Dougherty and Lister (2004).

became fully effective in 2005, and now means that anyone can ask for any information from a public body, e.g. the NHS, such as data relating to a complaint or staffing levels.

Confidentiality in records and documentation

Healthcare assistants must always be aware that information might be accessed by the patient, and in some cases friends or visitors, e.g. the TPR chart because it is often hanging on a patient's bed or wall. When patients are being admitted, they should be informed that the data (their personal details) would be shared with other members of the healthcare team as appropriate and relevant, to ensure that they receive the best care possible. NHS Scotland's *Working in Health* (2007) recommends maintenance of a professional attitude at all times when handling patient's information, and not to 'gossip' about patients to anyone. When passing on information to a colleague, as part of the job, take care to be accurate and clear in all that is said and written.

The patient should be reassured that these confidential notes are kept safe and, with the development of computerisation, given added reassurance that these are password protected, so only staff who have authorisation can access their records. Always consider the security of this information: do not leave a patient's records (e.g. nursing or case notes) lying around or walk away from a computer if on and still open at a patient record. Check what documents can be left safely at a patient's bedside, e.g. urine chart, peak flow chart. *Please check your local policy.*

Reflection point

Why are patient records necessary?

Types of documentation

The key aspect with regard to documentation is to *check your local practice area* and identify what is deemed acceptable and has been approved. In relation to clinical skills, focus would be on TPR, urinalysis, peak flow charts, charts for recording blood glucose levels, faecal occult blood (FOB) tests and patient care plan/case notes for recording, e.g. in peripheral intravenous cannulation: date, time, site, cannula gauge, reason for insertion, any issues and signature. The standard 12-lead ECG record is often noted on the recording itself and stored securely within the patient's record – local variations may apply. *Always check your local policy.*

Another type of documentation that may be used is a care pathway or integrated care pathway (ICP); Dougherty and Lister (2004) noted that these offer a consistent method of assessment, which enables communication among the various healthcare staff. The development of clinical protocols, care pathways, patient-held records or shared documentation emerged to help improve the patient's experience of care and service delivery (Dougherty and Lister 2004).

Middleton and Roberts (2000) describe a care pathway as an outline or plan of anticipated clinical practice for a group of patients with a particular diagnosis or set of symptoms (refer to Figure 4.1 for an example).

The following chapters explore a range of clinical skills; within each there is a review of the knowledge and skills necessary to perform the procedure(s) (clinical skill(s)) safely and competently. All require competent record keeping.

Reflection point

What clinical skills will you be required to undertake? Consider what types of records or documentation you will need to maintain in your practice area.

Legal aspects relating to documentation

The Department of Health (DH 2006) stipulate that all individuals who work for NHS organisations are responsible for any records that they create or use in the performance of their duties. Furthermore, any record that an individual creates is a public record. The DH (2006) guidance covers all NHS records (England):

- Information has most value when accurate, up to date and accessible when it is needed
- Information may be needed to support patient care and continuity of care
- Information must support patient choice
- Records must meet legal requirements (Data Protection and FOI Acts)
- Information must assist clinical and other types of audits
- Information may be needed to support evidence-based clinical practice
- Information may be needed to support decision-making
- Information is needed to support improvements in clinical effectiveness.

Birt (1998) noted that the main purpose of records is to provide good communication among health professionals, although it can also be extremely useful in defending a nurse (healthcare assistant) in the event of a complaint or claim.

Beech (2007) indicated that the Data Protection Act 1998 gives patients the right to access any personal information held about them, and for patients to do this they must apply to the designated authority (often a data controller within an organisation).

Reflection point

Who is designated to release patient records in your organisation?

Owen (2005) suggested that accurate records not only ensure quality of practice but also safeguard staff by providing evidence of their professional ability, because records can be used

Integrated Care Pathway for the Management of Diabetes in the Perioperative Period Site : RIE □ WGH □ St Johns □	UHD, NHS Lothian Addressograph or Name Dob Address Unit number CHI

INSTRUCTIONS *Insert information into appropriate spaces as required & complete 'Initial Key'*
Do not initial until actually done!

This ICP is an action checklist & a clinical record & requires a Kardex & SEWS chart

---

Date initiated: ___/____/___   **PRE-ASSESSMENT CLINIC**

PROPOSED DATE OF SURGERY   ...../......./.......

Type of Diabetes Type 1 □ Type 2 □   Usual treatment: Insulin □   Tablet(s) □   Diet □

HbA1c □   result................ : if HbA1c > 9%, discuss with Diabetes Specialist Nurse

Anaesthetist aware that patient has Diabetes Mellitus□

Ensure patient is first on the list when possible□
                        To be **Nil By Mouth** from:.......... on............

Patient on Metformin Yes □, No □   To be stopped on ..../........./.......

To be commenced on:
  SHORT Fast: when immediate post-operative resumption of oral intake is likely   □
  LONG Fast: when immediate resumption of oral intake after surgery not planned   □

Information leaflets provided □

DATE OF SURGERY   ...../......./....... **Peri-operative SHORT Fast**

When immediate post-operative resumption of oral intake is likely following protocol may be used

	initial
Omit breakfast & morning dose of insulin (and oral hypoglycaemic agents, if taking these) □	
Check blood glucose hourly from 8am□	
If blood glucose remains between 5-12 mmol/l, no action □	
If blood glucose is above 12 mmol/l, consider intravenous insulin □	
See Intravenous Insulin protocol sheet.	

---

	initial

DATE OF SURGERY   ...../......./.......   **Peri-operative LONG Fast**
The following protocol should be used for major surgery, when immediate resumption of oral intake after surgery is not planned:

The patient should be first on the operation list (preferably am)□

Omit breakfast & morning dose of insulin (and oral hypoglycaemic agents if taking these) □
                    [Note: oral hypoglycaemic agents = OHA]

Intravenous Insulin regime □

Time of commencement of Intravenous insulin: 8am □ , or, on arrival in theatre □

Note any Variances from Pathway with 'VAR' & explain fully

Name *sign* Profession designation	*print* date	initial

Figure 4.1 The diabetic care pathway. (Reproduced with kind permission of Suzanne Delaney, Diabetic Nurse Specialist, NHS Lothian.)

as evidence in a court of law. It is expected that records will demonstrate that the staff concerned understood and executed their professional and legal duty of care (Culley 2001; see also Chapter 1).

The approach to record keeping adopted by courts of law tends to be that, *if it is not recorded, it has not been done.*

Strategies to improve standards of record keeping

Dougherty and Lister (2004) indicated that use of a standardised format minimises confusion, gives uniformity and allows staff to record information in a recognisable way and order, and so is easy to locate and act upon.

Both unitary (single) patient records and electronic formats are becoming the 'norm' and allow information to be shared, reducing duplication and repetition. This is better for the patient, who does not have to repeat name, address, DOB, etc. over and over. Another advantage of electronic records is that they can be shared promptly across healthcare teams, e.g. a GP can send a patient's records when they are being admitted to hospital. This can allow data to be compared, e.g. the peak flow record of a patient with asthma will allow staff to monitor, and observe changes (e.g. deterioration from home/baseline) and response to treatment (Dougherty and Lister 2004).

The National Patient Safety Agency (NPSA 2005) explored risks in relation to patient identification and several aspects are relevant to clinical skills and documentation: identifying the correct patient, site (commonly associated with surgery) and procedure.

The NPSA (2005) noted that the main risks were caused by the misuse of address labels, mishearing, misspelling and misfiling. Other factors were illegible handwriting, use of abbreviations, unavailable records or failure to review records and distraction. Their following recommendations are relevant for clinical skills and records:

- Develop local guidance and policies and ensure that they are implemented
- Do not use abbreviations
- Always check patient identification (ID)
- Use positive patient identification, e.g. ask patient to state their full name, etc.
- Use double witnesses, e.g. two nurses for drug administration, and recording
- Consider the use of bar codes, e.g. to release drugs against patient ID.

Owen (2005) identified the following strategies to improve record keeping:

- Records should be subject to audit as a quality control and risk management measure, and Culley (2001) suggested informal peer review of records as a form of audit
- Adhere to the principles directed by the NMC (2005)
- Overcome attitudes regarding record keeping, reinforcing the importance of prompt recording and reporting.

 Reflection point

How could you audit your records?
Does your organisation have a formal audit process relating to record keeping?

Related aspects and terminology

Consent

Often a procedure will require written consent, and this would be carried out by a doctor or, in some cases, a registered nurse; however, it is important that healthcare assistants are aware of the key principles (covered in Chapter 1).

Scholefield et al. (1997) reviewed the principle of consent, and outlined the process of gaining legally valid consent:

- Patient must have capacity in law
- Patient has been properly informed beforehand
- Consent was given voluntarily.

Patient consent is essential for all procedures, so the healthcare assistant must ensure that written consent has been carried out, whenever appropriate. However, for most clinical skills, and those listed within this book, verbal consent is satisfactory for minor procedures, such as cannulation (Ingram and Lavery 2005). Dimond (2001) cited an example of verbal (spoken) consent, e.g. a patient is asked 'Are you ready to have your blood sugar test?' and, if responded to by a clear answer, 'yes', this is acceptable. Dimond (2001) noted that non-verbal consent (implied consent), where, instead of the reply, the patient nods their head or holds out a hand, also suggests agreement and consent. Therefore, when seeking verbal consent follow the same principles as for valid legal consent, ensuring that the patient understands all aspects of the procedure and can agree to participate fully.

Consent and children are often more complex, and this chapter reviews some basic principles. *Working in Health* (NHS Scotland 2007) stated that children under 16 years of age can give consent only if a qualified member of the medical team believes that:

- the child can understand the information given
- they can make an informed decision based on that information.

Fundudis (2003) proposed that, in general, adults are presumed to be competent under law, whereas children are presumed to be incompetent in many situations, and cited age-related studies around the ability to make informed decisions about treatment as:

- 14-year-old children did not significantly differ from an 18 year old
- 15-year-old children were no less competent than adults
- children under 14 years of age were found to have varying and less reliable levels of competence for making informed decisions about treatment.

Bray and Saunders (2006) noted that a child's rights can be ambiguous where procedures e.g. catheterisation, are to be done, because a parent or healthcare professional can override a child's wishes. They discussed the need for healthcare assistants to understand the child's level of understanding and, as some clinical skills can be unpleasant, to ensure that the child is involved, so that they feels some control over the situation.

Terminology

- Duty of care: standard of practice and duty to patients, colleagues, employer and self.
- Audit: a process for checking/monitoring, a 'snapshot' of what is actually happening in practice. Official examination of processes, e.g. financial audit.
- Ethics: the science of morals, moral principles, acting honourably.

Common problems

Birt (1998) and Culley (2001) identified the barriers to effective record keeping as:

- time constraints
- attitudes: staff do not perceive records as important or high priority
- duplication due to documentation systems and tools themselves
- poor example set by colleagues, which links to negative attitudes.

Owen (2005) cited information from the NMC (2003), which had stated that the biggest offence reported to the NMC was the failure to keep accurate records (30% of all charges made), due to the fact that most nurses did not see record keeping as a high priority activity. The time issue is often raised and Owen (2005) added that record keeping is seen as time-consuming, 'eating' into the time available to organise and deliver effective patient care.

Summary

As noted earlier by the NPSA (2005), many problems relate to poor communication, e.g. mis-hearing information, misspelling or poor handwriting, and misfiling data.

Birt (1998) advocated that good practice means that all records are factual, accurate and relevant, legible, dated, timed and signed. In addition, abbreviations should not be used and, if an alteration is necessary, e.g. entered BP in the wrong time, it should never be erased, overwritten or inked out, but rather the error should be scored out with one single line and the corrected entry written alongside, and dated/timed/signed.

McGeehan (2006) noted that record keeping was often thought of as a chore and done only at the end of a shift; effective record keeping is essential and *must be an integral part of nursing practice*.

The healthcare assistant must not only carry out the clinical skill in a timely and safe manner but also record their findings, as Dimond (2002), indicates contemporaneously (at the time).

Case study 4.1

John Simms is a healthcare assistant in your team, he reports to you that he was recording Mr Jung's urinalysis results in his records when he realised that he had written this information in the wrong record. He has been working in your clinical area for only 6 weeks and is unsure what he should do. What would you advise?

Table 4.2 Competency framework: record keeping

Competency	First assessment/Reassessment					Date/Competent signature
Steps	Demonstration/Supervised practice					
Record keeping	Date/signed	Date/signed	Date/signed	Date/signed	Date/signed	
	1	2	3	4	5	
Information was						
1 Held securely and confidentially						
2 Obtained fairly and efficiently						
3 Recorded accurately and reliably						
4 Used effectively and ethically						
5 Shared appropriately and lawfully						
Supervisors/Assessor(s):						

Permission granted and reproduced under the terms of the click-use licence.

Recommendation: the review of Skills for Health (2004a–c)

- HSC21: Communicate with, and complete records for individuals (Skills for Health 2004a)
- HSC224: Observe, monitor and record the conditions of individuals (Skills for Health 2004c)
- HSC 41: Use and develop methods and systems to communicate, record and report (Skills for Health 2004b).

These outline performance criteria and the knowledge and skills required to safely and competently perform these aspects of practice, and have been mapped to a knowledge skills framework process.

Hutchinson and Sharples (2006) described a model called HORUS, indicated within the NHS's Connecting for Health, which is used as the basis for a competency checklist (Table 4.2).

 ## Self-assessment

Assessment	Aspects	Achieved ✔
Records	*Have you considered all aspects of this section?*	
	Purpose and importance of accurate records	
	Access to and completion of appropriate records	
	Types of documentation in practice area	
	Ensuring security and safety of information	
Patient	*Have you considered all aspects of this section?*	**Achieved ✔**
	Consent aspects	
	Confidentiality	
	Patient education, e.g. access to health records	

References

Beech M (2007) Confidentiality in healthcare: conflicting legal and ethical issues. *Nursing Standard* 21(21): 42–46.

Birt G (1998) In defence of records. *Practice Nursing* 9(2): 14.

Bray L, Saunders C (2006) Nursing management of paediatric urethral catheterisation. *Nursing Standard* 20(24): 51–60.

Culley F (2001) The purpose and problems of record keeping. *Nursing and Residential Care* 3: 379–382.

Department of Health (2006) *Records Management: NHS Code of Practice, part 1–2*. London: DH.

Dimond B (2001) Legal aspects of consent 2: the different forms of consent. *British Journal of Nursing* 10: 400–401.

Dimond B (2002) *Legal Aspects of Patient Confidentiality*. Dinton: Quay Books.

Dougherty L, Lister S, eds (2004) *The Royal Marsden Hospital Manual of Clinical Nursing Procedures*, 7th edn. Oxford: Blackwell Publishing.

Evans D (2005) The Freedom of Information Act 2000 and the NHS. *Healthcare Risk Report* 11(5): 18–19.

Fundudis T (2003) Consent issues in medico-legal procedures: how competent are children to make their own decisions. *Child and Adolescent Health* **8**(1): 18–22.

Hutchinson C, Sharples C (2006) Information governance: practical implications for record-keeping. *Nursing Standard* **20**(36): 59–64.

Ingram P, Lavery I (2005) Venepuncture: best practice. *Nursing Standard* **19**(49): 55–65.

McGeehan R (2006) Best practice in record keeping. *Nursing Standard* **21**(17): 51–55.

Middleton S, Roberts A (2000) *Integrated Care Pathways*. Oxford: Butterworth-Heinemann.

National Patient Safety Agency (2005) *What We Know: Aspects of patient identification*. London: NPSA. Available at: www.saferhealthcare.org.uk/IHI/Topics/PatientIdentification/Whatweknow/ (accessed 3 August 2007).

NHS Scotland (2007) *Working in Health: Induction standards for healthcare support workers*. Available at: www.workinginhealth.com/workforce (accessed 5 January 2007).

Nursing and Midwifery Council (2005) *Guidelines for Records and Record Keeping*. London: NMC.

Nolan Y, Moonie N, Lavers S (2005) *Health and Social Science Care (Adults) S/NVQ level 3*. Oxford: Heinemann Educational Publishing.

Owen K (2005) Documentation in nursing practice. *Nursing Standard* **19**(32): 48–49.

Scholefield HA, Viney C, Evans J (1997) Expanding practice and obtaining consent. *Professional Nurse* **13**(1): 12–16.

Skills for Health (2004a) *HSC21: Communicate with, and Complete Records for Individuals*. Bristol: Skills for Health. Available at: www.skillsforhealth.org.uk/tools/view_framework.php?id=39 (accessed 27 February 2007).

Skills for Health (2004b) *HSC41: Use and Develop Methods and Systems to Communicate, Record and Report*. Bristol: Skills for Health. Available at: www.skillsforhealth.org.uk/tools/view_framework.php?id=39 (accessed 27 February 2007).

Skills for Health (2004c) *HSC224: Observe, Monitor and Record the Conditions of Individuals*. Bristol: Skills for Health. Available at: www.skillsforhealth.org.uk/tools/view_framework.php?id=39 (accessed 10 September 2007).

UNISON (2003) *The Duty of Care*. London: UNISON.

Section 2
Core clinical skills

Chapter 5

Pulse

Learning objectives

- Describe what a pulse is
- Explain how a pulse is initiated by the heart
- Name and describe the different locations where a pulse can be felt
- Describe common factors that can affect the pulse rate

Aim of this chapter

The aim of this chapter is to understand how a pulse is generated and felt within the body, the common sites and factors influencing its rate.

What is a pulse?

A pulse is felt where arteries are near the surface of the body, over a bone or another firm background and is the rhythmic expansion of the artery wall as it is stretched by a wave of blood pumped through with each heartbeat (Waugh and Grant 2001; Thibodeau and Patton 2007; Rawlings-Anderson and Hunter 2008). The heartbeat occurs when the ventricle of the heart (see 'Relevant anatomy and physiology' below) pumps blood into the already full aorta and out into the arterial system (Higham and Maddex 2005). Usually one heartbeat corresponds to one pulse beat, but if cardiac disease is present this may vary (Higham and Maddex 2005).

Reasons for performing a pulse reading

A pulse rate is often requested as part of 'routine' observations (observations to check wellbeing periodically) or as a baseline (a reading taken that acts as a reference for future readings). Other occasions include after a surgical intervention or to check that medication (drug) is working correctly (e.g. after administration of a medication to correct an abnormal heartbeat).

Relevant anatomy and physiology

The most common location for taking a pulse reading is the radial site (inside of the wrist). It is often the first choice because many patients may be familiar with this site and it is easily accessible and non-invasive. The pulse is strongest in the arteries closest to the heart, becoming weaker in the arterioles and then disappearing altogether in the capillaries (Tortora and Grabowski 2003).

The choice of site will often vary with the patient and the presenting clinical situation. If the patient was acutely unwell, perhaps with a condition that reduces blood volume e.g. shock, haemorrhage or a collapse with unknown cause, a pulse may not be easy to palpate at sites away from the heart because blood will be directed to the major organs. In such instances the radial pulse may be weak or difficult to find and the carotid or femoral site would be more appropriate (Figure 5.1). In children under the age of 2 the heartbeat is usually ausculated (listened to) via a stethoscope at the apex of the heart. The apex is located in the space between the fifth and sixth ribs (fifth intercostal space) on a line with the midpoint of the left clavicle (shoulder bone) (Thibodeau and Patton 2007) (Figure 5.1). This is deemed more accurate because movement by the child would make an accurate reading difficult to obtain (Higham and Maddex 2005). Pulses in the lower legs are usually palpated only when assessing the circulation (flow of blood) to the limbs, perhaps after surgery or trauma injury (Higham and Maddex 2005).

In some patients locating a pulse may prove challenging, despite them being clinically well. This can be due to slightly unusual anatomy or the presence of cardiovascular disease. It is also a skill that can prove difficult initially and practice is recommended, especially when accessing the carotid pulse, because locating this may be necessary in an emergency situation.

Reflection point

Ask your friends and family if you can practise taking their pulse at various sites. Note the difference in the pulses, including the rate, rhythm and strength (amplitude).

The heart generates an electrical impulse that causes the heart to contract (the muscles within the heart structure shorten and pulls inwards, compressing the chambers). Figure 5.2 shows the important structures involved in generating this impulse. The sinoatrial (SA) node is often described as the natural 'pacemaker' of the heart because it initiates impulses of contraction (Waugh and Grant 2001). This causes the atria (Figure 5.2) to contract, which then stimulates the atrioventricular (AV) node. The Purkinje fibres then convey this impulse to the apex of the myocardium, where the wave of ventricular contraction begins pumping blood into the pulmonary artery and aorta, resulting in a heartbeat and pulse (Waugh and Grant 2001).

Related aspects and terminology

Baillie (2005) suggests that the following be considered when obtaining a pulse.

The frequency of the pulse

This indicates the rate of contraction of the left ventricle and is affected by age, exercise, stress, injury and disease. Shock is a circulatory disturbance where there is usually a reduction in blood volume, and a rapid thready pulse is a characteristic sign of shock (Jevon and Ewens 2002).

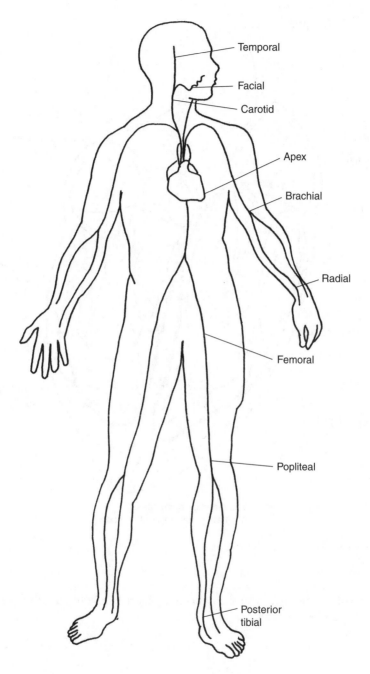

Figure 5.1 Sites for taking a pulse.

The volume

This indicates the strength of the ventricular contractions. A weak contraction may not generate a pulse at the limbs (peripheral) or, if present, it may be weak. It can also occur when there is a lack of blood volume, e.g. if the patient is bleeding heavily. A full bounding or throbbing pulse

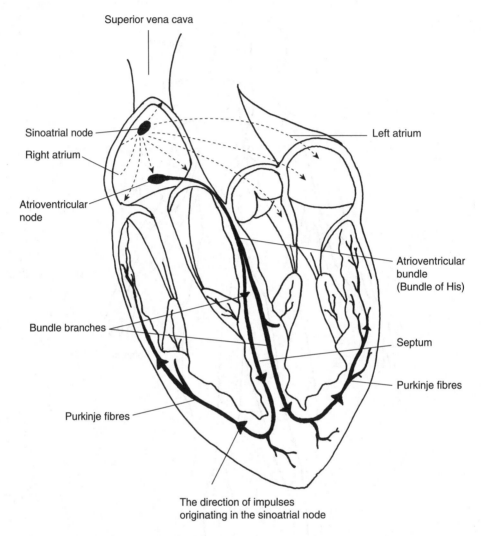

Superior vena cava

Sinoatrial node

Right atrium

Atrioventricular
node

Left atrium

Atrioventricular
bundle
(Bundle of His)

Bundle branches

Septum

Purkinje fibres

Purkinje fibres

The direction of impulses
originating in the sinoatrial node

Figure 5.2   Structure involved in initiation of a pulse.

may be indicative of complications such as anaemia, heart block, heart failure or early stages of septic shock (Jevon and Ewens 2002).

The rhythm

The rhythm of the pulse is determined by assessing the regularity of the pressure waves and can assist in establishing whether the heart is beating regularly (Rawlings-Anderson and Hunter 2008). This can be subdivided into a regularly irregular or irregularly irregular pulse. A regularly irregular pulse is noted when there is a pattern of irregularity, e.g. every third or fourth beat is not present, whereas an irregularly irregular pulse has no pattern and it cannot be anticipated when the next beat will occur (Rawlings-Anderson and Hunter 2008). An irregular pulse can indicate a possible abnormality in the heart's conduction system (Higham and Maddex 2005).

As anxiety can increase the pulse rate, before taking a pulse try to ensure that the patient is as relaxed as possible. Ensure that the patient is fully informed as to why the pulse is being taken and give reassurance if necessary. If the patient is unduly anxious consider a delay to provide them with time to settle into the surroundings and relax before the pulse is recorded.

The sound of the heartbeat comes primarily from blood turbulence caused by closing of the heart valves, although only the first two are loud enough to be heard through a stethoscope (Tortora and Grabowski 2003). The sounds are heard as 'lubb dupp', then followed by a pause, with the pause interval reducing when the pulse increases (Tortora and Grabowski 2003).

Factors affecting the pulse rate

Pulse rates can alter due to many factors, both physical and psychological, and may indicate conditions that are life threatening, e.g. cardiac arrest or long-term cardiac conditions, such as angina. Factors that increase and decrease pulse rates are the following:

- Exercise: this increases the heart rate (Marieb 2001)
- Anxiety: a patient's heart rate can increase due to anxiety
- Medication: some medication can both increase and decrease heart rates
- Trauma: in order to try to compensate for the injuries, the pulse reading may not be accurate
- Pain: this can cause an increase in heart rate
- Infection
- Cardiac abnormalities, e.g. if atherosclerosis (build-up of plaque) is present in the arteries this can influence the pulse rate (Higham and Maddex 2005)
- Circulation problems
- Temperature: increased body temperature (pyrexia) will increase the pulse rate (Jevon and Ewens 2002), whereas decreased body temperature (hypothermia) will decrease it (Waugh and Grant 2001)
- Sleep: the heartbeat reduces by 10–20 beats/min during sleep (Herbert and Alison 1996)
- Reduced consciousness: coma will decrease the pulse rate
- Fitness: if a person is very fit, the heart becomes very efficient and a lower pulse rate can deliver the required blood to the body
- Metabolic diseases: these affect the body's metabolic rate, e.g. over-/underactive thyroid
- Breathing pattern: in patients aged under 40 inspiration (breathing in) can increase the rate (Rawlings-Anderson and Hunter 2008)
- Age: see Table 5.3.

 Reflection point

Take your resting pulse rate. Now run on the spot for 2 minutes and take your pulse again.

What implications do you think this may have for patients attending the GP surgery or hospital? How would you ensure that you are measuring an accurate pulse rate for your patient?

Terminology

- *Irregular pulse*: this is a pulse that does not have a clear pattern and may have 'gaps' as if beats were being omitted. This cannot be detected on standard automated machines and is the reason why pulse readings should be taken manually.
- *'Normal' pulse*: the normal adult heart rate is between 60 and 100 beats/min, but at rest is usually between 60 and 80 beats/min (Waugh and Grant 2001). When assessing a patient's pulse it is important to look at what is considered 'normal' for every individual, bearing in mind the many factors discussed previously. Figure 5.3 shows the normal pattern of a pulse on an electrocardiograph (ECG) reading (see also Chapter 17).
- *Tachycardia*: this is an increased pulse rate of over 100 beats/min (Higham and Maddex 2005; Rawlings-Anderson and Hunter 2008). Atrial tachycardia relates to increased rate in the upper chamber of the heart. On an ECG this would show up as having an increased number of contractions on the strip (Figure 5.4).
- *Bradycardia*: a reduced heart beat of less than 60 beats/min (Higham and Maddex 2005, Rawlings-Anderson and Hunter 2008). This will result in a decreased number of contractions shown on the ECG (Figure 5.5).
- *Weak pulse*: this is when the pulse is not strong on palpation with two fingers placed over the site.
- *Thready pulse*: this is when the palpated pulse is weak and can be irregular.
- *Fibrillation*: a condition of rapid and irregular contractions (Dougherty and Lister 2004).
- *Sinus arrhythmia*: a harmless increase in the pulse rate due to inspiration (breathing in) in patients under 40 (Woods et al. 2005).

The contraction of the heart, which gives rise to a pulse, can be shown on ECG readings (see Chapter 17). The strips in Figures 5.3–5.5 show how normal, fast and slow pulses affect the

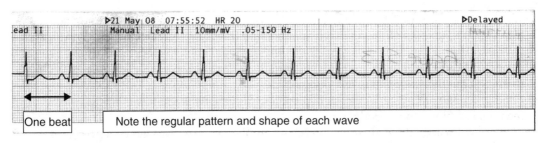

Figure 5.3 Rhythm strip for normal heart beat – 'sinus rhythm': note the regular pattern and shape of each wave. Reproduced with permission from NHS Lothian.

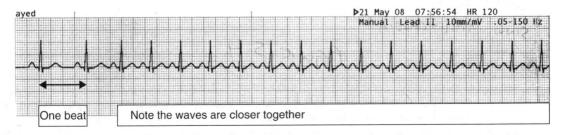

Figure 5.4 An increased heart rate – tachycardia: note that the waves are closer together. Reproduced with permission from NHS Lothian.

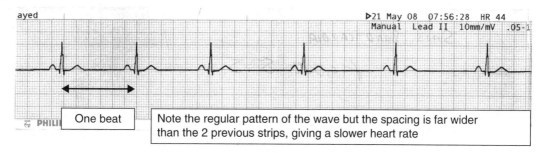

Figure 5.5 Bradycardia – slow heart beat: note the regular pattern of the wave, but the spacing is far wider than the strips in Figures 5.3 and 5.4, giving a slower heart rate. Reproduced with permission from NHS Lothian.

ECG. It is not the intention that individuals read ECGs (see also Chapter 17), merely to show how the pulse rate presents with different pulse values.

If a pulse is being taken manually a watch or clock with a second hand is required. The pulse should always be taken manually for a baseline, because use of an automatic monitor (e.g. Dinamap™, Critikon™) does not highlight the amplitude (depth), volume or whether it is regular (Dougherty and Lister 2004). Always seek advice as to which method of recording the pulse is being requested if not for a baseline recording. The procedure for taking a manual pulse is shown in Table 5.1 (note that for apex and radial pulse, this is shown in Table 5.5).

Table 5.1 Procedure for taking a manual pulse reading

Action	Rationale
Inform the patient and gain verbal consent (for children parent or guardian consent is required)	The patient is fully informed and has given consent voluntarily
Ensure access to a watch or clock with a second hand	To ensure accurate timing
Choose the site (usually radial) and, if necessary, explain the reasoning to the patient	Choose an appropriate site dependent on clinical presentation
	Children aged under 2 will require the apex site to be used (see Table 5.3)
For the radial pulse: place the first, second or third fingers along the appropriate artery and press gently (Figure 5.6)	The fingertips are sensitive enough to feel the pulse accurately
To record a manual pulse rate, count the number of beats for 60 seconds. The number counted will be the actual pulse rate, e.g. if 84 beats are counted in 60 seconds the pulse rate would be 84	This is more accurate than counting for 15 seconds and multiplying by 4 because it allows enough time for irregularities or other defects to be detected (Dougherty and Lister 2004)
Document the reading as per local policy and any other details, e.g. missed beats, irregular or thready pulse (Figure 5.7)	To ensure accurate records
	Patient may require further management
Report to nurse in charge	
Help patient to redress, where necessary	To maximise patient comfort
Reassure patient if necessary	Patient comfort

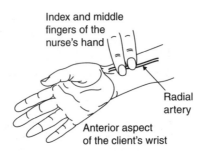

Index and middle
fingers of the
nurse's hand

Radial
artery

Anterior aspect
of the client's wrist

Figure 5.6   Taking a radial pulse.

Automated devices

Pulse recording is a feature on many machines including automated blood pressure machines (see Chapter 6) and pulse oximetry machines (see Chapter 8). The machine takes the reading automatically without the user needing to palpate (feel) the pulse. To ensure accurate readings the following points should be considered:

- The machine should be clean, appear undamaged and have been serviced regularly (usually annually but check local policy). When the machine is switched on it may do a self-test and if any error codes are displayed the machine should not be used.
- The machine must be used in accordance with the manufacturer's instructions and appropriate accessories used, where applicable, e.g. blood pressure cuff or finger probe.
- Competency-based training should be completed before using the device on a patient unsupervised to ensure correct placement of the accessories and competent use of the device.
- Some machines will have a time span in which they make an assessment before showing the pulse rate. This means that, in some instances, the pulse rate given by the machine will be the pulse rate 5–10 seconds before the reading is shown.
- If the pulse is very fast or irregular the pulse rate or abnormality may not be detected.
- Where patients have poor circulation to their arms or legs, e.g. peripheral vascular disease, an inaccurate reading may be obtained due to poor blood flow.
- If the patient moves while the reading is being taken, this may interfere with the signal, and movement may be wrongly interpreted as a heartbeat.
- A pulse should always be checked manually to ensure that it relates to the wave/pulse generated by the machine.

The procedure for taking a pulse rate using a machine is described in Table 5.2.

When taking a pulse reading, either manually or with a machine, it should also be remembered that the value of the pulse measurement should be done together with other observations of the patient, including the following:

- Assess the patient's circulation; if they are blue around the lips this would indicate poor circulation.
- Is the patient alert? If not they may have a degree of reduced consciousness.
- What are the values of other observations that have been performed, e.g. BP and temperature recordings? A correlation between these may indicate a more serious clinical condition e.g. shock or haemorrhage.

Table 5.2 Procedure for taking a pulse reading using an automated machine

Action	Rationale
Inform the patient and gain verbal consent	The patient is fully informed and has given consent voluntarily
Collect the appropriate machine and, where applicable, accessories. Ensure that the machine is clean and in good working order, and has been serviced as per local policy	To ensure machine is in good working order before use
	Correct accessories are essential for the machine to function accurately
Ensure that user has had competency training with the machine being used	To ensure that the machine is operated as the manufacturer intended
Apply the machine to the appropriate site, e.g. BP machine to arm, pulse oximeter probe to finger	To allow reading to be taken
Note the value of the recording, taking the patient's physical wellbeing and other observations into consideration, e.g. temperature, BP, pallor (colour) of patient	To assist in identification of incorrect recordings
Document the reading as per local policy (Figure 5.7)	To ensure accurate records
Report to nurse in charge if abnormal	Patient may require further management
Help patient to redress, where necessary	To maximise patient comfort
Reassure patient if necessary	Patient comfort

The role of the healthcare assistant will be to report findings, not to diagnose conditions, and therefore any reading that is unexpected or outwith the expected range should be reported to qualified staff to allow further investigation and/or management.

Fetal heartbeat

In both infants and children the normal heartbeat range is higher than that of adults (Rawlings-Anderson and Hunter 2008). Before being born, a baby's heartbeat can be heard by using a stethoscope or an electronic machine. The value is around 150 beats/min, which is significantly higher than in adults (Table 5.3).

Table 5.3 Pulse rates in relation to age

Age	Average heart rate (beats/min)
Fetus	160
Newborn	140
1–12 months	120
12 months–2 years	110
2–6 years	100
6–12 years	95
Young person	80
Adult	80

Adapted from Trimby (1989).

Neonates and young children

Once born, babies continue to have an increased heartbeat up until adolescence, with the pulse rate gradually decreasing until a more constant reading in adulthood (see Table 5.3). As mentioned earlier, to take the pulse of a child under the age of 2, a stethoscope is used to hear the apex heart beat because, if taken manually, the rapid pulse rate and small area for palpation result in inaccurate data (Dougherty and Lister 2004). The procedure for taking an apex beat is detailed in Table 5.4.

Table 5.4 Procedure for taking an apex pulse recording

Action	Rationale
Inform the patient and gain verbal consent (for children parent or guardian consent will be required)	The patient is fully informed and has given consent voluntarily
For very young children involving a play specialist may be helpful	Practising the procedure on, for example, a soft toy may reduce anxiety in the child and increase compliance
Collect equipment: watch/clock, and stethoscope; the stethoscope must be in good condition with clean, well-fitting earpieces. If required, clean as per local policy	So procedure can be performed without delay If the stethoscope is contaminated this presents an infection risk. If the stethoscope is broken it will not perform the function adequately
Draw the screens	Patient privacy
Check that the stethoscope is positioned correctly	Smooth and accurate facilitation of the procedure
Count the number of apex beats heard in 1 minute. The number counted will be the pulse rate, e.g. if 120 beats are counted in 60 seconds the pulse rate would be 120	This is more accurate than counting for 15 seconds and multiplying by 4 because it allows enough time for irregularities or other defects to be detected (Dougherty and Lister 2004)
Document the reading and any other details as per local policy, e.g. missed beats or irregular (Figure 5.7). Note that it may not be necessary to write apex or abbreviate to 'A' on individual readings as this may be documented at the top of the chart	To ensure accurate records Patient may require further management
Report to nurse in charge	
Help patient to redress, where necessary	To maximise patient comfort
Reassure patient if necessary	Patient comfort

Apex and radial pulse measurement

Where patients have a pulse deficit, i.e. the heartbeat does not match the heart rate at the radial pulse, apex (heart) and radial (wrist) pulses may be done together to assess the number of beats that are not transmitted. This will require two people to carry this out, with a watch that both individuals can see, and a stethoscope for the person assessing the apex beats. The procedure is shown in Table 5.5.

This is a skill that may require practice, especially when assessing the apex heartbeat, and competency should be achieved in this skill before performing it on a patient. The apex reading

Table 5.5 Recording apex and radial heart beats

Action	Rationale
Inform the patient and gain verbal consent	The patient is fully informed and has given consent voluntarily
Collect equipment: watch/clock, stethoscope – the stethoscope must be in good condition with clean, well-fitting earpieces. If required, clean as per local policy	Allow the procedure to be performed without delay
	If the stethoscope is contaminated this presents an infection risk. If the stethoscope is broken it will not perform the function adequately
Draw the screens	Patient privacy
Both individuals should be able to see the watch and agree when they will start counting beats	To ensure that the same time period is used to count the heartbeats.
Check that the stethoscope is positioned correctly and that a radial pulse is felt	Smooth facilitation of the procedure
Procedure commences with staff agreeing when counting will start, e.g. when the second hand gets to 12 we will count for a minute, or one person can also control the procedure by saying 'start' and 'stop'	To ensure that the same time period is used to count the heartbeats
Document the reading; this will involve using either different colours, e.g. blue/red, or different letters, e.g. A (for apex) or R (for radial) (see Figure 5.8)	To clearly identify which reading relates to apex and radial recording
Report to nurse in charge if abnormal	
Help patient to re-dress, where necessary	To maximise patient comfort
Reassure patient if necessary	Patient comfort

will always be higher because this is where the heartbeat is initiated from, and it is during the transmission to the radial pulse that beats are lost. Documentation is discussed next.

Documentation

The pulse may be recorded in the patient's notes (these may be held by the patient if they are in the community). In a hospital setting, the recordings will most probably be recorded on either a temperature, pulse and respiratory chart (TPR) or a variation; the readings often take the form of a graph (see Figure 5.7). As discussed earlier, where both the atrial and radial pulse are being taken it is useful to chart them in different colours to ensure that it is clear which reading relates to each site (Doucherty 2002), or write A (atrial) and R (radial) (Figure 5.8).

Common problems

Problems of ensuring an accurate pulse rate can be divided into technique, patient and equipment.

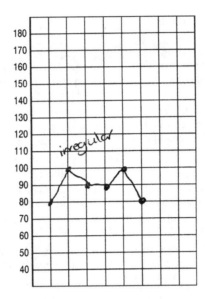

Figure 5.7   Observation chart with 'normal' and 'irregular' pulse charted. (Reproduced with permission from NHS Lothian 2008.)

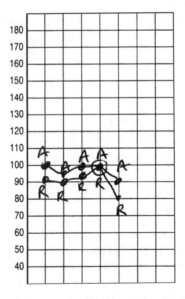

Figure 5.8   TPR (temperature, pulse and respiratory) chart with apex (A) and radial (R) pulse charted. (Observation chart reproduced with permission from NHS Lothian 2008.)

Technique

The technique is one that will require practice, especially when accessing sites other than the radial pulse. Using the thumb or forefinger is not recommended because these have pulses of their own and may confuse readings (Dougherty and Lister 2004). Recognising and having confidence to report an irregular pulse rate will also require practice and the healthcare assistant should seek help when unsure. Competency-based training should be completed before performing this task independently to ensure that the correct technique is performed.

Patients

Where patients have an underlying condition, e.g. poor circulation, the pulse may be more difficult to find at the radial site and other sites may prove more successful. If the patient is acutely unwell as a result, for example, of a major haemorrhage (blood loss) this will reduce the circulating blood volume and may make the radial site difficult to palpate. In preparation for a pulse rate being taken the patient should not have exercised or smoked before the procedure; if they have done so the reading may not be accurate (Rawlings-Anderson and Hunter 2008)

Equipment

Equipment being used should have been serviced, should be clean and when switched on should not display any error codes. Local policy will dictate when a machine can be used but it is not recommended if performing the reading for the first time on a patient because irregularity, depth and amplitude cannot be identified as mentioned earlier. If the reading obtained does not appear correct, the pulse rate should be taken manually to check.

Summary

A pulse should always be taken manually for the first time to feel its depth and ensure that it is regular. Subsequent readings can be taken using automated equipment if the pulse is regular and stable. As with all other clinical skills, users must be competent in a pulse measurement and understand the factors that influence its value before practising this skill independently on patients. Table 5.6 is an example of a competency framework for recording pulse.

Case study 5.1

Mr Gary Johnstone has been admitted for routine tonsillectomy (surgical removal of tonsils). He is 28 years old and enjoys playing sport competitively. He is fairly relaxed about his admission. His pulse rate is taken and it is 48. What factors do you think are influencing his pulse rate?

Table 5.6 Competency: recording a pulse rate

(Pulse)	First assessment/Reassessment*					Date/competent/signature
Steps	**Demonstration**					
	Date/sign	Date/sign	Date/sign	Date/sign	Date/sign	
	1	2	3	4	5	
Pulse – manual						
1 Describe what a pulse is and how the heart initiates this						
2 List the sites for taking a pulse with rationale						
3 Describe activities that affect the pulse rate						
4 State the difference in pulse rate for different age groups						
5 Collect equipment for manual or automated device						
6 Correctly identify the patient and explain procedure, and give an effective explanation about the procedure						
Recording pulse	**Demonstration**					Date/competent/signature
	1	2	3	4	5	
7 Demonstrate accurate recording for manual and/or automated machine						
8 Demonstrate tidying away of equipment if applicable						
9 Complete appropriate documentation applicable to the clinical area						

Case study 5.2

Mrs Celia Jones is 45 years old, married with two children and has come into hospital for investigations into suspected stomach cancer. She explains that she has had to rush here after dropping her children at school. Her pulse rate is 104. What factors do you think are influencing her pulse rate and what further actions would you take?

✔ Self-assessment

Assessment	Aspects	Achieved ✔
Patient	*Have you considered all aspects of this section?*	
	What initiates a heart beat?	
	The possible sites to take a pulse	
	The normal pattern of a pulse on an ECG and how a slow/fast heartbeat alters the pattern	
Procedure	*Have you considered all aspects of this section?*	**Achieved ✔**
	Factors that can affect the pulse reading	
	The factors that should be taken into consideration if using an automated device to take a pulse reading	
	Recording and reporting concerns	

References

Doucherty B (2002) Cardiorespiratory physical assessment for the acutely ill. *British Journal of Nursing* **11**: 800–807.

Dougherty L, Lister S, eds (2004) *The Royal Marsden Hospital Manual of Clinical Nursing Procedures*, 6th edn. Oxford: Blackwell Publishing.

Herbert RA, Alison JA (1996) Cardiovascular function. In: Hinchliff SM, Montague SE, Watson R (eds), *Physiology for Nursing Practice*, 2nd edn. London: Baillière Tindall, pp. 374–451.

Higham S, Maddex S (2005) In: Baillie L (ed.), *Developing Practical Nursing Skills*, 2nd edn. London: Hodder Education, Chapter 10. Monitoring vital signs, pp. 393–436.

Jevon P, Ewens B (2002) *Monitoring the Critically Ill Patient: Essential clinical skills for nurses*. London: Blackwell.

Marieb E (2001) *Human Anatomy and Physiology*, 5th edn. San Francisco, CA: Benjamin Cummings.

NHS Lothian (2008) *Observations Chart*. Edinburgh: NHS Lothian

Rawlings-Anderson K, Hunter J (2008) Monitoring pulse rate. *Nursing Standard* **22**(31): 41–43.

Thibodeau GA, Patton KT (2007) Anatomy and Physiology, 6th edn. St Louis, MO: Mosby Elsevier.

Tortora GJ, Grabowski SR (2003) *Principles of Anatomy and Physiology*, 10th edn. Chichester: John Wiley & Sons.

Trimby B (1989) *Clinical Nursing Procedure*. Philadelphia, PA: JB Lippincott.

Waugh A, Grant A (2001) *Ross and Wilson Anatomy and Physiology in Health and Illness*, 9th edn. London: Churchill Livingstone

Woods SL, Sivarajan Foelicher E, Underhill Motzer S, Bridges E (2005) *Cardiac Nursing*, 5th edn. Philadelphia, PA: Lippincott, Williams & Wilkins

Chapter 6
Blood pressure monitoring

Learning objectives

- Understand what blood pressure means, and how it relates to the anatomy and physiology of the body
- Discuss factors that affect blood pressure readings
- Discuss why lying and standing blood pressure readings are taken
- Measure and record blood pressure using equipment appropriately
- Demonstrate how to document blood pressure readings

Aim of this chapter

The aim of this chapter is to review the principles for undertaking blood pressure (BP) monitoring, the related anatomy and physiology, and the skills required to measure, record and report findings.

What is blood pressure?

Blood pressure can be defined as the force or pressure that the blood exerts on the walls of the blood vessels (Waugh and Grant 2001; Valler-Jones and Wedgbury 2005).

Reasons for monitoring blood pressure

Blood pressure is taken to obtain a baseline (a reading taken that acts as a reference for future readings) or as an ongoing measure of cardiovascular (heart) function in order to make comparisons, aid diagnosis and evaluate treatment of disease. It is also used to screen patients for underlying disease or complications, or as a precaution for side effects to certain medications (e.g. the contraceptive pill).

Who requests the test?

A BP reading can be requested in the community setting by a GP, practice nurse or community nurse. This may be part of patients' care when they are discharged from hospital, or to assess their health in relation to a long-term condition, e.g. hypertension (increased BP) as a result of heart disease. In the acute setting, such as a hospital, doctors or nursing staff may request blood pressure to be taken due to the patient's clinical presentation, or it may be part of a specific routine, e.g. admission procedure or after surgical intervention. Other professionals may also take a reading as part of an assessment, e.g. an occupational therapist or physiotherapist taking a reading to assess a patient after a history of frequent falls.

Who can take a BP reading?

Any healthcare professional can undertake BP measurement, the most important criteria being that they are competent in the skill. Incorrect recordings can result in inappropriate treatment or undiagnosed conditions that may have a severe effect on the patient's health. Accurate blood pressure, on the other hand, can give important clues about health and wellbeing (Valler-Jones and Wedgbury 2005).

What is done with the readings/information?

'Routine' BP recordings will be written in different documents, dependent on the purpose of the recording and whether in hospital, the GP surgery, the community or the patient's own home. The documentation may take the format of patient records (can be held by the patient, e.g. antenatal notes during pregnancy), admission documentation, care plans, integrated care pathways or on a specific chart for observations – commonly referred to as a TPR (temperature, pulse and respiratory rate) chart. The recording on the TPR chart is shown in Figure 6.4. If automated machines are used to take recordings, data may be stored by the machine and, in some critical care areas, it may be saved and 'sent' to a central computer station automatically. If the result is in any way unexpected or outwith 'normal' guidelines (see notes later) the reading must be verbally reported immediately to the nurse in charge.

Relevant anatomy and physiology

Structure of the heart

The heart is best described as a pump and to assist this function it is made almost entirely of muscle (Figure 6.1). This muscle works automatically; thus it does not need the brain to tell it to work but does so under what is known as 'involuntary action'. The heart is situated in the thorax (chest cavity) between and in front of the lungs (Waugh and Grant 2001). It is centrally placed but tilted, which is why the heartbeat is heard to the left and is roughly the size of a fist (Tortora and Derrickson 2006; Thibodeau and Patton 2007).

Within the heart, there are two top chambers known as the right and left atria and below two further chambers known as the right and left ventricles (Thibodeau and Patton 2007) (Figure 6.1). The right atrium receives blood from throughout the body via the superior vena cava, inferior vena cava and coronary sinus, and this blood does not contain oxygen (deoxygenated). The blood then passes into the right ventricle and the pulmonary arteries to go to the lungs to receive oxygen. Once the blood has combined with oxygen (oxygenated blood) it is returned to the heart via the pulmonary veins to the left atrium. The oxygenated blood is then expelled from the heart via the aorta to supply oxygen and blood to the tissues. This results in the left side of the heart having oxygenated blood and the right side deoxygenated blood. The two sides are completely separated by the septum so the blood cannot meet, resulting in the heart functioning as two pumps (Tortora and Derrickson 2006). An independent blood supply delivers blood to the heart muscle itself.

The amount of blood ejected from the ventricle in one contraction is called the 'stroke volume', and this volume is estimated to average 70 millilitres (mL) per beat in the average adult (Tortora and Grabowski 2003). To estimate the cardiac output, this is multiplied by the heart rate, giving the amount of blood ejected from the left ventricle in one minute (Box 6.1) (Jevon and Ewens 2002). Non-invasive blood pressure (involves a machine being applied externally) gives an early sign of a fall in cardiac output (Jevon and Ewens 2002).

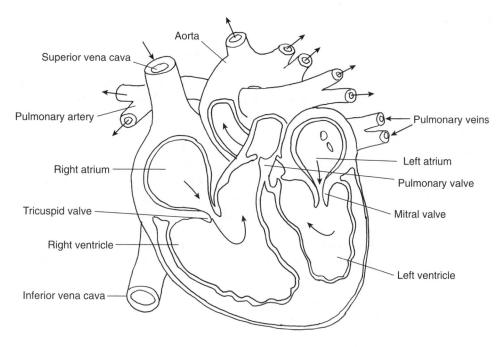

Figure 6.1 Internal structure of the heart.

Box 6.1 Cardiac output formula

Example
A man has a heart beat of 72 and a stroke volume of 70 mL (millilitres)
Cardiac output = Heart rate × Stroke volume
72 × 70
= 5040 mL/min or 5.04 litres per minute (L/min)

The role of valves within the circulatory system

There are four sets of heart valves, two sets guarding the openings between the atria and ventricles (the tricuspid and mitral valves), and two located inside the pulmonary artery and aorta (called the aortic and pulmonary valves or semilunar valves collectively). Thibodeau and Patton (2007) describe heart valves as mechanical devices that permit the flow of blood in one direction only. Degrees of valve incompetence will have a variable effect on the body, because some valve problems will result in no further actions being required, and in others valve replacement will be necessary.

Defective heart valves can cause heart murmurs and this leads to regurgitation (blood leaking backward through the valve when it should be closed). Diagnosis can result after unusual sounds are first heard through a stethoscope before, between or after normal heart sounds, or they may mask the normal heart sounds (Tortora and Derrickson 2006). These sounds are commonly known as 'innocent heart murmurs', because they do not present any health problems at all and the sounds are made by the blood circulating through the heart's chambers and valves, or through blood vessels near the heart. Heart murmurs can be common in children, often disappearing later in life (Tortora and Derrickson 2006).

The cardiac cycle

The heart maintains constant circulation by a series of events know as the cardiac cycle (Waugh and Grant 2001). The cycle consists of atrial systole, which is when the atrium contracts, and this lasts around 0.1 second, followed by ventricular systole, contraction of the ventricles that lasts around 0.3 s. Finally complete relaxation of both atria and ventricles occurs, lasting 0.4 s. It is this sequence of contraction and relaxation of the heart muscle that allows blood to flow around the body.

When the left ventricle contracts and pushes blood into the aorta, the resulting pressure is called the systolic blood pressure. This is the maximum pressure of the blood against the wall of the artery (Waugh and Grant 2001). It is expressed as the top figure when quoting blood pressure (think of a fraction: this is the first number above the line). When complete cardiac diastole occurs and the heart is resting following the ejection of blood, the pressure within the arteries is called diastolic blood pressure (the bottom number below the 'fraction' line). This is the minimum amount of pressure exerted against the wall of the artery, after closure of the aortic valve (Higham and Maddex 2005). An example of a blood pressure reading is shown in Box 6.2.

Box 6.2 Example of how a blood pressure is written

$\dfrac{132}{80}$ Systolic
            Diastolic

Arterial blood pressure is what is commonly referred to as blood pressure and is measured in millimetres of mercury (mmHg) using a sphygmomanometer or electronic device (O'Brien et al. 2001). Using the left arm for a blood pressure reading is a more accurate reflection of arterial blood pressure (Jevon and Ewens 2002) but blood pressure should be recorded in the arm with the highest reading (British Hypertension Society 2006). Wide discrepancies between arms can be indicative of an aortic aneurysm (Jevon and Ewens 2002), therefore good practice would be to take a reading in both arms initially and report any abnormalities to the nurse in charge. This should also be documented in the patient's records.

Normal blood pressure

Blood pressure can fluctuate within a wide range and still be considered within normal limits. Normal systolic pressure should be between 100 and 140 mmHg and diastolic between 60 and 90 mmHg (Waugh and Grant 2001). Often there can be variance in the definition of normal BP with individual BP fluctuating (Wallymahmed 2008). Systolic readings of around 120 mmHg and diastolic of about 80 mmHg are considered 'normal' (Joint British Societies 2005).

Related aspects and terminology

Maintenance of normal blood pressure

Blood pressure is maintained within normal limits through fine adjustments by the body with a number of factors affecting the value recorded; this is detailed in Box 6.3.

Box 6.3 Factors affecting blood pressure readings

- **Blood volume**: this relates to the amount of blood that is circulating around the body. Where the blood volume is reduced dramatically, such as haemorrhage (rapid blood loss), this causes a drop in BP. Tortora and Grabowski (2003) state that even losses of 10 per cent or more, e.g. in instances of trauma, haemorrhage or severe dehydration, can result in a fall in BP.
- **Peripheral resistance**: this relates to the pressure that is presented against the flow of blood and can reduce the efficiency of blood returning to the heart.
- **Elasticity of the artery walls**: this is how much 'give' the blood vessels have and, in cases of stenosis (narrowing of the artery) of the vessels, elasticity is lost (Waugh and Grant 2001). Atherosclerosis (build-up of fat deposits within the vessels) directly affects the elasticity of the arteries and it is thought that this may be influenced by a previous family history (Thompson and Webster 2000).
- **Respiratory centre**: when this centre is stimulated in the brain, particularly during inspiration, the blood pressure will rise (Jevon and Ewens 2002).
- **Nicotine**: as nicotine is a vasoconstrictor (reduces the diameter of the blood vessel), the BP increases (Jevon and Ewens 2002).
- **Age**: Marieb (2001) reports that BP increases from birth and throughout life, thus affecting the 'normal reading' for any specific patient. In addition, arteries harden with age and therefore an increase in BP is also expected.
- **Gender**: men generally have higher BP than women (Waugh and Grant 2001).
- **Weight**: increased weight tends to increase BP. This is due to the fact that an obese person's heart has to work harder, resulting in an increase in BP (Marieb 2001).
- **Emotional factors**: stress, fear, anxiety and excitement all increase the BP (Higham and Maddex 2005). The primitive 'fight or flight' response to fear affects BP because this is the body's preparation for survival. Relaxation has been shown to decrease BP (Leefarr 2000).
- **Diet/medications**: high salt and low calcium dietary intakes may lead to a rise in BP (Marieb 2001). Diuretics and tranquillisers can also reduce BP by decreasing blood volume (Tortora and Grabowski 2003).
- **Time of day**: BP is known to be lowest in the morning, rising throughout the day, reaching its peak in the afternoon, and then falling in the evening (Thompson and Webster 2000; O'Brien et al. 2003).
- **White coat hypertension**: this is when the individual's BP is consistently higher when measured in a hospital or medical setting rather than the individual's home, due to anxiety or fear of the medical environment (O'Brien et al. 2003). A study by Cappuccio et al. (2004) showed that patients who monitor their own BP at home have better BP control and are more likely to reach their target BP than those who do not, highlighting the importance of patient monitoring at home, as well as in the GP's surgery and clinic. If a patient has white coat hypertension often 24-hour monitoring can provide more accurate readings (see '24-hour monitoring').
- **Gravity**: if an individual moves from lying down to standing quickly the BP may fall; this known as 'orthostatic hypotension' (Marieb 2001). Baroreceptors, which are situated throughout the body and monitor changes in BP, raise the BP with increased stimulation (Valler-Jones and Wedgbury 2005). However, if this mechanism is lost, e.g. after prolonged bed rest, the patient may faint on standing (Jevon and Ewens 2002). This is also referred to as postural hypotension (the BP dropping when the person stands up suddenly) (see 'Lying and standing BP measurement').
- **Hormones**: there are also various hormones that affect BP and aid its regulation by altering cardiac output, changing systemic vascular resistance or adjusting the total blood volume, e.g. the hormones renin and aldosterone from the kidneys (Tortora and Derrickson 2006).
- **Family history**: this can be related to coronary heart disease, which can cause resistance to blood flow and increased peripheral resistance as mentioned earlier. Hypertension due to disease is called secondary hypertension (Higham and Maddex 2005) and examples include heart disease, kidney disease, endocrine disorders and neurological conditions (Marieb 2001).
- **Sleep**: this is when systolic BP is at its lowest (Marieb 2001).

Adapted from Higham and Maddex (2005).

Terminology

Hypertension

This is an elevation in the blood pressure and may be acute or chronic (Dougherty and Lister 2004). It is based not on one reading but on three or more readings taken at rest, several days apart, and where the value exceeds the upper limits of what is considered normal for the patient (Dougherty and Lister 2004). Hypertension increases the risk of having a stroke or heart attack and can be a result of stress, anxiety or recent strenuous activity. The National Institute for Health and Clinical Excellence (NICE) defines hypertension as elevated BP above 140/90 mmHg (NICE 2006) (see also British Hypertension Society guidelines 2004). If the BP reading is higher than 140/90 it is suggested that another reading be taken after giving the patient time to rest (Burton and Birdi 2006).

Hypotensive

This refers to when the systolic BP is below 100 mmHg and can be the first indicator of shock (where vital body processes shut down in response to a reduction in blood volume) (Jevon 2001; Marieb 2001; Dougherty and Lister 2004). It can also indicate that there is not sufficient pressure to pump blood to the head when a person is in a standing or sitting position, and can cause the individual to faint (see 'Postural hypotension').

Postural or 'orthostatic' hypotension

This is defined as low BP when the patient suddenly stands up (Jevon and Holmes 2007; Wallymahmed 2008). Symptoms may be dizziness and in some instances fainting. When this occurs BP is measured when the patient is both standing (erect) and lying (supine), to detect a deficit when the patient stands up. The procedure for measuring lying and standing blood pressure is shown later in Table 6.4.

The British Hypertension Society (2004), supported by the World Health Organization, classify blood pressure in Table 6.1.

Table 6.1 Blood pressure classification

Category	Systolic BP (mmHg)	Diastolic BP (mmHg)
Optimal blood pressure	<120	<80
Normal blood pressure	<130	<85
High normal blood pressure	130–139	85–89
Grade 1 hypertension (mild)	140–159	90–99
Grade 2 hypertension (moderate)	160–179	100–109
Grade 3 hypertension (severe)	>180	>110
Isolated systolic hypertension (grade 1)	140–159	<90
Isolated systolic hypertension (grade 2)	>160	<90

24-hour monitoring

Monitoring a patient's blood pressure over a 24-hour period can be done for various reasons that include where patients have:

- suspected white coat hypertension (as described earlier)
- fluctuating BP readings (Hypertension Influence Team 2007)
- BP that is not well controlled despite medication (Hypertension Influence Team 2007).

The device used is called an ambulatory monitor, which means that the patient is fully mobile while the device is recording the BP at regular intervals. This has the advantage of monitoring the patient's BP while that patient is participating in normal daily activities.

Korotkoff's sounds

When taking a BP reading manually, certain sounds known as Korotkoff's sounds are heard once you have inflated the cuff. The five phases are in Table 6.2.

In most instances all sounds will be heard; however, Williams et al. (2004) state that if, during phase 5, the reading reduces to zero phase 4 should be used. The British Hypertension Society (BHS 2006) states that this can occur in pregnancy; if so phase 4 sounds should be used for the systolic reading. It is essential that the skill of taking BP is both practised and assessed to ensure that the sounds are heard correctly, because this is important in obtaining an accurate reading.

Care must be exercised when taking patients' BP to ensure that efforts are taken to reduce anxiety, and that a period of time has elapsed after strenuous activity because they both influence the BP value.

Table 6.2 Korotkoff's sounds

Phase	Description
1	This is the systolic blood pressure. It is heard as repetitive, faint yet clear tapping sounds, which gradually increase in intensity
2	This is the softening of sounds, which may sound like blowing or swishing
3	This is the return of sharper and perhaps crisper sounds that do not regain the intensity of phase 1
4	This is where a distinct muffled sound is heard, which may become soft and blowing
5	No sounds are heard. This is the diastolic blood pressure

Adapted from O'Brien et al. (2003) and Trim (2005).

Equipment

Blood pressure is taken with a manual mercury sphygmomanometer, an aneroid sphygmomanometer or a fully automatic machine (see Table 6.3 for the procedure). When using any equipment, it is necessary before use to check that the machine has been serviced as per local policy and appears in good working order. It is also essential that the correct size of cuff be used to ensure accuracy of the BP readings. Table 6.5 shows correct sizing of cuffs.

If the cuff is too small, the reading could be falsely high and if too large a cuff is selected the reading could be too low (Gomersall and Oh 1997).

Table 6.3 Procedure to measure blood pressure with mercury, aneroid or electronic machines

Action	Rationale
1. The patient Explain the procedure to patients, paying particular attention to informing them of the tightness of the cuff and the need to stop eating, talking and moving during measurement (Dougherty and Lister 2004; Wallymahmed 2008)	To fully inform the patient, gain verbal consent and cooperation
The patient should not have been participating in strenuous activity for 30 minutes before taking the reading (Campbell et al. 1990; Jevon and Ewens 2002)	This would give an inaccurate reading
Let the patient rest for 5 minutes before the procedure (Wallymahmed 2008)	Anxiety will give an inaccurate reading
Wash and dry hands (Jevon and Ewens 2002)	Prevent the spread of infection
2. Equipment/accessories Ensure that the machine is in good working order, has been serviced as per local policy and is clean	To ensure accuracy of the machine
Choose an appropriate cuff (for both the type and model of the machine and the patient)	BP cuff should be appropriate for the patient (see Table 6.5) to ensure accuracy. The equipment should be in good condition
A stethoscope will be required for a manual reading and must be in good condition with clean, well-fitting earpieces	To ensure that it is fit for purpose and to prevent infection
Bladder length should be 80% of the arm's circumference but no more than 100% (Higham and Maddex 2005; Wallymahmed 2008)	To ensure accurate readings
For mercury position the manometer within 1 metre of the patient with the level of the mercury clearly visible and resting at the zero level (Wallymahmed 2008)	To ensure that the scale is easily visible (Wallymahmed 2008)
For aneroid, ensure that the dial can be seen when operating the machine	
3. Patient Expose the arm to the shoulder, removing tight or restrictive clothing (British Hypertension Society 2006; Jevon and Holmes 2007)	Restrictive clothing may produce inaccurate readings
The arm should be supported at the level of the heart; a pillow is ideal (Jevon and Holmes 2007; Wallymahmed 2008)	To ensure accuracy of the reading (see Box 6.1)
The same arm should be used each time to allow comparison	To ensure consistency if there is a variance between arms. The arm with the highest reading should be used (BHS 2006)
The bladder cuff should encircle the arm just above the antecubital fossa (crook of the elbow) 2.5 cm above the brachial artery (Higham and Maddex 2005). The centre of the bladder cuff should be positioned over the brachial artery at the point of maximum pulsation (Dougherty and Lister 2004). It is recommended that a space of two fingers should be evident between the cuff and where the stethoscope is placed	To ensure correct placement

Table 6.3 (*Continued*)

Action	Rationale
Connect the cuff tubing to the manometer tubing and loosen the valve of the inflation ball	To ensure smooth facilitation of the procedure
4. Procedure **For mercury/aneroid**: to estimate systolic blood pressure – palpate the brachial artery which can be located in the middle of the arm at the inner elbow, slightly inwards towards the body. By placing two or three fingers at this site the pulse can be found, as it is the site of maximum pulsation (Dougherty and Lister 2004). Inflate the cuff until pulsation disappears. Inflate a further 10 mmHg and release the valve slowly, taking a note of the reading on the mercury column when the brachial pulse returns	Provides an estimate of the systolic pressure
Deflate the cuff completely allowing all the air to escape	Residual air in the cuff many give an inaccurate reading
Palpate the brachial artery and place the bell of the stethoscope lightly over the site. Inflate the cuff to 30 mmHg above previous estimated systolic pressure	Excessive pressure can distort sounds or make them persist for longer
Listen through the stethoscope releasing the valve on the cuff by approximately 2–3 mmHg/s (Wallymahmed 2008)	At faster rates of deflation if using mercury it may fall too quickly, resulting in an inaccurate reading
When the first sound is heard the level should be noted; this is the systolic pressure. Continue to deflate the cuff and, at the point that the sounds disappear altogether, this is the diastolic pressure	Ensure knowledge of Korotkoff's sounds (see Table 6.2)
BP should be measured to the nearest 2 mmHg (Wallymahmed 2008)	Provides a more accurate reading
Electronic device: Switch on the device and press start	To obtain the reading
Read the systolic and diastolic blood pressure as displayed on the machine but ensure the reading is consistent with patient's overall general condition	To ensure that the reading is accurate and the machine functioning correctly
5. Documentation Document the systolic and diastolic BP on the appropriate chart (Figure 6.4)	To ensure record of BP reading is available
Report any abnormal readings to nurse in charge or medical staff	To allow further intervention where necessary
6. Remove equipment Remove the cuff and make the patient comfortable	Patient comfort
Return the equipment to appropriate store, cleaning as per local policy if required. Plug in electronic device	To allow equipment to be in good working order for next patient

Table 6.4 Procedure for lying (supine) and standing (erect) blood pressure recordings
First ensure that you follow the procedures detailed in Table 6.2 for the specific machine that you are using.

Action	Rationale
1. Explain the procedure and rationale to the patient	To fully inform the patient, gain verbal consent and cooperation
2. For lying (supine) blood pressure: Lie the patient down for 5 minutes (Jevon and Holmes 2007)	To prepare the patient for the procedure and ensure an accurate reading. It may also relax the patient
3. Complete the procedure as per Table 6.3 dependent on the device being used	To ensure that an accurate reading is obtained
4. Document the reading ensuring that you are recording it for lying (supine) reading (Figure 6.4) Leave the cuff in place	Accurate record of the BP reading Preparation for the next part of the procedure
4. Allow the patient to stand for 1 min, supporting the patient where necessary (Jevon and Holmes 2007)	To ensure that an accurate reading is obtained. Supporting the patient will ensure patient safety should they fall
5. Complete the procedure as per Table 6.3 Document the reading ensuring that you are recording it for standing (erect) reading (Figure 6.5)	To ensure that an accurate reading is obtained. Either a code of E (erect) and S (supine) or different colours can be used to record the different readings on an observations chart (Figure 6.5)
6. Explain the readings to the patients if they want this information	To ensure that the patient is fully informed and allow further information to be given, where necessary

Mercury sphygmomanometers

Standard mercury sphygmomanometers are becoming less common as mercury presents a health and safety hazard. Indeed, the Medical and Healthcare product Regulatory Agency (MHRA 2003) state that, where possible, mercury devices should be used only when there are no other alternatives, and staff should be trained appropriately in the procedure of dealing with a mercury leakage. This procedure should be detailed in local policies and procedures within organisations that use mercury sphygmomanometers. To ensure accurate readings using a mercury sphygmomanometer, it is important that the following points should be noted:

- Ensure that the measuring tube of the manometer is kept in a vertical position, because otherwise readings can be inaccurate (Campbell et al. 1990). The manometer should be clean to allow good visualisation and prevent the mercury sticking to the manometer which would over-estimate the BP reading (Markandu et al. 2000).
- The bladder (stored within the material cuff) must be in a good condition, intact and not leaking air (Beevers et al. 2001).

Table 6.5 Sizes of cuff

Indication	Bladder width × length (cm)	Arm circumference (cm)
Small adult/child	12 × 18	<23
Standard adult	12 × 26	<33
Large adult	12 × 40	<50
Adult thigh cuff	20 × 42	<53

From Williams et al. (2004).

- The control valve must tighten and loosen easily and not leak because this would cause an underestimation of the systolic pressure and overestimation of the diastolic pressure (Beevers et al. 2001).
- The rubber tubing should be intact and not perished (McAlister and Straus 2001).
- Deflation of the cuff should be slow (Dougherty and Lister 2004).

Aneroid sphygmomanometer

This device is commonly used in the community and sometimes patients may have these in their own homes. It works by measuring the cuff pressure using bellows connected to a cuff via rubber tubing, and the pressure is transferred to a dial to give the reading (Beevers et al. 2001). O'Brien et al. (2001) report that these machines can appear to be calibrated correctly and still cause inaccuracies due to damage that is not visible to the user. Therefore, the patient's clinical presentation should also be considered, and readings rechecked using another machine if they do not correlate with the BP reading obtained. To promote accurate readings in these machines it is recommended that:

- the indicators sit at the '0' correctly before use (Dougherty and Lister 2004)
- the faceplate is not damaged; commonly it can be cracked, which will affect readings (Dougherty and Lister 2004).

Automated devices

An alternative to the BP sphygmomanometer is the use of automated devices, which can be fixed or portable. An example of one model is given in Figure 6.2. They are sometimes referred to as monitors with some models capable of taking ECG (electrocardiograph), pulse and pulse

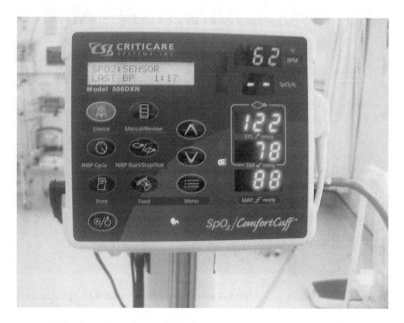

Figure 6.2 An automated blood pressure measuring machine.

oximetry readings. The machines can operate by battery, mains power or both. Some machines have functions allowing BP readings to be measured at regular intervals, e.g. every 15 minutes, and may have a facility to store the readings. It is essential that the machine is used in the way that the manufacturer intended, so individuals must ensure that they are taught how to use it correctly and refer to the manufacturer's instructions. The machine displays the systolic and diastolic values, and in some instances the mean value that is referred to as the 'mean arterial pressure'. The machine measures the blood pressure by detecting pressure oscillations (waves) in the cuff, which are generated by arterial wall movement, with each arterial pulsation beneath an occluding cuff. The amplitude (depth) of the oscillation depends on the relationship between the cuff pressure and the arterial BP, reaching a maximum when the cuff pressure equals the mean arterial pressure. Therefore, if the pulse is weak or thready, the reading may not be accurate and the reading should be checked with a manual sphygmomanometer (Beevers et al. 2001).

Sites for recording blood pressure

- Either arm using the brachial artery (most common)
- At the wrist where the radial and ulnar arteries are situated; this would not be expected from a healthcare assistant.
- The foot where the dorsalis pedis artery is situated; this would not be expected from a healthcare assistant.

Taking blood pressure

The cuff is usually placed on the upper arm at the heart level for both adults and children, with the thigh used only when the upper arm cannot be used, and this would not be expected of a healthcare assistant without further training. When using all BP measuring machines the arm

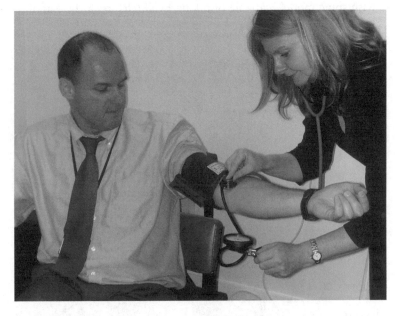

Figure 6.3   Inappropriate positioning for a blood pressure recording. The arm should be supported on a pillow and below heart level.

should be supported for optimum readings to be obtained (Jevon and Ewens 2002). Figure 6.3 shows inappropriate positioning for taking a BP reading.

Reflection point

Get someone who has completed competency-based training for blood pressure to take your blood pressure. Describe how it felt.

As mentioned earlier, where the patient has a variance in lying and standing BP a reading should be obtained for both lying and standing. Where the patient has a history of fainting or collapse when standing it is recommended that another person be available to ensure patient safety. Table 6.4 details the procedure for lying and standing BP measurement.

Reflection point

What factors would you consider when taking a blood pressure reading on a patient who is agitated and who has an intravenous infusion (drip) in place?

The British Hypertension Society (2004) summarise the main points regarding BP measurement using a standard mercury sphygmomanometer or semiautomated device as follows:

- Use a properly maintained, calibrated and validated device
- Measure sitting BP routinely: standing BP should be recorded at the initial estimation in patients who are older or have diabetes
- Remove tight clothing, support the arm at heart level, ensure that the patient's hand is relaxed and avoid talking during the measurement procedure
- Use cuff of appropriate size
- Read BP to the nearest 2 mmHg
- Measure diastolic BP during disappearance of korotkoff sounds (phase V)
- Take the mean of at least two readings; more readings are needed if marked differences between initial measurements are found
- Do not treat on the basis of an isolated reading.

Documentation

Charting blood pressure readings

Once the systolic and diastolic BP values have been obtained they should be recorded promptly. If they need to be charted on an observation chart, this takes the format of a graph. Despite variations of the chart being available, the principles are the same. The systolic pressure is marked by an arrow or cross at the top and the diastolic value by an arrow or cross at the bottom. The space between the readings is either drawn in a dotted or continuous line. Once various readings have been charted this method allows trends to be seen clearly. Figures 6.4 and 6.5 show examples of charts with BP readings recorded.

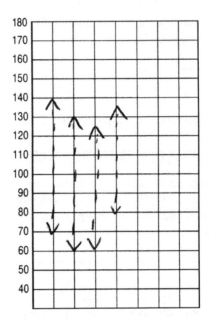

Figure 6.4   A TPR (temperature, pulse, respiratory rate) chart with blood pressure readings charted. (Observation chart reproduced with permission from NHS Lothian 2008.)

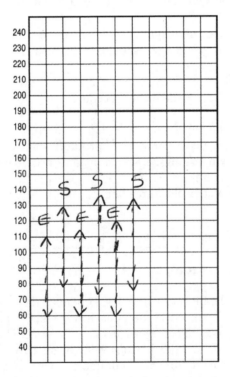

Figure 6.5   TPR (temperature, pulse, respiratory rate) chart with erect (standing: E) and supine (lying: S) blood pressure readings charted. (Observation chart reproduced with permission from NHS Lothian 2008.)

Reflection point

A blood pressure reading is taken with a cuff that is too large for the patient. How do you think this will affect the readings obtained?

Common problems

Common complications can occur when using non-invasive blood pressure devices and it is important to identify these promptly and then reporting them to the nurse in charge. Box 6.4 shows the common complications.

Box 6.4 Common complications of non-invasive blood pressure measuring devices

- Swelling at the site where the cuff is placed, known as limb oedema, can occur (Jevon and Ewens 2002)
- Friction blisters can occur if the blood pressure machine is used very frequently causing irritation at the site (Jevon and Ewens 2002)
- Nerve damage can occur to the nerves within the arm, known as ulnar nerve palsy (Jevon and Ewens 2002)
- Excessive bruising can result due the frequent or overinflation of the cuff, where the patient is receiving anticoagulant therapy that 'thins' the blood (e.g. heparin or warfarin) (Smith 2000)

Many patients who are having a BP recorded have underlying diseases or are receiving medical intervention that will need to be taken into account when considering the site suitable. Box 6.5 summarises some of the main considerations.

Box 6.5 Inappropriate sites and rationale

- **Intravenous infusion running**: taking blood pressure on this arm could interfere with fluid delivery.
- **Pulse oximetry machine being used**: taking BP on the same arm will alter the readings, because blood flow will be occluded
- **Fistula/shunt**: shunts are used for renal dialysis and taking BP at this site may cause damage to the shunt
- **Trauma**: where there has been injury to a site that could be used for BP measurement the cuff could cause further injury
- **Atrial fibrillation** (increased heart beat in the top chamber of the heart): some automated devices provide unreliable readings and in such instances another type of device should be used (O'Brien et al. 2003).
- **Previous stroke with residual damage to one side**: the patient's circulation may be affected or the arm is limited in movement or sensation
- **Lymphoedema**: this is swelling that can be due to many causes, e.g. mastectomy with lymph node removal, and taking a BP reading could damage an area that is already swollen
- **Arthritic limb**: the patient may have arthritis in the arm(s) resulting in correct positioning being problematic and causing discomfort and pain
- **Circulatory problems**: where circulation in the arms is affected this may result in inaccurate readings

---

To ensure accurate BP readings it is essential that the patient be prepared, the equipment be good working order and the healthcare assistant be competent in the skill. Table 6.6 summarises the common problems when taking a BP reading.

Table 6.6 Common problems when taking a blood pressure reading

Problem	Action to reduce inaccurate readings
Poor technique of the user (Beevers et al. 2001; Wallymahmed 2008)	Ensure that, before undertaking the procedure, competency-based training and assessment have been completed in line with local policy
Machine malfunction	Report to appropriate personnel (e.g. medical physics, servicing department or manufacturer). Do not use the machine
Equipment has tape applied to secure	Report and do not use the damaged piece of equipment
Use of an incorrectly sized cuff (Wallymahmed 2008)	This is essential for accurate readings and an appropriate sized cuff should be sought (see Table 6.5)
Failure to ensure that the mercury column is initially at zero (Wallymahmed 2008)	Always ensure that the mercury column is initially at zero before commencing the procedure
Patient has tight clothing on	This will give an inaccurate reading and clothing needs to be removed
The arm is not correctly supported	If the arm is unsupported the muscles may contract, leading to a rise in diastolic blood pressure (Wallymahmed 2008). If the arm is raised above heart level, this can lead to underestimation of blood pressure (MHRA 2006). Incorrect positioning during the procedure can lead to an error rate as high as 10% (Jevon and Ewens 2002)
Blood pressure cuff comes off when reading taken	This can be due to the wrong size of cuff and the arm circumference should be re-measured and the correct cuff used
	In other instances, the Velcro on the cuff may be worn and ineffective and will need to be replaced
Cannot 'hear' blood pressure sounds	Ensure that all equipment is working. Palpate pulse and ensure that the stethoscope is at the correct pulse point. Seek assistance if unsure.
Patient complains that it is sore to take blood pressure	Do not pump cuff up too high unless patient has hypertension. Use estimated systolic value (see Table 6.3) or previous readings to act as a reference
Movement causes noise and inaccurate readings	Ask the patient to remain still or if the patient cannot do this, ask colleague to assist you
Rounding up readings to the nearest 5 or 10 mmHg (Beevers et al. 2001; Wallymahmed 2008)	Document the exact reading that is obtained

Summary

An understanding of how the body controls blood pressure can help link theory to practice. It is essential that BP be taken with equipment on which the healthcare assistant has completed competency-based training because the recordings can affect patient management. Abnormal or unusual recordings for the patient should always be reported to ensure prompt management where necessary.

Blood pressure measurement is an area of healthcare assistant practice with the potential to make a real difference to the patient's quality of life and lifespan (Thornett 2007). Table 6.7 is an example of a competency framework for blood pressure measurement.

Table 6.7 Competency framework: recording a blood pressure

(BP)	First assessment/Reassessment					Date/competent/signature
Steps	**Demonstration**					
	Date/sign	Date/sign	Date/sign	Date/sign	Date/sign	
	1	2	3	4	5	
Blood pressure						
1 Describe what is blood pressure and the relationship with the heart						
2 State sites for recording blood pressure with rationale						
3 State examples of inappropriate sites for a healthcare assistant						
4 State the normal range for blood pressure readings						
5 Describe systolic and diastolic pressure						
6 Describe some factors affecting blood pressure						

(Continued)

Table 6.7 (*Continued*)

(BP) Recording blood pressure	First assessment/Reassessment					Date/competent/signature
	Demonstration					
	Date/sign	Date/sign	Date/sign	Date/sign	Date/sign	
	1	2	3	4	5	
7 Describe the procedure for manual, aneroid and automated devices, including choice of sites						
8 Describe maintenance of all pieces of equipment, including reporting faults						
9 Describe the procedure for dealing with mercury spillage (if applicable)						
10 State when to report/ask for assistance						
11 Collect all equipment						
12 Demonstrate correct identification of patient, effective explanation and communication in relation to blood pressure recording						
13 Demonstrate accurate recording using: (a) automatic blood pressure machine, (b) mercury sphygmomanometer and/or (c) aneroid sphygmomanometer						
14 Demonstrate correct documentation of the recording						
15 Demonstrate tidying away of equipment including cleaning						

Case study 6.1

Mrs Wooley has had an emergency appendectomy (removal of appendix). After surgery she is very restless and a little confused. An automatic machine is taking her blood pressure. However, the readings are inconsistent. Why do you think this may be the case and what actions could you take?

Case study 6.2

Mr Jones has lung cancer and is admitted for pain control and dehydration. He is emaciated (thin) and frail, and has an intravenous infusion running. His blood pressure is being taken with a mercury sphygmomanometer (and standard cuff), but the readings do not appear accurate. What actions would you take to ensure that the correct readings are taken?

 Self-assessment

Assessment	Aspects	Achieved ✔
Patient	*Have you considered all aspects of this section?*	
	What blood pressure actually measures in the patient	
	What the systolic and diastolic pressure represent	
	The factors that affect blood pressure	
	The role of the cardiac cycle	
Procedure	*Have you considered all aspects of this section?*	**Achieved ✔**
	Selecting equipment	
	Suitable sites	
	Patient information	
	Documenting and reporting concerns	

References

Beevers G, Lip GY, O'Brien E (2001) ABC of hypertension: Blood pressure measurement. Part II-conventional sphygmomanometry: technique of auscultatory blood pressure measurement. *British Medical Journal* **322**: 1043–1047.

British Hypertension Society Guidelines (2004) Guidelines for management of hypertension: report of the fourth working party of the British Hypertension Society, 2004 – BHS IV. *Journal of Human Hypertension* **18**: 139–185.

British Hypertension Society (2006) *Fact File 01/2006. Blood Pressure Measurement*. Available at: www.bhsoc.org/bhf_factfiles/bhf_factfile_jan_2006.doc (accessed 1 March 2008).

Burton NL, Birdi K, eds (2006) *Clinical Skills for OSCEs*, 2nd edn. London: Informa Healthcare.

Campbell NR, Chockalingam A, Fodor JG, McKay W (1990) Accurate, reproducible measurement of blood pressure. *Canadian Medical Association Journal* **143**(1): 19–24.

Cappuccio F, Kerry SM, Forbes L, Donald A (2004) Blood pressure control by home monitoring: a meta analysis of randomised trials. *British Medical Journal* **329**: 145.

Dougherty L, Lister S, eds (2004) *The Royal Marsden Hospital Manual of Clinical Nursing Procedures*, 6th edn. Oxford: Blackwell Publishing.

Gomersall C, Oh T (1997) Haemodynamic monitoring. In: Oh T (ed.), *Intensive Care Manual*, 4th edn. Oxford: Butterworth-Heinemann.

Higham S, Maddex S (2005) In: Baillie L (ed.), *Developing Practical Nursing Skills*, 2nd edn. London: Hodder Education, pp. 393–436.

Hypertension Influence Team (2007) *Let's Do it Well*. Nurse Learning Pack. Available at: www.bhsoc.org/pdfs/hit.pdf (accessed 16 October 2008).

Jevon P (2001) Measuring lying and standing BP – 1. *Nursing Times* **97**(1): 41–42.

Jevon P, Ewens B (2002) *Monitoring the Critically Ill Patient. Essential Clinical Skills for Nurses*. Blackwell: London.

Jevon P, Holmes J (2007) Blood pressure measurement. Part 3: lying and standing blood pressure. *Nursing Times* **103**(20): 24–25.

Joint British Societies (2005) Joint British Societies' guidelines on prevention of cardiovascular disease in clinical practice. *Heart* **91**(suppl 5): v1–52.

Leefar V (2000) Stress. In: Alexander M, Fawcett J, Runciman P (eds), *Nursing Practice in Hospital and Home: The adult*, 2nd edn. Edinburgh: Churchill Livingstone, pp. 613–633.

Marieb E (2001) *Human Anatomy and Physiology*, 5th edn. San Francisco, CA: Benjamin Cummings.

McAlister FA, Straus SE (2001) Evidence based treatment for hypertension – measurement of blood pressure: an evidence based review. *British Medical Journal* **322**: 908–911.

Markandu ND, Witcher F, Arnold A, Carnie C (2000) The mercury sphygmomanometer should be abandoned before it is proscribed. *Journal of Hypertension* **14**: 31–36.

Medicines and Healthcare products Regulatory Agency (MHRA) (2003) *Medical Devices containing Mercury*. London: MHRA. Available at: www.medical-devices.gov.uk (accessed 3 August 2007).

MHRA (2006) *Measuring Blood Pressure: Top Ten Tips*. London: MHRA. Available at: www.mhra.gov.uk/home/idcplg?IdcService=SS_GET_PAGE&useSecondary=True&ssDocName=CON2024207&ssTargetNodeId=386 (accessed 16 October 2008).

National Institute for Health and Clinical Excellence (NICE) (2006) *Hypertension: Management of Hypertension in Adults in Primary Care*. Clinical Guidelines No. 34. London: NICE.

NHS Lothian (2008) *Observations Chart*. Edinburgh: NHS Lothian.

O'Brien E, Waeber B, Parati G, Staessen J, Myers MG (2001) Blood pressure measuring devices: recommendations of the European Society of Hypertension. *British Medical Journal* **322**: 531–536.

O'Brien E, Asmar R, Beilin L et al. (2003) European Society of Hypertension recommendations for conventional, ambulatory and home blood pressure measurement. *Journal of Hypertension* **21**: 821–848.

Smith GR (2000) Devices for blood pressure measurement. *Professional Nurse* **15**: 337–40.

Thibodeau GA, Patton KT (2007) *Anatomy and Physiology*, 6th edn. St Louis, MO: Elsevier Mosby.

Thompson D, Webster R (2000) The cardiovascular system. In: Alexander M, Fawcett J, Runciman P (eds), *Nursing Practice in Hospital and Home: The adult*, 2nd edn. Edinburgh: Churchill Livingstone, pp. 7–58.

Thornett A (2007) New skills for healthcare assistants: taking a blood pressure. *British Journal of Healthcare Assistants* **1**(3): 133–135.

Tortora GJ, Derrickson B (2006) *Principles of Anatomy and Physiology*, 11th edn. Hoboken, NJ: John Wiley & Sons.

Tortora GJ, Grabowski SR (2003) *Principles of Anatomy and Physiology*, 10th edn. Chichester: John Wiley & Sons.

Trim J (2005) Blood pressure. Nursing times practical procedures. *Nursing Times* **101**(2): 32–33.

Valler-Jones T, Wedgbury K (2005) Measuring blood pressure using the mercury sphygmomanometer. *British Journal of Nursing* **14**: 145–150.

Waugh A, Grant A (2001) *Ross and Wilson Anatomy and Physiology in Health and Illness*, 9th edn. London: Churchill Livingstone.

Williams, B, Poulter, NR, Brown MJ et al. (2004) British Hypertension Society Guidelines. Guidelines for management of hypertension: report of the fourth working party of the British Hypertension Society 2004 (BHS IV). *Journal of Human Hypertension* **18**: 139–185.

Chapter 7

Thermometry

Learning objectives

- Describe the normal temperature range and how body temperature is controlled
- List some factors that affect heat production and heat loss
- Describe the symptoms and causes of increased and decreased temperature
- Describe the principles behind the different devices that record temperature and how they operate
- Describe how to take and record an accurate temperature

Aim of this chapter

To understand the body's role in temperature maintenance, the normal values and factors that influence its value.

What is temperature?

Warm-blooded animals, such as humans, control the body's internal temperature independent of normal environmental conditions (Tortora and Derrickson 2006). To ensure that a constant temperature is maintained, a fine balance is maintained between heat produced in the body and heat lost to the environment (Waugh and Grant 2001). The body's core temperature is the optimum temperature for the organs within the cranial (brain), thoracic (chest) and abdominal cavities to function, and the range varies between 36°C and 37.6°C (Brooker 1998). The shell temperature is the temperature near the body surface (Tortora and Grabowski 2003). Figure 7.1 shows the body temperature at different sites.

Reasons for measuring temperature

- To determine a baseline (a reading against which future readings can be compared) on admission to hospital (Dougherty and Lister 2004)
- To monitor fluctuations in temperature (Dougherty and Lister 2004)
- To identify deterioration in a patient's condition (Trim 2005)
- To diagnose pyrexia (increased temperature) or hypothermia (decreased temperature) (see later)
- To identify disease or infection (Trim 2005)
- To assist in deciding on a patient's treatment (Braun et al. 1998; DeVrim et al. 2007).

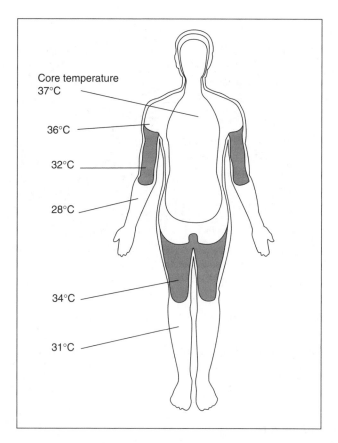

Figure 7.1 Body temperature at different sites on the body. (Adapted from Torrance and Semple 1998a.)

Normal limits

Temperature is maintained at an average of 36.8°C and is the optimum temperature for the many chemical processes in the body (Waugh and Grant 2001). However, temperature can safely range from 36°C to 37.6°C without these processes being affected (Brooker 1998). Accurate temperature recordings are essential because false readings can result in patients either receiving unnecessary or inappropriate interventions, or remaining untreated when intervention is required (Farnell et al. 2005).

Relevant anatomy and physiology

Temperature is controlled by both a temperature-regulating centre in the hypothalamus, which is responsive to the temperature of circulating blood, and the vasomotor centre in the medulla oblongata, which controls the diameter of blood vessels, controlling heat loss and gain (see later) (Waugh and Grant 2001). Figure 7.2 shows the location of the hypothalamus and medulla oblongata within the brain.

The body has thermoreceptors (sensors) in the skin and mucous membranes that report to the hypothalamus. The hypothalamus stimulates heat generating or reducing actions, resulting in a

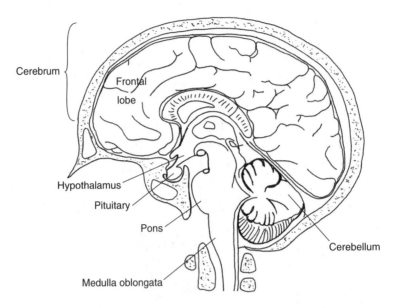

Figure 7.2   Location of the hypothalamus and medulla oblongata within the brain.

balance to maintain and regulate temperature. It is therefore vital that our body temperature be kept within fairly strict limits. This is done via a negative feedback system and is known as homeostasis (see Figure 7.5 later in text).

Related aspects and terminology

In order to understand temperature regulation, both heat production and loss need to be understood.

Heat production

All living cells produce heat during metabolism: in muscles when they are active and continuously by the liver. It can also depend on the body's metabolic rate (the rate at which the body uses energy). Factors that affect heat production are included in Table 7.1.

Reflection point

What effect do you think prolonged exposure to either a hot, humid desert environment or a cold, snowy, freezing climate would have on the human body?

When looking after patients many factors may influence the metabolic rate and temperature control. The skin can gain heat by radiation; this heat is then absorbed deep down into the subcutaneous layers and blood vessels. Figure 7.3 shows how the skin controls heat production and heat gain.

Table 7.1 Factors affecting heat production

Factor	Rationale
Metabolic rate	The basal metabolic rate produces heat, which in turn directly affects the body's temperature (Higham and Maddex 2005)
Exercise	Higham and Maddex (2005) report that exercise increases the metabolic rate. Furthermore, during strenuous activity the basal rate can increase by up to 15 times, increasing to 20 times for athletes (Tortora and Grabowski 2003). Immobility can have the opposite effect, with individuals needing to add layers of clothes for warmth (Higham and Maddex 2005)
Sweat gland activity	Reduced sweat gland activity preserves heat that would normally be lost by evaporation (see heat loss)
Goosebumps/Shivering	Goosebumps occur when the muscles surrounding the hair follicles contract causing the raising of the hair to trap a layer of air around the body and prevent heat loss. If this is ineffective shivering often follows
	Shivering involves intense, muscular contraction – a physiological response to cold, which produces heat, directly increasing the temperature (Brooker 1998)
Hormones/Disease	The main hormones relating to temperature control are those from the thyroid, predominantly thyroxine. Due to the nature of hormonal control, it may take some time for the hormones to take effect. In the case of an overactive thyroid, where there is increased hormone production, individuals may have a higher than normal body temperature (Edwards 1997). An underactive thyroid results in the opposite with a reduced metabolic rate and a reduced temperature (Higham and Maddex 2005)
	In times of stress adrenaline and other hormones may be released, which can also increase the metabolic rate and produce heat (Tortora and Grabowski 2003). Other conditions that affect temperature include hypoglycaemia (low glucose level in blood) and adrenal insufficiency (adrenal glands are situated on top of the kidneys)
Infection	The body responds to infection by increasing the temperature (Higham and Maddex 2005). For every degree centigrade increase in body temperature, the metabolism increases by around 10% (Tortora and Grabowski 2003)
Eating	Marieb (2001) states eating and digesting food can increase the metabolic rate up to 10–20%, with a higher increase for protein-based meals than that for carbohydrates and lipids (Tortora and Grabowski 2003)
Age	Neonates have an underdeveloped thermocentre in the brain and require intervention to ensure that heat loss is minimised, e.g. extra clothing, including a hat to reduce heat loss from the head (Higham and Maddex 2005). In children the metabolic rate (in relation to their size) is double that of an older person due to growth (Tortora and Grabowski 2003). In older people there is an increased sensitivity to cold and the body temperature is generally lower (Dougherty and Lister 2004)
Male/Females	Metabolic rates tend to be higher in males than females, which in turn increases the temperature (Tortora and Grabowski 2003)
Body shape	Larger individuals will have a higher basal rate due to an increase in surface area, therefore increasing the body temperature (Tortora and Grabowski 2003)
Pregnancy/Breast-feeding	Pregnancy and breast-feeding increase the basal metabolic rate and temperature (Tortora and Grabowski 2003)

(Continued)

Table 7.1 (*Continued*)

Factor	Rationale
Menstruation	Ovulation can elevate the body's temperature because it increases the metabolic rate (Tortora and Derrickson 2006). Temperature can also be raised during menstruation (Childs 2000)
Medications/alcohol	Some medications can increase the basal rate and temperature, e.g. amphetamines (Tortora and Grabowski 2003). Antidepressants, sedatives and tranquillisers have the opposite effect and can reduce the body temperature
	Alcohol does not promote heat production and may suppress the body's warning of low or high temperatures due to altered consciousness and awareness
Environmental factors	In a tropical region, a reduction in the basal rate occurs and the body reduces heat production in an effort to cool the body (Higham and Maddex 2005)
Time of day	The body's natural variance, which causes daily fluctuations, is known as the circadian rhythm, with the higher recording of temperature in early evening (Dougherty and Lister 2004)
	The metabolic rate reduces by around 10% during sleep, and body temperature is reduced (Edwards 1997)

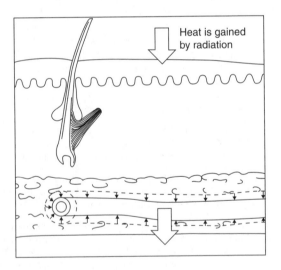

Figure 7.3   Heat production and heat gain from the skin.

Heat loss

Most heat loss from the body occurs through the skin (Figure 7.4), although small amounts are lost in expired air, urine and faeces (Waugh and Grant 2001). Heat is lost from the skin when heat is conducted to the skin surface. It is then lost by radiation, or mixed with sweat to be lost by evaporation.

The methods of heat loss are evaporation, conduction, radiation and convection, and each is described in turn.

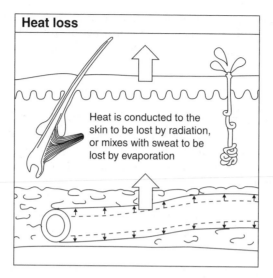

Figure 7.4 Heat loss from the skin.

Evaporation

Evaporation is the conversion of a liquid into a vapour. In the human body evaporation of water requires heat energy to be used, causing heat to be lost, primarily from the skin (Tortora and Derrickson 2006). An increase in temperature stimulates the sweat glands, which secrete sweat on the surface of the body via ducts. The sweat evaporating then loses heat (Waugh and Grant 2001).

Reflection point

List some instances of when your body sweated/shivered.

Evaporation is of particular importance at high environmental temperatures when it is the only method that cools the body (Tortora and Derrickson 2006). Loss of heat by evaporation can also occur from the deeper layers of the skin to the surface of the body, from mucous membranes and during breathing. Here the individual is unaware that evaporation is occurring, and it is known as insensible loss (Waugh and Grant 2001). Insensible loss is often used when calculating fluid balance charts to ensure that all fluid loss is considered (see Chapter 14).

Conduction

This is the transfer of heat to any substance in direct contact with the body (Tortora and Derrickson 2006). It accounts for a relatively small amount of heat loss and examples include clothes or jewellery taking up heat from the skin. Hot and cold drinks as well as hot and cold baths can also cause the body to conduct hot or cold (Tortora and Derrickson 2006).

Radiation

Radiation is the transfer of heat via infrared rays between a warmer and a cooler object without physical contact, e.g. the sun. In cool environments the body loses a greater percentage of heat loss from the skin by this method than by conduction and evaporation combined (Thibodeau and Patton 2007). In hot environments no heat is lost by this route, but may be gained by heat radiating to the skin (Tortora and Derrickson 2006).

Convection

This is movement of heat away from a surface by movement of heated air or particles (Tortora and Derrickson 2006). A cool fan or convection heater would fulfil this purpose by circulating and moving the air. Another example would be getting out of a hot bath, which would have provided heat to the body, and then the heat being quickly lost via a cool breeze from an open window (Tortora and Derrickson 2006).

Reflection point

What nursing actions are used to promote heat loss due to an increase in temperature in a patient and how do they work?

Temperature control is essential for the well being of the human body and this maintenance is done by constantly checking, and if necessary altering systems. This cycle is called a negative feedback mechanism and is shown in Figure 7.5.

Terminology

- **Core temperature:** the temperature deep within the body supplying the major organs (Tortora and Grabowski 2003).
- **Shell temperature:** the temperature near the body surface, skin and subcutaneous layer (Tortora and Grabowski 2003).
- **Hypothermia:** lowering of the body's core temperature to 35°C or lower (Torrance and Semple 1998a).
- **Pyrexia:** a temperature >37.2–38.9°C (Torrance and Semple 1998a)
- **Hyperthermia:** a core temperature >40.6°C (Torrance and Semple 1998a).

Hypothermia

This is when the body's temperature is <35°C (Brooker 1998) and mechanisms to increase heat production are ineffective (Dougherty and Lister 2004). The body reduces its metabolic rate and bodily functions to try to preserve heat (Trim 2005). The causes of hypothermia are shown in Box 7.1.

Patients may shiver due to being cold and a warming blanket or warmed fluids may be sufficient to raise the temperature (Trim 2005). If the temperature continues to drop shivering is replaced by muscle rigidity and cramps and blood pressure and heart rate become raised (Waugh and Grant 2001). Following this confusion, altered consciousness, coma or cardiac problems can occur, leading to death if the temperature falls to <25°C (Waugh and Grant 2001).

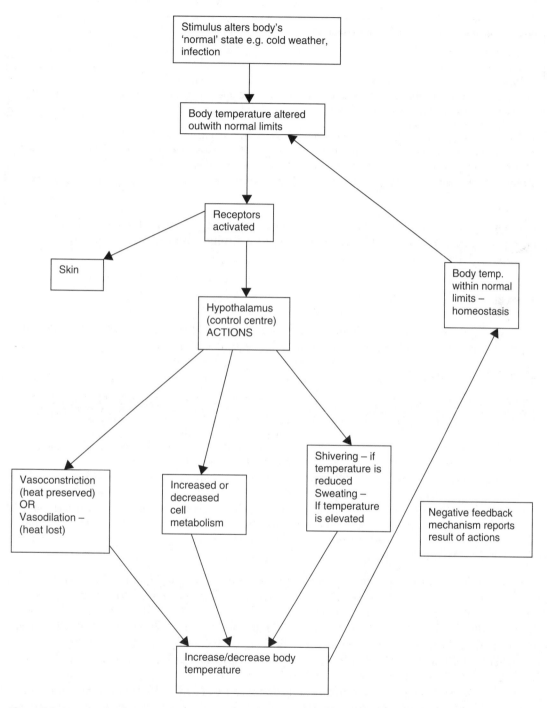

Figure 7.5 Negative feedback mechanism to control body temperature. (Adapted from Tortora and Grabowski [2003] and Dougherty and Lister [2004].)

Box 7.1 Summary of causes of hypothermia

- Renal dialysis (Trim 2005)
- Surgery (Trim 2005)
- Burns
- Extreme or overwhelming cold, e.g. exposure to a cold environment (Dougherty and Lister 2004; Trim 2005)
- Malnutrition (due to lowered metabolism)
- Blood transfusion (Trim 2005)
- Metabolic conditions, e.g. hypoglycaemia (low blood sugar) (Dougherty and Lister 2004)
- Medications that alter the perception of cold, increase heat loss by vasodilatation or inhibit heat generation, e.g. alcohol, paracetamol, antidepressants (Dougherty and Lister 2004)

Management of this patient may involve administration of warmed intravenous fluids via the abdominal (peritoneal) or bladder cavities in an effort to increase the core temperature, which allows essential organ function (Trim 2005).

Pyrexia

Pyrexia is a significant rise in core temperature (Dougherty and Lister 2004; Trim 2005). Patients may be red in the face and feel hot to the touch. Three grades of pyrexia are shown in Table 7.2.

Table 7.2 Grades of pyrexia

Grade	Temperature (°C)	Details
Low grade	37 to 38	Indicates an inflammatory response as a result of mild infection, allergy or disturbance of body tissue. Can also be due to trauma, surgery, malignancy or blood clots (thrombosis)
Moderate-to-high grade	38–40	Caused by a wound or other infections (e.g. respiratory or urinary tract)
Hypopyrexia	≥40	Bacteraemia (the presence of bacteria in the blood), damage to the hypothalamus or high environmental temperatures

Adapted from Dougherty and Lister (2004).

A sudden rise in temperature, sometimes referred to as a 'spike' in temperature, usually indicates infection, which can be caused by viruses or bacteria and their toxins (Torrance and Semple 1998a). If shivering is experienced, together with a high temperature, this is known as a 'rigor' (Marieb 2001). Where there is an increase in temperature but no infection evident, the causes for the increase in temperature are known as non-infective causes of pyrexia and hyperthermia (Dougherty and Lister 2004). Causes of non-infective pyrexia and hyperthermia are shown in Box 7.2.

Often the patients will be given medication to reduce their temperature (antipyrexial medication) and a fan (to promote air circulation), and be sponged with cool, slightly warm water (tepid sponging), which will aim to cool the surface of the skin. If the temperature continues to rise, dehydration can occur as a result of loss of fluid through sweating, and convulsions can occur (particularly common in the under-5 age group). Following this, body proteins (enzymes), which are involved in chemical reactions, are disrupted, affecting the chemical reaction in the body, leading to death at 44–45°C (Tortora and Grabowski 2003).

> **Box 7.2 Non-infective causes of pyrexia/hyperthermia**
>
> - Alcohol withdrawal
> - Medications (including recreational drugs such as ecstasy)
> - Allergic drug or transfusion reaction
> - Reaction to vaccines (common in neonates and children)
> - Exercise
> - Gout
> - Trauma
> - Heat stroke or heat exhaustion (Torrance and Semple 1998a)
> - Hyperthyroidism (overactive thyroid), this causes an increase in metabolic rate (Waugh and Grant 2001)
> - Malignancy (cancer)
> - Status epilepticus (constant fitting)
> - Stroke/Heart attack (myocardial infarction)
> - Central nervous system damage (Torrance and Semple 1998a)
> - Vasculitis (inflammation of a blood vessel)
> - Surgery
> - Environmental factors – hot and humid surroundings/too many layers of clothing
>
> (Adapted from Dougherty and Lister 2004)

Taking a temperature reading

There are various methods of taking a temperature reading and each is discussed in turn. The equipment that you use will often depend on whether it is suitable for the patient and availability in the clinical area. Recommended good practice is that the same site and method are used where possible and that this information is documented for future reference (Kiernan 2001). A summary of the advantages and disadvantages of each method is shown in Table 7.3. However, it should be noted that no one method or site is viewed as best, with many authors disagreeing about the accuracy of different methods and sites (Braun et al. 1998; Farnell et al. 2005; El-Radhi and Patel 2006; Mackechnie and Simpson 2006; DeVrim et al. 2007).

The main methods are the following:

- Mercury thermometer – oral/axilla or rectal
- Tympanic thermometer
- Electronic thermometer
- Chemical (dots)
- Temporal artery.

Mercury thermometer

This used to be the most popular method, and 'gold standard' (Mackechnie and Simpson 2006), but due to the health and safety risk of mercury, the Medicines and Healthcare product Regulatory Agency (MHRA 2003) states that these should be used only where there is no other alternative.

There can be different types of mercury thermometer, namely oral (for oral or axillary use) or rectal (for rectal use) and a low reading thermometer (for hypothermic patients), which can be used, at any site, but has a lower range, starting at 24°C.

Table 7.3 Summary of the advantages and disadvantages of different methods

	Advantages	Disadvantages
Mercury	'Gold' standard in terms of accuracy (Mackechnie and Simpson 2006)	Mercury is actively discouraged due to the health and safety risk – eventual replacement is planned (Mackechnie and Simpson 2006)
	Low cost and widely available (Higham and Maddex 2005)	
Electronic	Quick, easy to use	Cost implications re-disposables
	Disposable cover for each measurement, promoting infection control	Machine requires maintenance
		When using the machine with an oral probe, because of the weight of the probe it needs to be held in place
Tympanic	Quick, easy to use	Cost implications re-disposables
	Disposable cover for each measurement, promoting infection control	Machine requires maintenance and calibration
	Accepted alternative to mercury-in-glass thermometers (Mackechnie and Simpson 2006)	Not suitable for children under 1
		Can be used only in the ear for tympanic membrane use
	Can give true ear reading or equivalent core, oral, axillary or rectal readings	Virtually eliminates exposure to body fluids (Braun et al. 1998)
Chemical	Totally non-invasive	Cost implications re-disposables
	Disposable for each patient	Requires storage at below 30°C (Higham and Maddex 2005)
		Limited temperature range of 35.5–40.4°C (Farnell et al. 2005)
Temporal artery	Quick	Limited literature compared with other methods
	Accurate	
	Can be used on all age groups	

Tympanic thermometers

Tympanic thermometers operate by sensing body heat through infrared energy given off by the tympanic membrane in the ear (Carroll 2000; Mackechnie and Simpson 2006). The only site for this method is the ear canal. Ear canal size, presence of wax, operator technique and the patient's position can affect the accuracy of the readings (Carroll 2000; Kiernan 2001; Knies 2003). DeVrim et al. (2007) report that, as the tympanic membrane and the hypothalamus share a common blood supply, it is a valid indicator of core temperature. An exception to this would be in children, in whom temperatures >38°C should be checked by either the oral or the rectal route to confirm the elevation (Kiernan 2001). In children aged under 1 year, reliable measurements are shown to be difficult to obtain because of the small ear canal, and other methods should be sought (Wilshaw et al. 1999).

In addition, maintenance of the machines is essential and it is particularly important that they are calibrated correctly, because failure to do so results in the reading being unreliable, with measurements continually becoming less accurate as more readings are taken (Mackechnie and Simpson 2006). The thermometer can calculate the temperature at the tympanic membrane, but can also convert it into the reading at the skin surface, oral or core by using the 'mode' button.

To ensure that accurate readings are obtained it is essential that healthcare assistants understand this function. Models and manufacturers do vary, so check locally with regard to the model used in practice.

Electronic thermometer

This is an electronic or digital machine with a probe, which can be used orally, rectally or in the axilla. Kiernan (2001) states that digital thermometers are easier and faster to use than standard mercury ones, and can be adapted to oral, axillary or rectal use by placing plastic sheaths over the tip. Most machines give an audible 'beep' when the reading has been taken either by a pre-set time or when the maximum temperature has been reached, taking away the need for the user to time the procedure (Carroll 2000). Maintenance and knowledge of how to use the machine is essential. Figure 7.6 shows an electronic thermometer.

Chemical thermometer

These are thin plastic strips that have 50 small dots of thermosensitive chemicals, which change colour with increasing temperature (Higham and Maddex 2005). They should be stored at below 30°C and can be used orally or per axilla (Higham and Maddex 2005). It is essential to ensure that they are placed correctly; where the axillary route is being used, the dots must placed next to the inner part of the body, in contact with it. For either oral or per axilla use it is essential that the thermometer be left in place for the correct amount of time (Farnell et al. 2005). They are disposable for each patient and non-invasive.

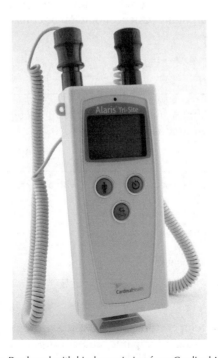

Figure 7.6 Electronic thermometer. Produced with kind permission from Cardinal Health.

Temporal artery thermometer

This is a hand-held thermometer that takes a reading after the probe has been scanned along the forehead and behind the ear. Both sites are used to ensure the most accurate reading, as sweat may be present on the forehead, which cools the skin, giving a lower reading. The machine uses an 'arterial heat balance method' to take a reading by measuring the temperature of the skin surface over the artery and the ambient temperature, and then calculating the arterial temperature (Roy et al. 2003). The method is thought to work well because the temporal artery is located in the forehead, both close to the skin's surface and directly connected to the heart through the carotid artery (Roan 2001). Disposable caps and sheaths are available for single use. It has been shown to be better than tympanic thermometry in infants, especially when a rectal temperature reading is required (Greenes and Fleisher 2001).

As mentioned previously there is some dispute as to the best method of taking a temperature recording. In reality the healthcare assistant will not have a wide choice because most clinical areas have only one or two pieces of equipment.

In summary, there are many methods of taking a temperature recording. However, all equipment must be used as intended by the manufacturer, including correct placement and timing, otherwise inaccurate recordings will be obtained.

Route

The choices of sites for temperature measurement are oral, rectal, axilla, tympanic membrane and temporal artery. A summary of the advantages and disadvantages of each site is given in Table 7.4.

When deciding on the site for recording temperature factors such as previous sites, the equipment available and an assessment of the patient should all be considered. The procedure to obtain recordings is given next.

Taking a temperature reading

First, taking a temperature reading using a mercury thermometer is discussed at oral, rectal or axillary sites. The equipment required is shown in Box 7.3.

Box 7.3 Equipment needed to take a temperature recording with a mercury thermometer

- Vessel containing thermometer
- Alcohol swabs
- Tissue (for rectal use)
- Lubricant (for rectal use)
- Watch that is capable of timing in minutes

The procedure for taking a temperature reading using a mercury or electronic thermometer device is shown in Table 7.5, taking a tympanic temperature reading is shown in Table 7.6 and temporal artery thermometer is shown in Table 7.7.

Table 7.4 Summary of the advantages and disadvantages of different sites for measuring body temperature

Sites	Advantages	Disadvantages
Oral: requires the probe tip to be placed in the mouth in the sublingual pocket, which is under the tongue (Braun et al. 1998)	Easily accessible, no undressing required	Sublingual pocket must be used or inaccurate results will be obtained
		The patient cannot talk while the procedure is being performed and it is not suitable for breathless patients because it is important that the lips close around the thermometer (Higham and Maddex 2005)
		It is also unsuitable for patients who have disease or pain/discomfort in the oral mucosa because the thermometer may cause further pain or discomfort
		Not suitable for children, confused or unconscious patients because they may bite the probe or be unable to hold in place
		When timing the duration, the thermometer must remain in place for an accurate reading; this is a source for error because it is often not left *in situ* for long enough, giving inaccurate readings (Carroll 2000)
		When using mercury thermometer, if the glass breaks this causes a hazard (O'Toole 1998)
		This route is unsuitable for patients who have recently had a hot or cold food or drink, or smoked. Torrance and Semple (1998b) suggest waiting 15 minutes
Rectal: involves placement of the probe 4 cm into the rectum in adults (Dougherty and Lister 2004)	Useful if the patient has peripheral shut-down (poor circulation at extremities)	Invasive and can be embarrassing for patients
		Not suitable for neonates because of incidence of rectal perforation (DeVrim et al. 2007)
	Useful if other sites are not possible	The presence of soft stools can alter recordings (Dougherty and Lister 2004)
		Not suitable if any rectal disease or irritation is evident (Dougherty and Lister 2004)
Tympanic: the probe is inserted into the ear canal (see Table 7.3)	Non invasive	Correct placement not always achieved
	Very quick – takes 3 seconds	Localised temperature can affect results, e.g. cool air or placement against a pillow (which will generate heat) before measurement can affect results
	Suitable for most adults (Higham and Maddex 2005)	
	Value not influenced by food, drink or smoking	
Axilla: where the thermometer is placed under the arm	Non-invasive	Often not left in for sufficient time (Carroll 2000)
	Patient can talk while in place	Vasoconstriction (blood vessels narrow) or chilled skin gives inaccurate readings (Higham and Maddex 2005)
		Thin people often cannot hold it in the correct place (Higham and Maddex 2005)
		Can prove difficult to hold in place for the required duration, especially for children, confused patients and the elderly

(Continued)

Table 7.4 (*Continued*)

Sites	Advantages	Disadvantages
Temporal artery: requires the device to be 'stroked' across the centre of the forehead from the midline to the lateral hairline and then placed behind the earlobe, in the soft depression below the mastoid	Non-invasive Quick Value unaffected by eating, drinking or smoking	Correct placement will require some education Limited research available currently

Table 7.5 Procedure for taking a temperature reading using either a mercury or electronic thermometer

Action	Rationale
1. Explain the procedure to the patient fully, including reason for test and to gain verbal consent	Patient fully understands why test is being performed and the procedure, and has agreed to participate
2. Check whether the patient has had food or drink or has smoked in past 20–30 minutes. *Oral only*	To ensure accurate reading
3. Wipe thermometer with alcohol swab. Check that mercury is at base of thermometer	Prevent cross infection To ensure accurate reading
4. Place the thermometer **For oral:** place the bulb of the thermometer in patients' mouths under the tongue in the sublingual pocket and ask them to close their lips around it **For axillary:** place the bulb fully under the arm of the patient with the arm across the chest to hold it in place **For rectal:** lubricate the thermometer with lubricating jelly; place 4 cm into the rectum (Dougherty and Lister 2004)	To ensure correct positioning of the thermometer for accurate reading
5. Leave in place for 3–5 min, minimum of 2 min (Torrance and Semple 1998b) Electronic thermometer will beep.	Duration variable but 3–5 min is the average (Higham and Meddex 2005). To ensure accurate reading
6. Remove the thermometer Immediately wipe both the patient's rectum and the thermometer with tissue for rectal site Document and/or report reading	Patient comfort Report abnormal findings immediately to nurse in charge as further care may require planning. Documentation provides a legal record
7. Wipe with alcohol – start at the end held by the nurse and wipe in a rotating manner towards the bulb end Shake the thermometer so that the mercury returns to the base Replace probe in correct position for storage (electronic)	Prevent cross-infection Thermometer ready for use next time

Table 7.6 Procedure for taking a temperature reading using a tympanic thermometer

Action	Rationale
1. Explain the procedure to the patient fully, including the reason for test and to gain verbal consent	Patient fully understands why test is being performed and procedure, and has agreed to participate.
	Note that not suitable for children under 1 year (Wilshaw et al. 1999)
2. Ensure that the patient is not positioned in a draught or that the ear has been against a pillow	May affect readings
3. Do not use ears that have been reported as sore, have known disease present or wax present	May affect placement and accurate readings
4. Apply a new probe cover each time the machine is used	As per manufacturer's instructions
	Prevent cross-infection
	Provide accurate readings
5. 'Tug' the ear to insert probe where advised by the manufacturer (Kiernan 2001)	Not required for all models of tympanic thermometers
Position thermometer as per manufacturer's instructions	Optimal reading
6. Scan the ear, and then listen for audible beep	Confirms reading has been taken. Kiernan (2001) suggests three successive readings, using the highest reading but local policy should be checked
	A measurement may not be the same in the left and right ear due to physiological differences so record which ear the reading has been taken from
7. If reading is not valid, repeat	Wait at least 2 min before repeating a measurement in the same ear to reduce an artificially low reading from 'draw down', caused by placing the probe tip into the ear canal and reducing its internal temperature
8. Report any abnormal findings	To plan further management

Reflection Point

Which methods and sites do you think would be suitable for the following patients: a frail, thin older patient, an unconscious patient, a baby of 11 months and a child aged 6 years?

The temperature recorded at different sites will give various different readings, rectal measurements giving the highest because it is deeper in the body, followed by tympanic, with oral methods recording the lowest value. Table 7.8 summarises the variance in temperature dependent on the site.

Documentation

Document the temperature recording in the patient's case notes or on an observation chart. Temperature recordings on an observation chart are usually documented in a graph (Figure 7.7). A baseline recording, often done on admission to hospital, will act as a reference for what is

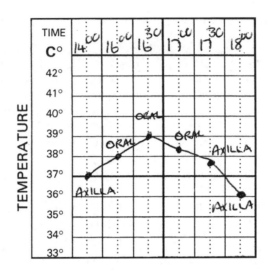

Figure 7.7   TPR (temperature, pulse and respiratory rate) chart with temperature recordings. (Observations chart reproduced with permission from NHS Lothian 2008.)

'normal' for that patient. As temperature can vary due to the site, documenting the site where the temperature is taken from, as well as the actual reading, is recommended (Braun et al. 1998).

Abnormalities should always be reported to the nurse in charge, so further management can be planned where necessary. However, the reading should also be taken together with how the patient looks and feels, e.g. is the patient feeling hot/clammy, are they red in the face, hot or cold to the touch, shivering or is the body rigid? This helps ensure that inaccuracies are identified and, if necessary, checked by another method or route.

Common problems

Problems relating to thermometry can be split into three areas: the patient, the equipment and the technique.

The patient

Specific routes have disadvantages and limitations as mentioned in Table 7.4. If there is any doubt as to where exactly the thermometer should be placed, e.g. sublingual pocket, further advice should be sought. Where possible the patient should also be actively involved in using any specific routes that may improve patient comfort, e.g. rectal route would not be a preference for most people unless it was specifically indicated.

The equipment

As with all pieces of equipment the thermometer should be clean, in good working order and serviced (where applicable). Only dedicated disposables should be used and multi-use of, for example, probe covers should never occur.

Table 7.7 Procedure for taking a temperature reading using a temporal artery thermometer

Action	Rationale
1. Explain the procedure to the patient fully, including reason for test, and gain verbal consent	Patient fully understands why test is being performed and procedure, and has agreed to participate
2. Run or 'stroke' the scanner across the centre of the forehead from the midline to the lateral hairline, depressing the button constantly throughout. A disposable cover may be used in some models	To record an accurate temporal artery temperature Prevention of cross-infection
3. Touch behind the ear lobe, in the soft depression below the mastoid	To account for any differences in the temperature in the temporal artery due to sweat (the temperature would be lower)
4. Release the button and read the temperature from the display window	To view reading
5. Report any abnormal findings	To plan further management. Patient safety
6. Dispose of cover if being used or clean as per manufacturer's instructions	Prevent contamination Ready for use

Table 7.8 Variance in temperature range dependent on site

Body site	Normal temperature range (°C)
Oral	36.5–37.5
Core (tympanic)	36.8–37.9
Rectal	37.0–38.1

The technique

The specific technique in relation to both the type of thermometer and the route should be fully understood before proceeding with the procedure. Competency-based training should also be undertaken in line with local policy.

Summary

It does not matter which route or site is used to record temperature, the most important factor is that it is accurate. As mentioned earlier the way that the patient looks and feels should also be taken into consideration when assessing the patient's temperature, thus ensuring that the recording obtained represents the true clinical symptoms. Table 7.9 gives an example of a competency framework for recording temperature.

Table 7.9 Thermometry competency: practical assessment form

Competency: record temperature	First assessment/reassessment					
Steps	**Demonstration**					**Date/competent signature**
	Date/sign	Date/sign	Date/sign	Date/sign	Date/sign	
	1	2	3	4	5	
Recording temperature						
1. State normal range for body temperature (°C)						
2. Define the terms pyrexia and hypothermia						
3. State different sites for recording temperature						
4. Describe different types of thermometers used and rationale						
5. Describe the common problems with each type						
6. Describe how you would prepare a patient for each method and gain consent						
Steps	**Demonstration**					**Date/competent signature**
	Date/sign	Date/sign	Date/sign	Date/sign	Date/sign	
	1	2	3	4	5	
Recording temperature						
7. Describe the procedures for the models of thermometer being used in your practice						
8. Identify and justify the use of documentation						
9. State when to ask for assistance/report findings						
10. Describe safe disposal and cleaning of the equipment following use						
11. State when to ask for assistance/report findings						

Supervisors/Assessor(s):

Case study 7.1

Archie is an active 12-month-old boy. His temperature is taken with a tympanic thermometer and shows that it is within the normal range. However, he is very hot and clammy.
You suspect the reading may be incorrect. Why?

Case study 7.2

Mrs Jones had abdominal surgery 2 days ago. She has a temperature of 39.5°C. What actions do you think you should take and what are the possible causes of the increased temperature (pyrexia)?

Self-assessment

Assessment	Aspects	Achieved ✔
Patient	*Have you considered all aspects of this section?*	
	Why is temperature recorded?	
	What mechanism does the body have to control temperature?	
	Give some causes of increased/decreased temperature	
	List some factors that affect heat loss and gain in the body	
Procedure	*Have you considered all aspects of this section?*	**Achieved ✔**
	Describe the different methods of recording temperature	
	List the sites and rationale for each	
	Documentation	

References

Braun S, Preston P, Rae N (1998) Getting a better read on thermometry. *Nursing Journal for Registered Nurses* **61**(3): 57–60.

Brooker C (1998) *Human Structure and Function*, 2nd edn London: Mosby.

Carroll M (2000) An evaluation of temperature measurement. *Nursing Standard* **14**(44): 39–43.

Childs C (2000) Temperature control. In: Alexander M, Fawcett J, Runciman P (eds), *Nursing Practice in Hospital and Home: The adult*, 2nd edn. Edinburgh: Churchill Livingstone, pp. 719–735.

DeVrim I, Kara A, Ceyhan M et al. (2007) Measurement accuracy of fever by tympanic and axillary thermometry. *Pediatric Emergency* **23**(1): 16–19.

Dougherty L, Lister S, eds (2004) *The Royal Marsden Hospital Manual of Clinical Nursing Procedures*, 6th edn. Oxford: Blackwell Publishing.

Edwards S (1997) Measuring temperature. *Professional Nurse* **13**(2): 55–57.

El-Radhi AS, Patel S (2006) An evaluation of tympanic thermometry in a paediatric emergency department. *Emergency Medicine Journal* **23**: 40–41.

Farnell S, Maxwell L, Tan S, Rhodes A, Philips B (2005) Temperature measurement: comparison of non-invasive methods used in adult critical care. *Journal of Clinical Nursing* **14**: 632–639

Greenes, DS, Fleisher GR (2001) Accuracy of a noninvasive temporal artery thermometer for use in infants. *Archives of Pediatric and Adolescent Medicine* **155**: 376–381.

Higham S, Maddex S (2005) Monitoring vital signs. In: Baillie L (ed.), *Developing Practical Nursing Skills*, 2nd edn. London: Hodder Education, pp. 393–436.

Kiernan B (2001) Ask the expert. Taking a temperature: which way is best? *Journal for Specialists in Pediatric Nursing* **6**: 192–195.

Knies R, ed. (2003) Temperature measurement in acute care. In: *Research Applied to Clinical Practice*. Available at: www.enw.org/Research-Thermometry.htm (accessed 16 October 2008).

Mackechine C, Simpson R (2006) Traceable calibration for blood pressure and temperature monitoring. *Nursing Standard* **21**(11): 42–47.

Medicines and Healthcare products Regulatory Agency (2003) *Medical Devices containing Mercury*. London: MHRA. Available at: www.medical-devices.gov.uk (accessed 3 August 2007).

Marieb E (2001) *Human Anatomy and Physiology*, 5th edn. San Francisco, CA: Benjamin Cummings.

NHS Lothian (2008) *Observations Chart*. Edinburgh: NHS Lothian.

O'Toole S (1998) Temperature measurement devices. *Professional Nurse* **13**: 779–86.

Roan S (2001) High fever, Meet high-tech thermometer. *Los Angeles Times* 9 April 2001. Available at: www.exergen.com/medical/newsarch/latimes04092001.htm (accessed 16 October 2008).

Roy S, Powell K, Gerson LW (2003) Temporal artery temperature measurements in healthy infants, children, and adolescents. *Clinical Pediatrics* **42**: 433–437.

Thibodeau GA, Patton KT (2007) *Anatomy and Physiology*, 6th edn. St Louis, MO: Mosby Elsevier/

Torrance C, Semple M (1998a) Practical procedures for nurses. Recording temperature 1, no 6.1. *Nursing Times* **94**(2): insert 2p.

Torrance C, Semple M (1998b) Practical procedures for nurses. Recording temperature 2, no 6.2. *Nursing Times* **94**(3): insert 2p.

Tortora GJ, Derrickson B (2006) *Principles of Anatomy and Physiology*, 11th edn. Hoboken, NJ: John Wiley & Sons.

Tortora GJ, Grabowski SR (2003) *Principles of Anatomy and Physiology*, 10th edn. Chichester: John Wiley & Sons.

Trim J (2005) Monitoring temperature. *Nursing Times* **101**(20): 30–31.

Waugh A, Grant A (2001) *Ross and Wilson Anatomy and Physiology in Health and Illness*, 9th edn. London: Churchill Livingstone.

Wilshaw R, Beckstrand R, Waid D, Schaalje B (1999) A comparison of the use of tympanic, rectal and axillary temperature in infants. *Journal of Paediatric Nursing* **14**: 88–93.

Chapter 8

Pulse oximetry

Learning objectives

- Describe how a pulse oximetry machine operates and produces a reading
- State the indications for pulse oximetry
- List the conditions and factors that can affect readings
- Identify suitable sites for the probe
- Describe how to take and record an oxygen saturation level

Aim of this chapter

The aim of this chapter is to understand how pulse oximetry measures the oxygen saturation levels in blood, its significance and its application in practice.

What is an oxygen saturation reading?

Pulse oximetry is a non-invasive method of measuring the oxygen saturation of arterial blood. Oxygen saturation is the percentage of haemoglobin (a component of red blood cells, see below) that is saturated with oxygen (Booker 2008).

Who can perform the test?

Only individuals who are taught how to use the machine correctly and have obtained a clinical competency should undertake this clinical skill. Local guidelines and policies should also be followed. Abnormal findings, or a change in the patient's 'normal' reading, should be reported immediately to the nurse in charge.

Reasons for recording an oxygen saturation level

- As part of general respiratory management in patients with long-term pulmonary (lung) disease (Higgins 2005)
- To monitor unstable cardiac conditions (e.g. cardiac failure or heart attack) (Keenan 1995, Booker 2008)
- When transporting patients who are unwell and require oxygenation assessment (Higgins 2005)
- To diagnose respiratory illness (e.g. asthma, chronic obstructive pulmonary disease) (Place 2000)

- To monitor the effectiveness of oxygen/respiratory therapy (Allen 2004, Higgins 2005)
- During and after procedures that may require sedation/anaesthesia, or potential respiratory depression (Allen 2004, Higgins 2005)
- During the administration of medications that may cause respiratory depression, such as patient-controlled analgesia (Dougherty and Lister 2004)
- To reduce the need for frequent arterial blood sampling (see later) in acute care (Booker 2008).

When measuring the oxygen saturation levels in a patient, the overall condition and other vital signs should also be considered. This then allows review of the entire clinical presentation and not just the value of the reading in isolation. Casey (2001) and Woodrow (1999b) support this, stating that pulse oximetry should not replace traditional observations but complement them. In relation to respiratory symptoms or disease, Allen (2004) states that pulse oximetry cannot replace frequent, comprehensive respiratory assessment.

Pulse oximetry is very useful in the detection of cyanosis (where there is a reduction of oxygen to the skin and mucous membranes, leading to bluish coloration, e.g. in the lips and nailbeds), and this will result in an oxygen saturation reading of below 89%. Without this reading, even experienced practitioners have been known to find this diagnosis difficult (Jevon and Ewens 2002). Fox (2002) noted that early identification of hypoxia (reduced oxygen to the tissues) can also be identified by pulse oximetry, and can allow intervention that prevents further deterioration in the patient's condition. However, reduced oxygen in arterial blood (hypoxaemia) can still occur without reduced oxygen to the skin and membranes (cyanosis). This occurs where the concentration of haemoglobin is low or the capillaries do not receive enough blood, sometimes referred to as not being well perfused (Jevon and Ewens 2002).

Reflection point

Have you seen a pulse oximeter used in your clinical area? If so can you remember the purpose of recording the oxygen saturation level in a specific patient?

Relevant anatomy and physiology

Haemoglobin is the efficient and active oxygen-carrying part of red blood cells (Woodrow 1999a). Oxygen is transported to the body's tissues in the blood, by red blood cells that contain haemoglobin, combining to form oxyhaemoglobin, which releases oxygen to the tissues (Dougherty and Lister 2004). The red blood cells are specifically designed by having a biconcave shape, which is a round curved shape to maximise the available surface area. Under normal conditions, 99% of oxygen is carried in the body by combining with haemoglobin to form oxyhaemoglobin (Hinchcliffe et al. 1996). The rest is carried in plasma, a component of blood and this is a less effective method.

The amount of haemoglobin that combines with oxygen can be influenced further by various factors, including blood pH, temperature and carbon dioxide levels (Higgins 2005). When certain levels of these substances are present, the oxygen will be at its optimum, i.e. the best possible level for oxygen uptake. This is known as the oxygen dissociation curve. The oxygen saturation reading is a measure of the percentage of haemoglobin molecules saturated with oxygen, but does not indicate the actual number of red blood cells (Dougherty and Lister 2004).

Related aspects and terminology

- Hypoxia: diminished oxygen in tissues.
- Cyanosis: bluish or purple coloration of the skin and mucous membranes due to excess carbon dioxide and insufficient oxygen in the blood.
- Hypoxaemia: insufficient oxygenation of blood (Baillie et al. 2005).
- Haemoglobin: the pigment contained in red blood cells, which is used to carry oxygen.
- Oxyhaemoglobin: haemoglobin combined with oxygen molecules.
- Plethysmographic waveform: the visual representation of the pulse wave on a pulse oximeter machine. This represents the quality of the pulse at the point where oxyhaemoglobin saturation is being measured (Jevon 2000)

The mechanics of pulse oximetry

Beer's law states that the concentration of an unknown solute dissolved in a solvent can be determined by light absorption (Lynne et al. 1990). Therefore, pulse oximetry works on the principle that blood saturated with oxygen is a different colour from blood depleted of oxygen (Dougherty and Lister 2004; Higgins 2005). Thus, oxygen saturation can be estimated by measuring the difference between light absorption of full and empty capillaries (Woodrow 1999b). To assist this process, the pulse oximeter probe consists of two light-emitting diodes (one red and one infrared) on one side of the probe. These transmit red and infrared light through body tissue, usually a fingertip or ear lobe, to a photodetector on the other side of the probe (Jevon and Ewens 2002). A microprocessor filters the signals received and provides a digital display of oxygen saturation symbolised by the abbreviation SpO_2 (Jenson et al. 1998). Figure 8.1 shows an adult pulse oximetry probe. The difference in light absorption is calculated over a number of pulses, usually 5 (Harrahill 1991). However, an assumption is made that anything that pulses and absorbs red

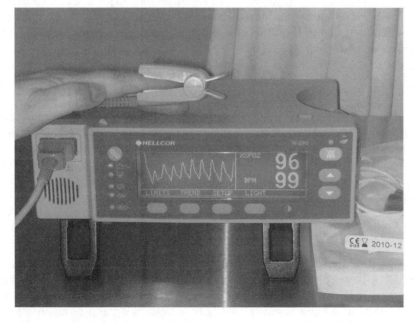

Figure 8.1 A pulse oximeter with probe *in situ*.

and infrared light between the light detector and the light source must be arterial blood, which can cause potential inaccuracies (Lowton 1999).

Advantages of pulse oximetry

Previously the only method of measuring the concentration of arterial blood would have been arterial blood gases. Despite this being seen as the 'gold standard' it is invasive, time-consuming, costly and provides only intermittent information (Jenson et al. 1998). Sampling arterial blood either involves drawing blood from an arterial line, a line that is inserted into the main vessel of the heart (often used in the intensive care unit), or sampling from an artery using a needle. Sampling from an artery is a highly skilled procedure, mostly carried out by medical staff; carries complications of increased risk of infection and bruising, and is often painful (Baillie et al. 2005). A sample from an arterial line is pain free for the patient but also carries the risk of infection. It is not expected that a healthcare assistant would undertake this procedure, but check local policy. The arterial blood sample is injected into a blood gas analyser, so a prerequisite is access to a blood gas analyser (Baillie et al. 2005). If the machine is within a unit or clinical area, it requires personnel to be trained in both its use and the interpretation of its findings.

Limitations of pulse oximetry

As pulse oximetry measures only haemoglobin oxygen saturation and not haemoglobin concentration, the patient can still have a depleted amount of oxygen (hypoxia) despite a 'normal' pulse oximetry reading (Higgins 2005). A further limitation is that pulse oximetry does not provide an indication of the adequacy of ventilation, carbon dioxide retention, partial pressure of oxygen or respiratory rate (Jevon 2000; Fox 2002; O'Neill 2003). Despite this, it is still an invaluable monitoring tool in a variety of clinical settings as long as its uses and limitations are fully understood (Jevon and Ewens 2000). The accuracy of the machines is usually within 2–3% for saturations >80%, with the accuracy dropping at lower saturation levels (Higgins 2005). Baillie et al. (2005) report that most pulse oximetry machines become inaccurate below 70%, but medical intervention is usually required before levels become this low, making inaccuracies of limited practical significance (Woodrow 1999a).

Equipment

Pulse oximeters are either non-invasive units or fully integrated into a patient monitoring system, such as those found in critical care areas. Some may record the pulse rate and this may be seen visually as a waveform. It is highly unlikely that a pulse oximeter would be used as a method to take a pulse because the reading would give a pulse rate only at the probe site and this may not always be accurate due to reduced blood flow. Therefore, use of a pulse oximeter is predominantly to measure haemoglobin oxygen saturation (Booker 2008).

Normal readings

Normal levels are usually between 95% and 100 %, but depend on individual patients (Jevon 2000). Alarms can be set depending on individual patients' clinical presentation, but guidance should be sought as to both the levels that should be set and whether local policy allows healthcare assistants to do this. Jevon and Ewens (2002) advise that, in general terms, oxygen saturation <90% is of concern. It is essential always to record the oxygen therapy being received by the patient together with the readings, and assess the clinical condition of the patient. A sustained trend of falling oxygen saturation levels is clinically important, even if the precision of individual readings is poor (Hutton and Clutton-Brock 1993). Some diseases can affect readings, so the patient's medical history should be considered before carrying out the procedure (see Box 8.1 for possible factors).

Box 8.1 Factors affecting oxygen saturation readings

Poor circulation

This can be due to peripheral vascular disease or vasoconstriction (narrowing of blood vessels), low temperature (hypothermia) or low blood pressure (hypotension) (Casey 2001; Dougherty and Lister 2004). All can give low readings due to the reduced blood flow. which results in a decreased pulsatile flow upon which the pulse oximeter relies to calculate the reading (Baillie et al. 2005). Arterial constriction or shock would also affect readings (Keenan 1995). To ensure accurate readings it is recommended that the probe be placed where there is a good blood flow.

Carbon monoxide

The presence of carbon monoxide (CO) in blood gives erroneously high readings because the CO combines with O_2 to form carboxyhaemoglobin. This substance is bright red, similar to oxyhaemoglobin; as both compounds have a similar absorbence, this results in over-estimation. This can be a result of cigarette smoking, exhaust fumes or exposure to fire smoke (Moyle 1996; Woodrow 1999a). In these instances pulse oximetry should not be used (Baillie et al. 2005).

Tricuspid incompetence (heart valve failure)

Inaccurate readings are obtained due to the machine not being able to differentiate between arteriolar and venous pulsation (Baillie et al. 2005). Further advice should be sought as to whether pulse oximetry should be used.

Anaemia

High oxygen saturation can be recorded but inadequate oxygen is actually perfusing (getting into) the tissues due to the reduced number of haemoglobin molecules (Woodrow 1999a; Dougherty and Lister 2004). Advice should be sought to identify the appropriateness of pulse oximetry for these patients.

Atrial fibrillation

This is a fast heartbeat from the top chamber of the heart that interferes with the pulsatile signal (Baillie et al. 2005). If this is an intermittent problem it may still be possible to obtain accurate readings, so further advice should be sought.

Parkinson's disease or seizures

An incorrect reading may be obtained due to the tremor associated with Parkinson's disease or the irregular movement caused by seizures or shivering (Baillie et al. 2005; Moore 2007). Both cause interference and artefact (disturbance), and in such an instance, the use of an ear probe has been reported to reduce the interference or alternatively support the probe when *in situ* (Carroll 1997. Moore 2007).

Altered red blood cell shape

As mentioned earlier, blood cells are biconcave in shape to promote oxygen uptake. Sickle cell disease and some medications (e.g. anaesthetic agents) alter the shape of red blood cells and will alter readings. Therefore caution and further advice should be sought both in the interpretation of these readings and as to whether pulse oximetry is appropriate for these patients (Woodrow 1999a).

Using a pulse oximeter

Before performing the skill, ensure that you have received approved training and undertaken supervised practice in line with local policy (Higgins 2005). It is also advisable to consult the manufacturer's directions for the make and model in use.

It is essential that the correct cable and probe be used with the appropriate machine (see later) for accurate recordings. The machine should have been serviced in the past year (usually a sticker will be in place with a date), should be visibly clean and, when switched on successfully, should go through a series of self-tests with no error codes (see 'Common problems'). If an error code or abnormality is noted, report the fault and use another machine. Likewise, if there are problems getting a reliable trace or reading, and the probe has been changed with no success, try another machine (Jevon 2000). Furthermore, Moore (2007) suggests that you test the machine on yourself before the patient, to test that it is working; and the added advantage of showing patients who are new to the procedure that it is painless.

Reflection point

Set up a pulse oximetry machine on yourself, rotating the site and type of probe where possible.

Pulse oximetry probes

There are multiple sites where a probe can be placed, which depend on both the probe being used and the individual patient. Moyle (1999) stresses the importance in children of using the correct size of probe for the size of the child and that special probes for neonates, babies and small children are available, which are often applied to the palms, feet or arms. Woodrow (1999a) also describes a probe that uses the bridge of the nose in infants. In adults the probe is dependent on the site intended by the manufacturer, but possibilities include probes suitable for fingers or toes, and specialist ear probes. Ear probes are applied to the ear lobe but care should be taken not to position the sensor over a pierced area because this may adversely affect the reading (GE Healthcare 2005). GE Healthcare (2005) also suggest that the site be massaged for 20–30 seconds using an alcohol pad or cream (but not a vasodilator because this would falsely increase blood flow to the site). This action acts to increase perfusion (blood flow) and improve the trace. The cable should also be loose, so movement will not disrupt the sensor and the clip should be attached to the shoulder of the patient. Finally, a headband is also available and this requires the cable to be looped around an ear and tucked in. This may not be available in every clinical area.

If the pulse oximetry reading requires continuous monitoring, the patient's preference may be taken into account or, in the case of confused or agitated patients, a site that is out of vision may be best.

Whatever site is chosen, only an appropriate probe for the machine being used should be in place. Tape, to hold the probe in place, should be used only where it is essential, because Moyle (1999) has reported that using tape to secure the probe can cause pressure or thermal (heat) damage to the extremity. The site should be checked and rotated at least 2-hourly to prevent any pressure damage resulting from prolonged use at any one site (Medical Devices Agency 2001; Fox 2002). Where the patient is unable to flex the fingers voluntarily, this may result in stiffness, and the site may need to be changed more frequently (Jevon and Ewens 2002).

Particular care when using pulse oximetry probes is advised for children, patients with poor perfusion, older people, patients who are confused or unconscious due to reduced sensations, or the patient who is unable to report discomfort (Jevon 2000; Baillie et al. 2005).

The probe should be visually examined before use to ensure that it is not broken or dirty (Baillie et al. 2005). Replace the probe if it is faulty and always refer to manufacturer's recommendations for cleaning. If it is proving difficult to obtain a trace, warm and rub the skin to improve the circulation (Jevon 2000). Table 8.1 describes the procedure for recording an oxygen saturation level using a pulse oximeter.

Table 8.1 Procedure for recording an oxygen saturation level

Action	Rationale
1. Explain the procedure to the patient and gain verbal consent. Document	The patient will fully understand the procedure and agree to participate
2. Check that the equipment has been serviced, is in good working order and clean, and has designated accessories (lead/probe)	The machine should be serviced as per local policy to ensure that an accurate reading is obtained
	A clean probe will prevent cross infection
	Correct accessories essential for accurate readings
3. Ensure the patient is warm and comfortable	If the patient is cold they could have decreased peripheral blood flow that can reduce blood flow (and give a low reading). If the patient is shivering this can interfere with the signal
	If the patient is comfortable they will be more relaxed, especially if having continuous monitoring (Dougherty and Lister 2004)
4. Wash hands and put on a clean apron (Higgins 2005)	Prevent cross-infection
5. Select a suitable site for the probe and place as per manufacturer's instructions	Ensures accuracy of reading
6. Switch the machine on and check function; should beep with each detected pulse or waveform (Dougherty and Lister 2004)	Accurate pulse detection
	Shows the patient that the procedure is painless and checks the machine
7. Record both the oxygen therapy (where applicable) and SpO_2 reading – reporting any abnormal readings. This may be a change for the patient or out with 'normal' limits	To provide a legal record of the measurement
	The nurse in charge may want to reset alarms/parameters to identify changes in recorded saturation levels (Higgins 2005). If set incorrectly, alarms can be a nuisance if constantly activated
8. Remove the probe, if using for routine or intermittent observation (and when appropriate for continuous monitoring)	Patient comfort
When continuously monitoring, ensure that cable is positioned as safely as possible and probe secured if necessary	For health and safety round the bed space
Return to check probe is not causing any complications. Rotate site every couple of hours	To prevent damage to the probe site (Higgins 2005)
9. Clean the equipment, in line with local policy Return to equipment store; plug in to re-charge if appropriate.	Prevent cross-infection
	To recharge the machine ready for use

Documentation

Ensure that any oxygen therapy that the patient is receiving is recorded together with the pulse oximetry reading. If the oxygen saturation readings are high the patient may be receiving unnecessary oxygen, and prolonged use can be harmful (Woodrow 1999b). Likewise, avoid taking oxygen saturation levels when the patient has just been suctioned (a catheter inserted into the windpipe to remove secretions), because this will give a false reading (see Chapter 9).

Pulse oximetry recordings may be documented in the patient's case notes if the patient is in the community or on various charts if in hospital.

Common problems

Errors in pulse oximetry readings can be due to many different variables, some of which can be reduced to promote a more accurate trace. They have been split into three different areas, namely those causes by light transmission, pulse detection and actual use of the equipment.

Light transmission/absorption

As mentioned previously and shown in Figure 8.1, the finger probe consists of two parts, with one side receiving the light source and the other being a photodetector. If bright light, either artificial or sunlight, is picked up readings can be affected (Baillie et al. 2005). If the reading is an intermittent recording (i.e. not continuously in place), consider closing a curtain or switching off the fluorescent lights until the reading has been taken. In instances where the light is necessary for treatment, e.g. phototherapy to treat jaundiced babies, the probe needs to be covered to ensure accurate readings (Stoddart et al. 1997). Nail varnish also causes problems with the transmission of light and the darker the nail polish the more problematic it is (Baillie et al. 2005). Patients who have nail varnish in place should be asked if they would mind removing it. Interestingly, unpolished acrylic nails do not affect pulse oximetry measurements and these can be left in place (Peters 1997).

Other factors that affect the transmission of light, and cause low readings, include the presence of dried blood on the skin (Jevon 2000), presence of bilirubin or substances such as engine oil on the hands (Dobson 1993; Booker 2008). Keenan (1995) noted that intravenous dyes used in imaging affect light transmission, and individuals using pulse oximetry should seek advice about how long these agents are active for, should be sought to enable measurements to be taken when they are no longer active.

Pulse detection

Baillie et al. (2005) identified that movement, including shivering, may present a problem due to artefact causing a 'noisy signal' (Woodrow 1999b), or the probe to become dislodged (Moore 2007). In some instances another site may produce a better trace, e.g. an ear or toe. If it is an intermittent reading, supporting the probe in place may be beneficial, and for continuous monitoring taping the probe to the back of the hand can reduce problems (Baillie et al. 2005). Interference from other equipment or mobile phones has also been identified as a potential problem (Baillie et al. 2005).

Equipment use

As with all pieces of equipment, the pulse oximeter should have been serviced as recommended by the manufacturer and local policy. When the device is switched on it should perform a self-test and not display any error codes; this ensures the accuracy and reliability of the machine (Booker 2008).

If the machine is dropped or broken, as with other pieces of equipment, qualified staff should check it – local policy will dictate whether this is an in-house department or the manufacturer.

The correct accessories, e.g. probes, should be used for each specific machine and the accessories checked to ensure that they are clean and for signs of damage.

Measuring oxygen saturation levels on the same arm as a BP cuff or venous line can disrupt the machine's ability to measure the pulse (Jevon and Ewens 2002; Newman 2005; Moore 2007).

Table 8.2 Practical assessment form: competency framework for recording SpO$_2$

Steps	First assessment/reassessment Demonstration					Date/competent signature
	Date/sign	Date/sign	Date/sign	Date/sign	Date/sign	
	1	2	3	4	5	
Recording oxygen saturation levels (SpO$_2$)						
1. State normal range for SpO$_2$ as a percentage						
2. State what oxygen saturation levels actually measure and the limitations						
3. Define the terms cyanosis and hypoxia						
4. State different sites for recording oxygen saturation						
5. List common causes of inaccurate recordings, caused by disease processes and the equipment						
6. Describe different types of models in use						
7. Describe appropriate sites and the reasons for these choices						
8. Describe how you would prepare a patient for obtaining an oxygen saturation reading and gaining consent						
9. Describe the correct procedure for recording oxygen saturation						
10. Describe safe disposal and cleaning of the equipment following use						
11. Identify and justify the use of documentation						
12. State when to ask for assistance/report findings						

Supervisors/Assessor(s):

Indeed the pulse reading should match with the patient's heart rate; if this is not the case it may indicate that not all pulsations are being detected and another machine should be sought (Moore 2007).

Summary

Pulse oximetry, when used appropriately, is a good way of accurately measuring oxygen saturation levels. If the role of the healthcare assistant involves taking these readings it is essential that competency-based training is undertaken in accordance with local policies and procedures for the specific device that is in use. Table 8.2 provides a competency framework for recording SpO_2 levels.

Case study 8.1

Mrs Semple is a frail 86-year-old woman who has been admitted to hospital with hypothermia (low temperature) and shivering. She requires her oxygen saturation levels to be monitored.
What equipment would you consider for her and what factors affect your decision?
Describe some of the reassurances and special precautions that should be taken for her.

Case study 8.2

Baby Ben is aged 8 months and has been admitted with a respiratory problem (suspected pneumonia). He is to be started on a pulse oximeter for continuous monitoring.
What factors affect the equipment and site choices for him? What special precautions should also be taken for him to ensure that no harm comes to him during his treatment?

Self-assessment

Assessment	Aspects	Achieved ✔
Patient	*Have you considered all aspects of this section?*	
	The purpose of the red and infrared lights used to measure oxygen saturation	
	The diseases that can affect pulse oximetry readings	
	Advantages and disadvantages of pulse oximetry	
	The indications for pulse oximetry use	
Procedure	*Have you considered all aspects of this section?*	✔
	What the normal limits for pulse oximetry are	
	The possible sites and types of probe available	
	Documentation of readings	

References

Allen K (2004) Principles and limitations of pulse oximetry in patient monitoring. *Nursing Times* **100**(41): 34–37.

Baillie L, Corben V, Higham S (2005) Respiratory care: assessment and interventions. In: Baillie L (ed.), *Developing Practical Nursing Skills*. London: Hodder Arnold, Chapter 11.

Booker R (2008) Pulse oximetry. *Nursing Standard* **22**(30): 39–41.

Carroll P (1997) Pulse oximetry – at your fingertips. *Nursing Journal for Registered Nurses* **60**(2): 22–27, 43.

Casey G (2001) Oxygen transport and use of pulse oximetry. *Nursing Standard* **8**(15): 46–53.

Dobson F (1993) Shedding light on pulse oximetry. *Nursing Standard* **7**(46): 4–11.

Dougherty L, Lister S, eds (2004) *The Royal Marsden Hospital Manual of Clinical Nursing Procedures*, 6th edn. Oxford: Blackwell Publishing.

Fox N (2002) Pulse oximetry. *Nursing Times* **98**: 40.

GE Healthcare (2005) *OxyTip Ear Sensor information sheet*. Helsinki, Finland: GE Healthcare.

Harrahill M (1991) Pulse oximetry, pearls, and pitfalls. *Journal of Emergency Nursing* **17**: 437–439

Higgins D (2005) Pulse oximetry. *Nursing Times* **101**(6): 34–35.

Hinchcliffe SM, Montague SE, Watson R (1996) *Physiology for Nursing Practice*. London: Baillière Tindall.

Hutton P, Clutton-Brock T (1993) The benefits and pitfalls of pulse oximetry. *British Medical Journal* **307**: 457–458.

Jenson LA, Onyskiw JE, Prasad NGN (1998) Meta-analysis of arterial oxygenations saturation monitoring by pulse oximetry in adults. *Heart and Lung* **27**: 387–408.

Jevon P (2000) Pulse oximetry – 2. *Nursing Times* **96**(27): 43–44.

Jevon P, Ewens B (2000) Pulse oximetry. *Nursing Times* **96**(26): 43–44.

Jevon P, Ewens B (2002) *Monitoring the Critically Ill Patient*. Oxford: Blackwell Publishing.

Keenan, J (1995) Pulse oximetry (cardiology update). *Nursing Standard* **9**: 35–55.

Lowton K (1999) Pulse oximeters for the detection of hypoxaemia. *Professional Nurse* **14**: 343–350.

Lynne M, Scnapp MD, Neal H et al. (1990) Pulse oximetry: uses and abuses. *Chest* **98**: 1244–1250.

Medical Devices Agency (2001) *Tissue Necrosis caused by Oximeter Probes SN 2001 (08)*. London: MDA.

Moyle J (1996) How to guides. Pulse oximetry. *Care of the Critically Ill* **12**(6): insert.

Moyle J (1999) Step by step guide. Pulse oximetry. *Journal of Neonatal Nursing* **5**: insert.

Moore T (2007) Respiratory assessment in adults. *Nursing Standard* **21**(49): 48–56.

Newman A (2005) Understanding pulse oximetry principles can improve practice. *Nursing Times* **101**(2): 43.

O'Neill D (2003) An introduction to blood gas analysis. *Nursing Times* **99**: 11.

Peters SM (1997) The effect of acrylic nails on the measurement of oxygen saturation as determined by pulse oximetry. *Journal of the American Anaesthetic Nurses Association* **65**: 361.

Place B (2000) Pulse oximetry: benefits and limitations. *Nursing Times* **96**(26): 42.

Stoddart S, Summers L, Platt MW (1997) Pulse oximetry: what it is and how to use it. *Journal of Neonatal Nursing* **3**(4): 10, 12–14.

Woodrow P (1999a) Pulse oximetry. *Emergency Nurse* **7**(5): 34–39.

Woodrow P (1999b) Pulse oximetry. *Nursing Standard* **13**(42): 42–46.

Chapter 9

Respiratory care

Learning objectives

- Discuss the anatomy and physiology relating to respiration
- Explore how and why a respiratory rate is assessed and recorded
- Identify when to measure a peak flow and discuss how to safely carry out the procedure
- Discuss suctioning techniques and safety aspects
- Have an understanding of related terms and complications of respiratory care and their role

Aim of this chapter

The aim of this chapter is to identify the anatomy and physiology relating to respiration, and explore the recording of a respiratory rate and a peak flow. It also discusses suctioning techniques.

What do we mean by respiratory care?

The respiratory system is made up of the nose, pharynx, larynx, trachea, bronchi and lungs (Bennett 2003) (Figure 9.1).

If there is a problem at any point in the system this may result in the patient feeling breathless. This chapter describes the role of a healthcare assistant in assessing and assisting a breathless patient through their observation, recording and reporting of respiratory rate and/or peak flow.

The treatments commonly associated with respiratory care, e.g. oxygen therapy, are explored briefly in Chapter 15, because for many healthcare assistants this might not be an accepted role.

Relevant anatomy and physiology

The main function of the respiratory system is to supply the body with oxygen and remove carbon dioxide through the process of inspiration (breathing in) and expiration (breathing out) (Baillie et al. 2005). The gas exchange takes place in the alveoli (clusters that have been likened to a bunch of grapes and have a surface area of 70 m^2 in an adult, and if placed out flat are equivalent to the surface area of a football pitch) (Tortora and Derrickson 2006).

Thus, breathing is the movement of air in and out of the lungs, entering through the mouth and nose, and passing via the pharynx (throat), larynx (voice box), trachea (windpipe), bronchi and bronchioles into the lungs (Tortora and Derrickson 2006). The respiratory system is in two sections: the upper respiratory system refers to the nose, pharynx and associated structures, whereas the lower respiratory system refers to the larynx, trachea, bronchi and lungs.

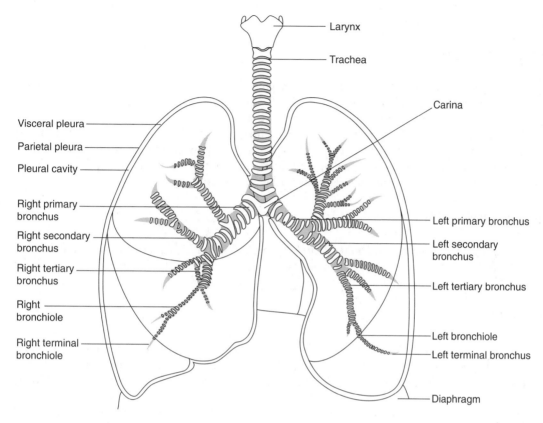

Figure 9.1 The respiratory system.

Upper respiratory system

The nose has two parts: external and internal (Tortora and Derrickson 2006):

(1) External: a supporting framework of bone and cartilage, covered with muscle and skin and lined by mucous membrane
(2) Internal: the nasal cavity is split by the nasal septum, which divides into a right and left side.

When air enters the nostrils it passes through the vestibule (just inside the nostrils), which is lined by skin containing coarse hairs that filter out large dust particles. Air that is passed through the nose is filtered, but also warmed and moistened (humidified).

The pharynx (throat)

This is a funnel shaped tube about 13 cm (5 inches) long, which lies behind the nasal and oral cavity, above the larynx and just in front of the cervical vertebrae. The pharynx functions as a passageway for air and food, provides a resonating chamber for speech sounds and houses the tonsils, which help eliminate foreign invaders (Tortora and Derrickson 2006).

Lower respiratory system

Larynx (voice box)

This is a short passageway that connects the pharynx with the trachea, and the wall of the larynx is made of cartilage (Tortora and Derrickson 2006). When small particles, e.g. dust, smoke, food or liquids, pass into the larynx a cough reflex occurs to expel the material.

However, normally the epiglottis (a large leaf-shaped piece of elastic cartilage) is able to move up and down like a trap door (leaf portion), so during swallowing the larynx rises and allows the free edge of the epiglottis to move up and down and form a lid; therefore liquids and foods are routed into the oesophagus and kept out of the larynx and lungs.

Trachea (windpipe)

This is a tubular passage for air, about 12 cm (5 inches) long and $2^1/_2$ cm (1 inch) in width (Tortora and Derrickson 2006). It is found in front of the oesophagus, and extends from the larynx to the bronchi, which then split into a right and left primary bronchus.

Bronchi

When the trachea divides, a right primary bronchus (windpipe) goes into the right lung and a left primary bronchus goes into the left lung. The right main bronchus is more vertical, shorter and wider than the left, so any aspirated object, e.g. foodstuff, is more likely to enter and lodge in the right primary bronchus.

On entering the lungs, the primary bronchi divide to form smaller bronchi.

The right lung has three lobes, whereas the left has two lobes and the smaller bronchi branch further to smaller bronchi until they divide into bronchioles. This extensive branching from the trachea resembles a tree trunk with its branches and is commonly called the bronchial tree (Tortora and Derrickson 2006).

Lungs

These are a pair of cone-shaped organs lying in the thoracic (chest) cavity, separated from each other by the heart. The lungs have two layers of serous membranes called the pleural membrane which enclose and protect each lung. Within the lungs are alveoli where gas exchange takes place; it is estimated that the lungs contain 300 million alveoli.

To aid breathing we have muscles of respiration (Figure 9.2).

Many breathless patients may prefer to sit upright to help and they may need to use accessory muscles of respiration, e.g. the neck and abdominal muscles (Baillie et al. 2005).

Breathing is regulated in the brain and has both conscious and unconscious control. Conscious control is when a patient takes an extra breath or a deeper inspiration, whereas most breathing is unconscious – we just do it without thought. The regulation of breathing is managed by a respiratory centre, which responds to the gas levels in the blood, usually oxygen and carbon dioxide, and also hydrogen. The centre monitors gas levels, and in normal respiration is driven by the increase in the carbon dioxide level, which triggers nerve impulses down to the respiratory muscles and stimulates respiration.

In patients with a chronic lung disease, e.g. chronic bronchitis, over time the body adapts to a constantly elevated level of carbon dioxide (CO_2) and therefore the respiratory centre switches

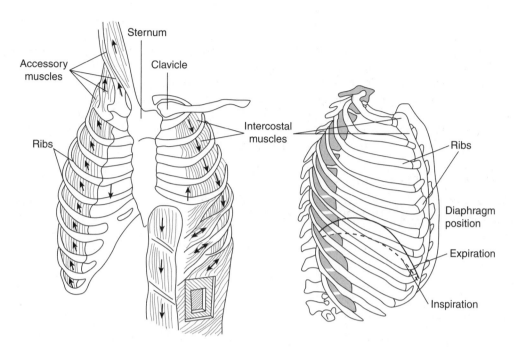

Figure 9.2   Muscles of respiration.

to respond to a drop in the oxygen (O_2) level. This is one reason why any respiratory patient needs careful observation and monitoring of blood gases, and accurately and carefully titrated (dosed) O_2 therapy. Too high a level of O_2 would remove the respiratory drive in these patients, e.g. the respiratory centre fails to trigger the respiratory muscles and the patient stops breathing.

Breathing can be affected by many factors: disease, e.g. infection, lung cancer, asthma; emotional state, e.g. stress, fear leading to hyperventilation (overbreathing); position, e.g. cramped or slouched will restrict breathing; trauma, e.g. accident to the brain or chest, or surgery; and exercise.

Recording a respiratory rate

Why and when a respiratory rate is observed, assessed and recorded

- On admission – to provide a baseline record
- Before procedures, e.g. surgery; again baseline
- When a patient's condition suggests it, e.g. feeling unwell, breathless, complaining of pain or injury
- To monitor response to treatments/medications, e.g. oxygen, morphine
- Before specified medications for baseline, e.g. blood administration
- To monitor changes in oxygenation or respiration, e.g. someone with asthma.

What do you observe?

Bennett (2003), Dougherty and Lister (2004) and Baillie et al. (2005) discuss rate, depth, pattern, sound, regularity/rhythm and colour.

Rate

When assessing the respiratory rate, you need to know the expected normal rate for a person's age group (Baillie et al. 2005). The baseline rate on admission or before procedures/medications will allow comparison. However, the respiratory rate varies according to age, size (build) and gender, and other demands, e.g. exercise; discussed in more detail below.

The normal adult respiratory rate in a man is 14–18 breaths/min and in a woman 16–20 breaths/min (Dougherty and Lister (2004)). Bennett (2003) and Baillie et al. (2005) suggest a range from 10 breaths/min to 16 breaths/min, whereas children's rates vary with age (Table 9.1).

Table 9.1 Children's respiratory rate and age

Age (years)	Respiratory rate (breaths/min)
Newborn	30–80
<1	25–35
1–5	20–30
5–12	20–25
>12	15–25

Adapted from Dougherty and Lister (2004) and Baillie et al. (2005).

Stress, fear, anxiety and exercise will increase the respiratory rate and this is normal. Let us consider a patient on admission; they may be anxious, have rushed to get to the appointment on time or be in pain, and these factors may have affected the respiratory rate. Therefore this recording may not be a true baseline.

Bennett (2003) advocates resting a patient for at least 5 min before any respiratory measure, because a rise in the respiratory rate is the most sensitive indication of deterioration in a patient.

A raised respiratory rate (tachypnoea) in an adult would therefore be over 20 breaths/min and a decreased respiratory rate (bradypnoea) is considered if the rate is below 10 breaths/min.

We have noted that some factors, e.g. stress and exercise, can increase rate, but if you recorded a respiratory rate of 40 and over, and the patient is resting and not having exercised, e.g. running, this must be reported immediately.

Bradypnoea can be caused by certain conditions, e.g. brain tumour, or treatments, e.g. morphine, which is known to depress (reduce) the respiratory rate, and is the reason why a patient newly started on any opioid, i.e. morphine, will have their respiration monitored. A rate of 10 or below must always be reported promptly.

A good rule of thumb to apply is 'if in doubt, shout' (report) (Baillie et al. 2005). Bear in mind that you would also be monitoring a patient's pulse, blood pressure and probably temperature too. In healthy people the relationship between the pulse and respiratory rate is fairly constant, with one breath to 4–5 heart beats, so, in an adult with a respiratory rate of 15 breaths/min, you would expect a pulse rate of 60–75 beats/min.

Reflection points

Mrs Winifred Johnson is 57 years old and has been admitted for a bronchoscopy to investigate her persistent cough.
You are asked to admit her and while recording her respiratory rate you measure her rate at 38 breaths/min.
What factors might you need to consider?
What action might you take?

Depth

Does the chest rise and fall – shallowly, deeply or evenly? This observation is crucial (Baillie et al. 2005).

Deep rapid breaths (hyperventilation) are often associated with anxiety or panic attacks. If prolonged, a patient will start to feel dizzy and faint; this is a result of a drop in the CO_2 level, and you can help by encouraging the patient to breathe slowly in and out of a paper bag (this allows the patient to re-breathe the exhaled CO_2 and so stabilises them). Slow shallow breaths (hypoventilation) can occur with some drugs, e.g. morphine, and will also lead to poor gas exchange and insufficient oxygen. Dougherty and Lister (2004) stated that normal breathing is effortless, automatic and regular. The depth is the volume of air moving in with each respiration, and in an adult is about 500 ml.

Pattern

As noted before, normal breathing is effortless, so, if a patient is struggling to breathe (dyspnoea), you might observe irregular, noisy breaths and also possibly the use of the accessory muscles of respiration (neck and abdominal muscles). Changes in the pattern of respiration are often found in disorders of the respiratory centre in the brain (Dougherty and Lister (2004)).

Therefore, assessment should include the pattern of breathing, e.g. mouth breathing, when a patient tries to gulp air in. This happens because there is less resistance to air flow through the mouth than the nose: noses can often block, e.g. with a common cold, but this can cause the mouth to become dry and so mouth hygiene is essential to help keep the mouth moist and the air humidified.

People with asthma, caused by narrowing of the airways, cannot 'shift' air and in some cases you might observe minimal movement of breathing, e.g. little rise or fall in the chest, which is serious and must be reported promptly. If you are unsure of a patient's breathing pattern, you can place a hand gently over their lower chest and see if you can feel the movement of the ribs as the patient breathes (Baillie et al. 2005). In general, you would observe the chest rise and fall to measure the respiratory rate and, to prevent a patient altering the respiratory rate, you can continue to hold the wrist as though still counting the radial pulse rate. This ensures that the respiratory rate is not altered consciously.

Sound

As noted earlier, breathing should be quiet, so, if it can be heard, there may be a problem (Baillie et al. 2005).

A loud harsh, almost rasping sound (stridor), usually heard on inspiration, is frequently due to a partial or blocked larynx (airway) from injury, foreign body or illness, e.g. tumour, and must be reported immediately.

A wheeze, characterised by a noisy, musical sound (Bennett 2003), often on expiration, is usually found in people with asthma (during an asthmatic attack) and is caused by swelling, which leads to narrowing of the airways. Patients with chronic bronchitis and emphysema may also have a wheeze.

A 'rattly' chest is caused by the presence of fluid (e.g. sputum, blood) in the upper airway.

Snoring breathing, especially in the unconscious patient, may be caused by the tongue blocking the airway (Bennett 2003). Prompt checking and action are required here.

Finally whooping cough causes a distinctive whoop sound, usually when coughing, and is most commonly found in children.

Regularity/rhythm

This might be considered similar to pattern, so breathing should be regular and rhythmic and any period without breathing (apnoea) must be reported immediately. Some children experience apnoea in tantrums (Baillie et al. 2005), whereas in adults it can be associated with some brain injuries or illnesses. Bennett (2003) described Cheyne–Stokes respirations as a 'pattern' of breathing where the patient has periods of apnoea alternating with periods of overbreathing (hyperpnoea); it is often associated with left ventricular failure (heart failure) or brain injury.

Colour

As well as assessing rate, depth, pattern, sound and regularity, you should also be observing the patient's colour, to identify any abnormality. If patients are not getting enough oxygen they become cyanosed, which manifests as a bluish dusky colour of the mucous membranes, and can be observed in the skin and nailbeds, which is why patients are asked to remove nail polish/varnish. It is often most noticeable around the lips, earlobes, mouth and fingertips. In dark-skinned patients it is most noticeable in the lips and nailbeds, which become dusky in colour (Bennett 2003). This is also why we ask patients to remove lipstick, especially before procedures, e.g. surgery. The patient's condition will probably be poor by the time that you observe cyanosis, but it is one aspect that you should always consider whenever checking a patient's pulse and respiratory rate.

How to measure and record a respiratory rate accurately

Baillie et al. (2005) suggest that you have a watch with a second hand; the patient should be comfortable and relaxed, preferably sitting or lying, and you can watch the chest, although not too obviously, because this may cause embarrassment with females or an altered pattern of breathing.

Start counting as you observe each rise and fall of the chest, and if regular you could count the number in 30 seconds and double. However, if the pattern is irregular it is better to count for the full 60 seconds, so that there is no risk of error. In children, it is recommended that you always count the full minute, especially in babies aged under 1 year (Baillie et al. 2005).

How often you record will depend on the patient's condition, treatment and monitoring requirements. A patient with acute asthma might need the respiratory rate measured every 15 minutes, so always follow your local policies and practice. A patient who is stable will have measurements gradually reduced, maybe from 4-hourly to twice a day, or less. Any changes however, would need to be quickly monitored, recorded and reported.

Now that we have explored measuring respiration and rate, let us consider another means of monitoring a patient's respiration – measuring and recording a peak expiratory flow rate (PEFR).

Measuring and recording a peak expiratory flow rate

This is achieved by use of a meter called a peak flow meter; this simple device can be a very useful tool to monitor a patient's breathing, and is very commonly used for monitoring asthma. It

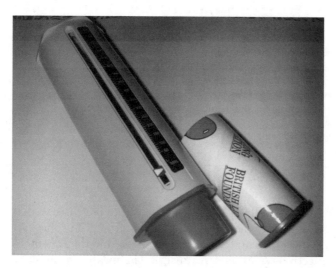

Figure 9.3   Peak flow meter with disposable one-way mouthpiece. (Photograph by I Lavery.)

provides a simple quantitative (measurable), reproducible (repeatable) and objective measurement of airway function (Kennedy et al. 1998).

The peak flow measures, in litres per minute, the maximum flow rate that a patient can blow out when starting from full inhalation (bit like blowing out those birthday candles!). This measure allows monitoring of a patient with any lung disease; it is easy, quick and cheap, but technique is crucial to ensure accuracy (Baillie et al. 2005). It allows monitoring of ongoing treatments and can be very useful for someone who has difficulty recognising that their condition is worsening, e.g. asthma. Booker (2007) suggests limited usefulness in other respiratory diseases and in children aged under 5–6 years. It can be used in children, but if younger than 5 years they can often confuse suck with blow, so it is recommended for use only once a child understands 'suck' for inhale.

To measure a peak flow, a meter is commonly used (Figure 9.3) and this comes with a disposable mouthpiece for each patient. Peak flow meters dispensed on prescription are labelled for single patient use; however, in clinics or hospitals some may be labelled for multiple patient use, but are always used with a disposable one-way mouthpiece (Booker 2007).

Cleansing and disinfection are important (see Addendum for manufacturer's advice). Booker (2007) further advises: in hospitals a log is kept of each meter's cleansing and disinfection; disposable one-way mouthpieces are used (one way to prevent patient inhaling through meter); and there is an annual replacement of meters.

The patient should be sitting or standing upright, to allow full chest expansion. Kennedy et al. (1998) suggest that it be used at least twice daily over 2–3 weeks to establish a patient's personal best score.

Higgins (2005) advocates that the patient first be given information about the procedure and so they can give consent and understand it. This is important to encourage compliance and understanding of what must be done with the scores. Booker (2007) proposes that the nurse demonstrate the technique first to help the patient understand the procedure. The nurse must ensure that their hands are washed and an apron is put on before assembling the meter. Box 9.1 outlines the technical aspects.

The frequency will depend on each patient's condition. For maintenance (to monitor ongoing treatment), the patient may measure the peak flow once in the morning, or in some cases twice daily, and so also record an evening peak flow.

Box 9.1 Technique

- Patient holds meter level, and ensures their fingers don't obstruct the scale
- Flow indicator is set to zero/lowest reading on the scale
- With mouthpiece fitted securely, the patient should take a deep breath, clamp the lips tightly round the mouthpiece and then blow out as hard and fast as possible, e.g. like blowing out candles
- Check the flow indicator position and record the score, e.g. 370 l/min
- It is recommended to do the best of three, so a further two attempts are made, ensuring that indicator is zeroed each time, then recording the best score

Adapted from Baillie et al. (2005), Higgins (2005) and Booker (2007).

During any acute episode of illness, the frequency would increase, so that any treatments and their effectiveness, e.g. nebuliser therapy, would be monitored. In some cases measurements are taken pre-treatment, e.g. asthma and nebuliser treatment, and then again 30 min after treatment (this monitors the effectiveness of any treatment). The measurement should be recorded, and some recommend recording before and after measurements in different colours to differentiate these two measures consistently (Baillie et al. 2005).

Normal peak flow measure

A peak flow measurement will vary depending on gender, age and height (Higgins 2005):

- Gender: adults usually achieve 400–700 l/min, but males achieve higher readings.
- Age: children would be lower, e.g. 9 year old expect 175 l/min, but height is a factor too. The normal range in children is 100–400 l/min.
- Height: this increases the lung capacity and so increases the peak flow scoring, so a tall 9 year old might score slightly higher.

Other variations are due to timings; morning readings tend to be lower, with highest readings usually in the early evening, hence the usual twice daily readings for people with asthma to monitor and compare scores. Scores are plotted and trends can be spotted early, because one lower score may not be meaningful. However, it is best to report this, remembering that other recordings will be monitored as well, e.g. temperature, pulse and blood pressure, and these can support findings. In people with asthma the pulse rate will increase, and if due to an infection they may also have a raised temperature.

Other circumstances can affect readings, e.g. cold air, cats' hair acting as a trigger (allergies); and again, by keeping a record, these trends can be observed and identified.

Regular monitoring can therefore allow the patient to manage their breathing/condition, e.g. asthma, and respond quickly to any deterioration:

- If the rate falls below 80% of individual's best level, then refer to doctor as they would likely increase preventative treatment, e.g. inhaler
- If the reading falls below 50% of their usual reading, alert medical staff immediately.

Again, if in doubt refer to a professional colleague. Ask yourself – was the patient relaxed and rested? If the patient has just got back from the toilet with maybe more demands on their breathing, they may be tired resulting in a lower reading, so wait 5 minutes and repeat.

Reflection point

Jenny Wilkinson is a 15 year old with asthma; you are supervising her peak flow measurement and notice that her technique is poor.
Explain what advice you might give her to help improve her technique.

Performing suctioning

Suctioning techniques are now considered; depending on your local policy it may be an accepted role with supervised training, *so please check before undertaking any aspect of a suctioning role.*

Bennett (2003) noted two types of suctioning relevant to this book: oropharyngeal and nasopharyngeal suctioning.

Oropharyngeal

This is oral suction, which is used to help a patient clear the airway when too weak to cough sputum (expectorate) from the pharynx. Other indications include:

- Unconscious or semi-conscious patient, e.g. after surgery
- No gag reflex, e.g. drug overdose, alcohol poisoning
- Oral surgery or trauma.

Nasopharyngeal

This may be indicated when the oral sucker (suction tube) cannot pass to the back of the pharynx, as a result of teeth clenching, dental/oral surgery or trauma, or if the patient cannot tolerate a 'sucker' at the back of the pharynx, because it can often induce gagging. It is particularly useful for patients with a lot of secretions at the back of the throat who are unable to cough and expectorate.

Both procedures require skilful practice, because some patients may be at risk of hypoxia (low oxygen level), causing cardiac arrhythmias (irregularities) if suctioning occurs for more than 10 seconds (Bennett 2003).

Perry and Potter (1994) describe three assessment aspects for suctioning (Table 9.2).

Having confirmed your assessment, you would plan for the procedure:

(1) Assemble the necessary equipment, e.g. Yankauer (sucker) and suction tubing of appropriate size, suction machine (if not wall mounted), gloves, apron, water and container, and clinical waste bag.
(2) Wash your hands and apply non-sterile gloves to minimise risk of transmitting infection.
(3) Turn on suction – machine or wall mounted – to appropriate level (Table 9.3).
(4) Connect one end of plastic suction tubing to the machine and the other to suction piece, e.g. Yankauer (rigid short plastic tube). Test working by applying Yankauer to container with water and ensure that sucking water.
(5) Remove any oxygen mask, if present on patient.

Table 9.2 Assessment for suctioning

Assessment	Rationale
Patient's airway	Check if obstructed? Any obvious secretions, e.g. vomit?
Patient's knowledge	Have they had before? Offer explanations to reassure
Risk factors	Does the patient have:
	Impaired cough or swallowing?
	Impaired gag reflex?
	Decreased level of consciousness?

Adapted from Perry and Potter (1994).

(6) Insert the Yankauer catheter into the mouth, along the gum line to the pharynx; move the catheter gently around the mouth until all the secretions are cleared. This may take several repeated suctionings. Also, if possible, encourage the patient to cough and check if there are any more secretions. Remember to take only a few seconds, and as Bennett (2003) advises no more than 10 seconds per attempt to ensure that oxygen levels do not drop too low (hypoxia).

(7) Replace the patient's oxygen mask, if present, after each suctioning and allow the patient time to recover breath between suctions, if required.

(8) Clear the tubing by sucking more water, until tubing is clear of secretions, e.g. sputum.

(9) Switch off the suction.

(10) Dispose of tubing and Yankauer as per local policy, and gloves and apron into clinical waste.

(11) Wash your hands.

(12) Ensure that patient is comfortable; check respiratory rate and colour, to ensure that patient is stable before leaving.

(13) Ensure that the procedure is documented in patient records as per local policy.

(14) Ensure monitoring after the procedure to check that patient does not develop any unexpected side effects, e.g. increasing breathlessness (Perry and Potter 1994).

Care of suction equipment is also important, and Perry and Potter (1994) recommend that the suction bottle or collection chamber be cleaned every 24 hours or more frequently, depending on the volume of secretions, and also that it is disinfected every 24 hours to prevent any bacteria growing in the moist environment. Many practice areas now use plastic disposable suction units, so the entire suctioning equipment is disposed of after each use. *Please check local equipment and guidance.*

Perry and Potter (1994) note that nasopharyngeal suctioning may require a local policy for this practice, *so please check and ensure that any training is carried out before either aspect of suctioning, but specifically the use of nasal suctioning.*

Table 9.3 Suction pressures

Wall-mounted suction (mmHg)			Portable machine (mmHg)		
Adult	Child	Infant	Adult	Child	Infant
120–150	100–120	60–100	7–15	5–10	3–5

Adapted from Perry and Potter (2004).

Reflection point

Miss Barbara Jones, 34 years old, has returned from knee surgery. You observe that she is still very drowsy and is sounding chesty. If you were considering suctioning as an option how would you assess her? Is suctioning appropriate here?

Related aspects and terminology

- Apnoea: cessation (stopping) of breathing
- Cyanosis: due to low oxygen levels and presents as a dusky bluish colour of the mucous membranes, e.g. lips, nailbeds
- Tachypnoea: raised respiratory rate, usually if rate above 20/min
- Bradypnoea: decreased respiratory rate, if rate below 10 breaths/min
- Dyspnoea: difficulty breathing, patient struggles to get air in so they might open their mouth and gulp air in, and heave shoulders up in an effort to get more air in
- Hyperventilation: deep rapid breaths
- Hypoventilation: slow shallow breaths, often associated with drugs, e.g. morphine, an opioid that acts on the respiratory centre
- Cheyne–Stoke respirations: often associated with brain injury and leads to a gradual increase in the depth of respirations, in turn leading to hyperventilation, followed by a gradual decrease in depth, and then a period of apnoea of 15–20 seconds, before the cycle starts again.

Common problems

A common problem when recording a respiratory rate is not allowing the patient to rest before measuring, so that the recording can be inaccurate (Bennett 2003). Also, if the patient becomes aware of the monitoring, they may alter their breathing pattern (Baillie et al. 2005). Finally, make sure that the patient is relaxed and sitting or lying comfortably so that they can breathe properly, and that the time is checked accurately with a watch with a second hand.

Bennett (2003) identified some common problems with a peak flow measure:

- Poor seal between lips and mouthpiece, so air leaks out
- Forgetting to zero indicator between peak flow measures, leading to an inaccurate reading
- Obstructing indicator with fingers, so blocking the movement of indicator
- Poor position for recording, e.g. lying down, so hindering breathing.

Booker (2007) noted some additional points:

- Failure to take maximum inhalation
- Holding the breath at maximum inhalation and delaying blowing into meter
- Blocking the mouthpiece with tongue or teeth
- Poor technique, e.g. coughing or spitting into meter.

Higgins (2005) also noted that, when a patient is acutely breathless, measuring the peak flow rate might have little success, because the procedure requires some physical effort. Therefore, you will need to decide, using your observational skills, if the patient is fit physically and able mentally to undertake this procedure. As noted before, a peak flow measure is simple and quick, but a wrong reading may have a serious effect if any treatment is based on a peak flow result.

Tables 9.4–9.6 are competency frameworks for recording a respiratory rate and PEFR and for suctioning.

Please ensure that you have undertaken supervised practice, in your clinical area and follow any local policy.

Problems with suctioning might relate to faulty or poorly maintained equipment, or poor suctioning technique. Perry and Potter (1994) indicate that regular checking and maintenance of the equipment are essential, e.g. cleaning collection chamber every 24 hours. When suctioning observe the patient and time, because Bennett (2003) suggests that each attempt should take no longer than 10 seconds, and allow the patient to recover between. If the patient is becoming distressed or tired, stop and, if they are on oxygen therapy, replace the mask or prongs and allow the patient to rest, before considering further attempts.

Please ensure that you have undertaken supervised practice and follow your local policy.

Summary

In this chapter the skills of recording a respiratory rate, measuring a peak flow and suctioning technique were explored. Observation and communication are essential skills, as well as effective recording and reporting.

Case study 9.1

Melanie Jones is a 14-year-old girl admitted with an acute asthmatic attack. This is her first admission to hospital and she is very frightened.
  What factors should you consider when admitting her and recording her respiratory rate?
  Discuss what you might expect, in her rate, depth, pattern, sound, regularity and colour.

Case study 9.2

Mr Adjit Singh, a 24-year-old man, is admitted for monitoring and stabilisation of his asthma. You are asked to start monitoring his peak flow rate; when you approach him, he tells you that he has never done this before.
  Describe how you explain the procedure to him and how you will carry out the procedure.
  His best score is 245 l/min. Describe your actions.

Case study 9.3

Jane Sackler is a 78-year-old woman admitted with a chest infection. She is very frail and is finding it hard to cough and expectorate sputum. She becomes very distressed and you can hear that her chest is very noisy (rattly).
  Discuss possible actions that may aid her breathing.
  If you are asked to undertake oropharyngeal suctioning, consider whether you are trained and competent in this procedure.
  If yes, describe your actions in undertaking suctioning on Miss Sackler.

Table 9.4 Competency framework: recording a respiratory rate

First assessment/reassessment						
Steps	**Demonstration/Supervised practice**					**Date/competent signature**
Recording a respiratory rate	Date/sign	Date/sign	Date/sign	Date/sign	Date/sign	
	1	**2**	**3**	**4**	**5**	
1. Identify need for respiratory check						
2. Ensure that patient is in best position (e.g. upright)						
3. Consider if patient is rested, so true baseline						
4. Explain to patient, reassure, get consent						
5. Have watch with second hand ready						
6. Note time and start counting for appropriate time						
7. Observe chest rise and fall, and if necessary place hand lightly on patient's lower chest						
8. Note depth of breaths						
9. Observe pattern of breathing						
10. Note sounds of breathing						
11. Consider how regular/rhythmic breathing is						
12. Observe patient's colour						
13. Record rate on appropriate chart, note any abnormalities, e.g. irregular, noisy breaths						
14. Report any abnormalities promptly and appropriately						

Supervisors/Assessor(s):

Table 9.5 Competency framework: recording a peak expiratory flow rate (PEFR)

Steps	First assessment/reassessment					Date/competent signature
	Demonstration/Supervised practice					
Recording a PEFR	Date/sign	Date/sign	Date/sign	Date/sign	Date/sign	
	1	2	3	4	5	
1. Patient is upright, sitting or standing						
2. Patient is ready for procedure, so rested and consented						
3. Ensure that patient is able to undertake procedure, check understanding						
4. Peak flow assembled with clean mouthpiece secure						
5. Ensure that patient holds device level and fingers (nurse/patient) don't obstruct scale						
6. Flow indicator set to zero reading on scale						
7. Ensure that patient follows correct technique						
8. Check flow indicator position, record score						
9. Ensure that patient performs three, and record best score						
10. Check and compare with previous scores						
11. Report score and any variances promptly						
12. Store peak flow meter correctly, cleaning or disposing of mouthpiece as per local policy						

Supervisors/Assessor(s):

Table 9.6 Competency framework: suctioning

		First assessment/reassessment					
Steps		**Demonstration/Supervised practice**					**Date/competent signature**
Suctioning		Date/sign	Date/sign	Date/sign	Date/sign	Date/sign	
		1	**2**	**3**	**4**	**5**	
1.	Undertake risk assessment pre-procedure						
2.	Assemble the necessary equipment						
3.	Wash hands and apply non-sterile gloves						
4.	Turn on suction to required level						
5.	Connect and test equipment, by ensuring that sucking water appropriately						
6.	Remove oxygen mask, if present on patient						
7.	Commence suctioning correctly, noting time and patient comfort						
8.	Replace patient's oxygen mask, if present, and allow time to recover breath between suctions, if required						
9.	Clear the tubing by sucking more water, until tubing is clear of secretions						
10.	Switch off the suction						
11.	Dispose of equipment as appropriate						
12.	Remove gloves and wash hands						
13.	Ensure patient comfort, and check respiratory rate and colour after procedure						
14.	Ensure that documented in patient records						
15.	Ensure that monitoring after procedure is in place, e.g. pulse and respiratory checks						
16.	Report outcome to appropriate person						

Supervisors/Assessor(s):

✔ Self-assessment

Assessment	Aspects	Achieved ✔
Respiration	*Have you considered all aspects of this section?* Patient assessment: rate, depth, pattern, sound, regularity/rhythm and colour Recording the results Reporting concerns or results Problem solving	
Peak flow	*Have you considered all aspects of this section?* Measuring a peak flow – technique aspects Cleansing/disinfection of equipment Recording the results Reporting concerns or results Problem solving	
Suctioning	*Have you considered all aspects of this section?* Assessment of patient – risk assessment Procedure Maintenance and cleansing of equipment. Recording the results Reporting concerns or results Problem solving	

References

Baillie L, Corben V, Higham S (2005) Respiratory care: assessment and interventions. In: Baillie L (ed.), *Developing Practical Nursing Skills*, 2nd edn. London: Hodder Education, Chapter 11.

Bennett C (2003) Nursing the breathless patient. *Nursing Standard* **17**(17): 45–53.

Booker R (2007) Peak expiratory flow measurement. *Nursing Standard* **21**(39): 42–43.

Dougherty L, Lister S, eds (2004) *The Royal Marsden Hospital Manual of Clinical Nursing Procedures*, 6th edn. Oxford: Blackwell Publishing.

Higgins D (2005) Measuring PEFR. *Nursing Times* **101**(10): 32–33.

Kennedy DT, Chang Z, Small R (1998) Selection of peak flowmeters in ambulatory asthma patients: a review of the literature. *Chest* **114**: 587–592.

Perry AG, Potter PA (1994) *Clinical Nursing Skills and Techniques*, 3rd edn. St Louis, MO: Mosby-Year Book Inc.

Tortora GJ, Derrickson B (2006) *Principles of Anatomy and Physiology*, 11th edn. Hoboken, NJ: John Wiley & Sons Inc.

Addendum

Wright meter cleaning information

Reproduced with kind permission from Clement Clarke International.

How to disinfect the Mini-Wright Standard Peak Flow Meter, the AFS Low Range Mini Peak Flow meter and the Mini-Wright Digital

The Mini-Wright Peak Flow Meter was designed as a portable device to help healthcare professionals monitor lung function; to minimise the risk of cross-infection, it has an integral one-way valve that prevents the patient from breathing in any of the previous patient's exhaled breath that could remain in the meter (the Mini-Wright Digital does not have a one-way valve).

The importance of peak flow monitoring results in many patients receiving their own personal meter for home monitoring of lung function, by prescription or recommended purchase. Doctor's surgeries and hospitals may also wish to issue peak flow meters on a loan basis and therefore need a means of reprocessing each device before reissue. The following instructions have been prepared to facilitate multiple-patient use.

Note that we would recommend that, if the last user was diagnosed or suspected of having a serious communicable disease, the meter should be disposed of.

Devices used for multiple patients may need to be replaced more often than those used by only one person.

Frequency of disinfecting the Mini-Wright range of peak flow meters

The following recommendations for disinfecting peak flow meter frequencies are presented as a guide only. In practice, the person responsible for the clinical wellbeing of the patient should consider the specific circumstances of the next patient and the risk posed by cross-infection.

Mouthpiece type	Disposable one-way cardboard mouthpieces (single use device[a])	Disposable bacterial filters (single-use device[a])	Disposable cardboard mouthpieces (single-use device[a])	Sterilisable plastic mouthpieces
Frequency	WEEKLY	WEEKLY	Between patients	Between patients

[a] Single use device means 'do not reuse' (EN 980:2003). Clement Clarke International Ltd consider that multiple measurements being made by the same patient in one consultation can be considered as 'single use' as long as the mouthpiece/filter is not damaged between measurements. This interpretation cannot be applied to all devices marked as 'single use'.

Reprocessing: sterilisable plastic mouthpiece

- Clean using an automatic dishwasher (2 min pre-wash, 3 min detergent wash, dry).
- Autoclave in saturated steam (max. 134–137°C) for 3 minutes (refer to autoclave manufacturer's instructions for details of cycles available).
- Alternatively, the method below can be used to disinfect the mouthpiece.

Cleaning and disinfection

(1) Inspect the unit for signs of damage or wear; if any is evident replace meter.
(2) Prepare a solution of detergent in accordance with the manufacturer instructions in a container large enough for the peak flow meter(s) to be totally submerged.
(3) Agitate the meter while in the solution to ensure that any trapped air is expelled. Do not use any mechanical aids such as brushes or cloths.
(4) Rinse and dry as recommended.
(5) Prepare a quantity of your chosen disinfectant in a suitable container.
(6) Immerse the peak flow meter; again agitate the meter to ensure that air is expelled and leave it in the solution for the recommended time.
(7) Rinse as stated, shake gently to remove any excess water and allow to dry naturally; do not use hot air or a drying cupboard.

Detergents

The following detergents have been tested for compatibility with Clement Clarke International Ltd's peak flow meters.

Name	Solution strength	Comments
Lancerzyme	40 ml in 5 litres of water	Enzymatic cleaner
Cidezyme		Enzymatic cleaner
Hospec		

Disinfectants

The following disinfectants have been tested for compatibility with Clement Clarke International Ltd's peak flow meters.

Chemical type	Examples	Solution strength	Comments
Chlorine dioxide generator	Tristel one day	20 ml in 1 litre water	Safety data sheet and further information available from www.tristel.com
ortho-Phthalaldehyde	Cidex OPA	Undiluted	
Sodium hypochlorite (NaOCL)	Milton	1000 p.p.m.	Ensure thorough rinsing, as corrosion of the metal parts will occur if exposed to chlorine for long periods.
Sodium dichloroisocyanurate (NaDCC)	Presept, Actichlor, Sanichlor, Haz-Tab	1000 p.p.m.	
Hydrogen peroxide and peroxygen compounds	Pera Safe	1.62% w/v	

Clement Clarke International Ltd accepts no liability for damage caused to products if the above procedure and recommended solutions are not used.

It is the user's responsibility to choose which of the recommended solutions are used within their establishment or hospital and we stress that the infection control nurse/department should be consulted when making the choice.

It is the responsibility of the user to keep up to date with the latest information from the relevant disinfectant manufacturer concerning instructions, effects, concentrations and immersion times.

If your preferred cleaner/disinfectant is not on the recommended list, please contact our customer service advisers on 01279 414969 or fax 01279 456 304 or email resp@clement-clarke.com.

References

Medical Healthcare product Regulatory Agency (MHRA). *Chemical disinfection in hospitals – PHLS, Sterilization, disinfection and cleaning of medical device equipment (MAC Manual)*. London: MHRA.

Chapter 10

Urinalysis and faecal occult blood testing

Learning objectives

- Describe when and how to undertake urinalysis testing
- Outline faecal occult blood testing and when this is performed
- Consider problems and how to manage or prevent them

Aim of this chapter

The aim of this chapter is to describe how to undertake urinalysis and faecal occult blood (FOB) tests, and to discuss why these are performed within the clinical environment.

Reasons for performing urinalysis and FOB tests

Urinalysis is a simple non-invasive clinical procedure, which is quick and easy and can give clues as to the health status of the person (Cook 1996). Baillie and Arrowsmith (2005) state that this is the reason why all newly admitted patients must have their urine tested.

Faecal occult blood tests involve the testing of a specimen of stool, to identify whether there is any blood present that is not visible to the naked eye. It is useful in helping to diagnose many bowel conditions, e.g. colorectal (bowel) cancer (Kyle and Prynn 2004). The procedure is simple and non-invasive and requires a small sample of faeces to smear onto a specimen card; it is quick and easy to carry out. Kyle and Prynn (2004) noted evidence from the National Screening Committee, which indicated that, if FOB testing were available to those aged 50 years and over, there would be a 15% reduction in mortality from colorectal (bowel) cancer.

Relevant anatomy and physiology

The urinary system has two kidneys, two ureters, one urinary bladder and one urethra (Tortora and Derrickson 2006) (Figure 10.1).

Tortora and Derrickson (2006) describe the two kidneys as reddish organs shaped like kidney beans, which filter blood and restore selected amounts of water and solutes (materials) to the bloodstream, with the remaining water and solutes becoming urine. Dougherty and Lister (2004)

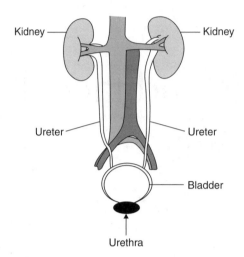

Figure 10.1 Urinary system.

note that urine is formed in the kidneys, and these process approximately 180 litres of blood-derived fluid a day.

The two ureters, one for each kidney, connect the kidneys with the bladder and are hollow tubes of length approximately 25–30 cm (10–12 inches).

The urinary bladder is a hollow muscular organ lying in the pelvic cavity, in males directly anterior (in front) to the rectum, and in females anterior to the vagina and inferior to (below) the uterus (Tortora and Derrickson 2006).

It is worth briefly reviewing the process of digestion, because from this we get the formation of faeces. Food is consumed through the upper gastrointestinal tract, and broken down into molecules small enough to enter cells; this process is called digestion. The organs that perform this are called the digestive organs, and include the mouth, pharynx, oesophagus, stomach, and small and large intestine (Tortora and Derrickson 2006) (Figure 10.2).

Tortora and Derrickson (2006) note that the small intestine begins at the pyloric sphincter (circular muscle that constricts an opening) of the stomach and coils round the abdominal cavity, before opening into the large intestine. The small intestine is 2.5 cm (1 inch) in diameter and around 3 m (10 feet) long, and is divided into three sections: duodenum, jejunum and ileum; most digestion and absorption of nutrients occurs here.

The large intestine described by Tortora and Derrickson (2006) is 1.5 m (5 feet) long and 6.5 cm (2½ inches) wide, and the overall function of the large intestine is to complete the absorption process, manufacture certain vitamins, form faeces and aid the expulsion of faeces from the body.

Urinalysis testing

Elimination of urine is an essential bodily function and urinalysis is a vital nursing assessment tool (Pellatt 2007). Timing of urine testing is important, and Baillie and Arrowsmith (2005) and Rigby and Gray (2005) advocate that the first voided sample (early morning urine) that has been stored in the bladder for at least 4 hours provides the most accurate results, because it is the most concentrated.

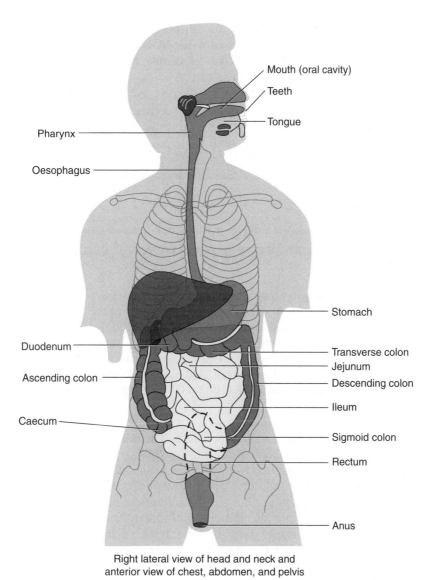

Mouth (oral cavity)

Teeth

Tongue

Pharynx

Oesophagus

Stomach

Duodenum

Transverse colon

Jejunum

Ascending colon

Descending colon

Ileum

Caecum

Sigmoid colon

Rectum

Anus

Right lateral view of head and neck and
anterior view of chest, abdomen, and pelvis

Figure 10.2   Digestive system.

Rigby and Gray (2005) outlined that specimen collection must be in a dry clean container and suggest five options:

1. A random (clean) sample at any time of day, e.g. on admission, although in women it may contain vaginal contamination during menstruation (monthly bleeding).
2. An early morning sample – first sample after sleep (as above).
3. A midstream urine (MSU) sample, usually taken for laboratory sampling so needs careful collection.

4. A catheter specimen of urine (CSU) sample, usually only if there is a catheter *in situ* and under special circumstances, e.g. patient unable to provide MSU as unconscious
5. A suprapubic catheter sample provides the purest sample, but is rarely used.

However, any sample collected must be tested as soon as possible after collection, so that any bacteria present will not have time to increase and therefore affect results. The presence of bacteria, whether or not causing an infection, can cause changes in the pH or affect other constituents of the urine (Rigby and Gray 2005).

Reflection point

How are you going to collect a specimen of urine from a patient on admission?

Before testing the urine using reagent test strips, there are useful observations that you can undertake, including the colour of the urine, the smell (odour) and the clarity.

Baillie and Arrowsmith (2005) and Dougherty and Lister (2004) describe urine as typically clear, pale to deep yellow in colour and slightly acidic (pH 6), although they add that the pH can change as a result of metabolic processes or diet (e.g. beetroot). Cook (1996) suggested that some laxatives could change urine to an orange colour, whereas diet, e.g. rhubarb, can change urine to a red colour. Baillie and Arrowsmith (2005) also noted that some medicines, e.g. various antibiotics, can affect urine colour.

The composition of urine can change dramatically as a result of disease and may contain red blood cells, proteins, glucose, bile or white blood cells. The presence of these abnormalities in the urine is an indicator of illness (Dougherty and Lister 2004).

Dougherty and Lister (2004) state that freshly voided urine smells faintly aromatic, although Cook (1996) indicated that urine could develop an ammonia smell if left standing. Rigby and Gray (2005) advocate consideration not only of the colour of urine, but also of the smell and presence of debris, because these are also indicators of illness. They describe infected urine as having a fishy smell, whereas acetone excreted by patients with diabetic ketoacidosis gives urine a sweet smell. Cook (1996) added that eating fish, curry or other strongly flavoured foodstuffs could also make urine smell.

Urine that is cloudy or has sediment (debris) is often caused by infection, so observation is important. Cook (1996) described cloudiness as being caused by suspended particles, e.g. white and red cells, which will settle on standing to leave a deposit.

Cook (1996) discussed the need to ensure that any patient providing a sample of urine for testing gets the following:

- An explanation of the reason for testing
- Instruction in the method of collection
- Provision of suitable equipment, e.g. container for specimen
- An appropriate environment, e.g. privacy and space.

Cook (1996) noted a debate around the necessity of cleaning the genital area. Baillie and Arrowsmith (2005) describe the theory that the first part of the urine stream flushes away microorganisms from the first part of the urethra, and that the urine does not flow over the perineum, as long as there is enough urine in the bladder to produce a good stream. Rigby and Gray (2005), however, outlined cleansing when collecting an MSU, and they noted that it is easier to obtain a clean specimen of urine from males, but that cleansing is still essential.

Male cleansing includes patients first washing their hands, then retracting the foreskin and cleansing the meatus with soap and water, or as per local policy. To collect the sample the patient passes the first part of the urine stream (15–30 ml) into the toilet, and then collects the next part (50–100 ml) in a clean dry container, and finally finishes emptying the bladder into the toilet. The container cap must be replaced immediately and the hands washed.

For females, again patients wash their hands, then clean the vulval and urethral meati with soap and water, or as per local policy, then separate the labia (this might be difficult for some patients, e.g. patient with arthritis) and continue as above.

In young children or babies, a sterile collection bag placed over the genitalia to catch the urine may be necessary (Pellatt 2007). Steggall (2007) suggests four main ways to collect samples from infants and young children:

1. 'Bagged sample' using a perineal collection bag; however, this is the least favoured method because it carries a risk of contamination from the perineum and rectum.
2. 'Clean catch' where the child or infant is sat over a sterile container and urine collected as they passes urine.
3. MSU sample: most reliable for testing; however, not always possible in young children. Females should be encouraged to part the labia and males should retract foreskin and then pass urine into a sterile container
4. Suprapubic bladder aspiration would be performed only in urgent situations because it carries the risk of bladder puncture and is not suitable in children aged under 2 years.

Once the sample has been collected and you have observed, and recorded, the colour and noted the presence, if any, of odour, or if the urine is cloudy, you proceed to test the urine. Reagent test strips allow testing of a range of factors: leucocytes (white cells), nitrites, urobilinogen, protein, pH, blood, specific gravity, ketones, bilirubin and glucose (Baillie and Arrowsmith 2005). Check the strips in your area and check which substances are tested (Table 10.1). (Figure 10.3 is an example of a recording slip.)

Cook (1996) proposed that, if urine is not going to be tested within 1 hour of collection, it be refrigerated; however, allow it to return to room temperature once removed before testing.

Procedure for testing

This procedure is taken from Dougherty and Lister (2004):

1. Check that reagent strips are correctly stored (discussed later)
2. Explain and discuss the procedure with the patient – discussed earlier
3. Obtain fresh sample
4. Dip reagent strip fully into the urine, remove immediately and tap strip against the side of the container to remove any excess urine
5. Hold stick at an angle, so urine does not run from square to square and mix reagents (could alter results)
6. Wait the specified time interval for each square as noted per bottle
7. Read and record your findings as per local policy

Table 10.1 Significance of substances in the urine

Substance	Causes
Glucose: not normally detected in urine	Diabetes mellitus, acute pancreatitis, pregnancy, glycosuria
Bilirubin (stale urine may give a false positive)	Liver cell damage: viral/drug induced, hepatitis, paracetamol overdose, cirrhosis; Biliary tract obstruction – gallstones, cancer of pancreas
Ketones	Due to excessive breakdown of body fat – fasting, specially with fever/vomiting, some high protein diets, diabetic ketoacidosis, starvation/excessive dieting
Specific gravity: normal 1.001–1.035	High: concentrated urine due to dehydration or chronic renal failure Low: high fluid intake, renal disease
Blood: haematuria	Kidney disorders: urinary tract infection (UTI), stones, tumour, severe burns, transfusion reaction, trauma
pH: normal 4.5–8.00	High: stale urine, UTI, Low diabetic ketoacidosis, starvation
Protein: test may not be sensitive to presence of all proteins	UTI, fever, pre-eclampsia, heart failure, high-protein diet, severe hypertension In men may be due to sperm after sex
Urobilinogen: normally present in urine	Increased secretion: viral hepatitis, cirrhosis Decreased secretion – gallstones, pancreas cancer, medicines, e.g. neomycin
Nitrite: not usually found in urine	UTI
Leucocytes	Renal or bladder infection

UTI, urinary tract infection.
Adapted from Baillie and Arrowsmith (2005), Dougherty and Lister (2004), and Pellatt (2007).

8. Dispose of urine in sluice or toilet and test strip into clinical waste
9. Report findings and results as per local policy
10. Ensure that the patient is comfortable, and where appropriate given results; please discuss this role locally before proceeding.

Rigby and Gray (2005) noted the debate over the reliability of near patient testing and urinalysis, and suggest that reports are only 85% reliable, so its use in screening is questionable. Therefore, it is important that you complete the test correctly without interruption, to ensure that it is as accurate as possible.

Reflection point

Emily Boyd, aged 22 years, has been admitted in labour, and requires a urine test. What aspects will you observe and test for?

From the test results, any action taken may depend on other results (e.g. blood tests); however, your action must be to report any abnormalities immediately. If the specimen is old and has

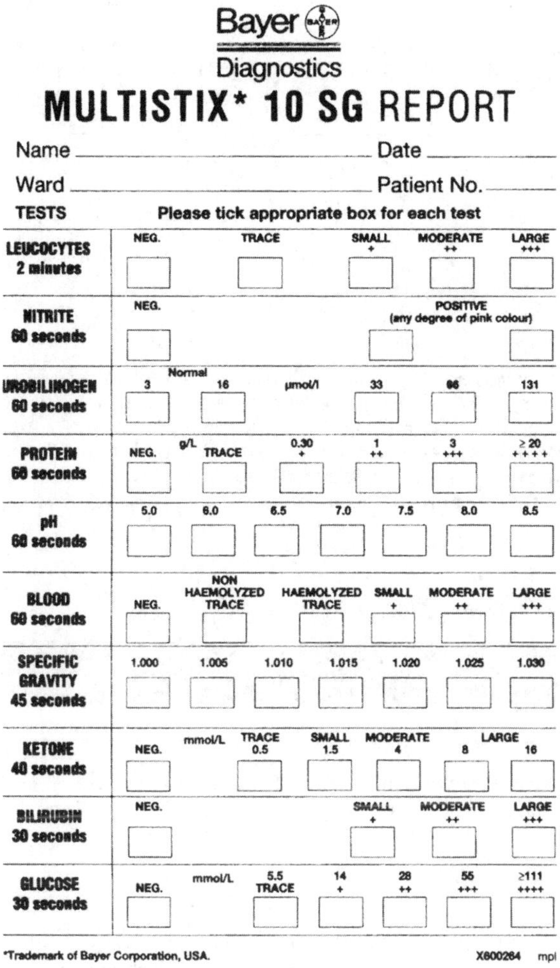

Bayer
Diagnostics

MULTISTIX* 10 SG REPORT

Name _____ Date _____

Ward _____ Patient No. _____

TESTS   **Please tick appropriate box for each test**

LEUCOCYTES 2 minutes	NEG.	TRACE		SMALL +	MODERATE ++	LARGE +++

NITRITE 60 seconds	NEG.			POSITIVE (any degree of pink colour)		

UROBILINOGEN 60 seconds	Normal 3	16	µmol/l	33	66	131

PROTEIN 60 seconds	NEG.	g/L TRACE	0.30 +	1 ++	3 +++	≥ 20 ++++

pH 60 seconds	5.0	6.0	6.5	7.0	7.5	8.0	8.5

BLOOD 60 seconds	NEG.	NON HAEMOLYZED TRACE	HAEMOLYZED TRACE	SMALL +	MODERATE ++	LARGE +++

SPECIFIC GRAVITY 45 seconds	1.000	1.005	1.010	1.015	1.020	1.025	1.030

KETONE 40 seconds	NEG.	mmol/L	TRACE 0.5	SMALL 1.5	MODERATE 4	LARGE 8	16

BILIRUBIN 30 seconds	NEG.			SMALL +	MODERATE ++	LARGE +++

GLUCOSE 30 seconds	NEG.	mmol/L	5.5 TRACE	14 +	28 ++	55 +++	≥111 ++++

*Trademark of Bayer Corporation, USA.   X800264   mpl

Figure 10.3   Example of a test recording slip. (Photograph by I Lavery.)

been lying for a while, suggest a repeat test with a fresh sample of urine. In most cases further laboratory tests may follow, e.g. urine for microscopy, culture and organism (Rigby and Gray 2005), and/or blood tests. So ensure accurate testing, recording and prompt reporting. If in doubt, report.

Accurate testing leads us to consider storage of the reagent strips. Baillie and Arrowsmith (2005) advise that we should check that strips are in date, and stored and used correctly because, otherwise, this can affect results.

Cook (1996) and Rigby and Gray (2005) also noted the following:

- Store reagent strips out of direct sunlight
- Keep strips at a constant temperature, usually cool and dark, not in the fridge
- Use strips according to manufacturer's guidance
- Strips should be stored in the bottle supplied
- Replace cap on the bottle as quickly as possible after each test
- Never remove desiccant (some manufacturers place this in the lid).

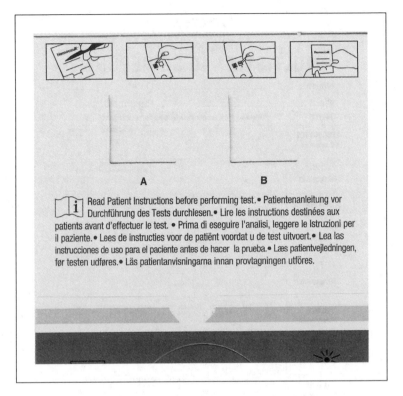

Read Patient Instructions before performing test. • Patientenanleitung vor Durchführung des Tests durchlesen. • Lire les instructions destinées aux patients avant d'effectuer le test. • Prima di eseguire l'analisi, leggere le Istruzioni per il paziente. • Lees de instructies voor de patiënt voordat u de test uitvoert. • Lea las instrucciones de uso para el paciente antes de hacer la prueba. • Læs patientvejledningen, før testen udføres. • Läs patientanvisningarna innan provtagningen utföres.

Figure 10.4   A faecal occult blood (FOB) specimen card. (Photograph by I Lavery.)

Faecal occult blood testing

Faeces consist of the unabsorbed endproducts of digestion: bile pigments, cellulose, bacteria, epithelial cells, mucus and some inorganic materials (Dougherty and Lister 2004). Stools are normally semi-solid in consistency and contain about 70% water. Baillie and Arrowsmith (2005) noted that normal stools are brown, soft and formed, so, when collecting a specimen for FOB testing, the colour, smell and consistency should be noted and recorded as part of the bowel assessment. Some areas use the Bristol Stool Scoring to classify faeces (see Addendum at end of chapter).

Baillie and Arrowsmith (2005) discussed smell as part of a bowel assessment. Fatty, offensive-smelling stools can indicate bowel disease, e.g. gallbladder disease. Stools that are covered with mucous and /or blood indicate disease such as ulcerative colitis. Black tarry stools can indicate digested blood and have a distinctive smell, often due to upper tract disorders, e.g. stomach ulcer. Finally, stools with fresh blood often indicate haemorrhoids. All these require prompt reporting.

Kyle and Prynn (2004) discuss the FOB test as part of a bowel examination and state the need for a specimen card (Figure 10.4) and chemical additive to ensure that the sample is tested or correctly sent to the laboratory, promptly. Ouyang et al. (2005) identified the most common test as the guaiac-impregnated Haemoccult.

Ouyang et al. (2005) gave advice on diet and other aspects for patients having a FOB test for 4 days before the first sample and during the test period; these are outlined below. However, in acute hospital settings, it may not be possible to follow dietary advice if specimens are urgently required. Kyle and Prynn (2004) also state that gastrointestinal bleeding may be intermittent, so two or three FOB tests should be carried out on two or three different separate samples of faeces from the patient on different days, e.g. collected over three consecutive days.

Kyle and Prynn (2004) offered advice for patients before having an FOB test; this may be a useful guide for staff to discuss with each patient, and suggests that patients:

- eat a diet rich in roughage (helps stimulate bleeding if any lesions present)
- avoid alcohol and aspirin or other non-steroidal anti-inflammatory drugs, and vitamin C or iron tablets (could worsen bleeding or affect results)
- avoid fish with dark meat, e.g. salmon, tuna, sardines, mackerel
- avoid red meat and blood products, e.g. black pudding, kidneys or liver
- avoid tomatoes, cauliflower, horseradish, turnip, melon, bananas and soybeans
- are asked if menstruating (if female), have diarrhoea or had a recent nose or throat bleed (as could affect result); if yes postpone the test
- ask staff if they have any concerns or queries.

Ouyang et al. (2005) note that, with guaiac (FOB) tests, false positives can occur with red meats and some fruits and vegetables, e.g. turnip, and also false negatives can occur with high doses of vitamin C.

Reflection point

Wendy Williamson is to have FOB tests, *and you have been asked to give her advice about the procedure and preparation. What advice might you offer?*

Kyle and Prynn (2004) also offer advice for staff:

- Test specimen within 12 hours of collection, otherwise it can degrade and lead to false negatives.
- Do not use a sample from digital (manual) removal of faeces, because this may contain blood from trauma during the procedure.

Equipment for the FOB test

- Sample card (see Figure 10.4) and wooden stick
- Chemical solution
- Non-sterile gloves and apron
- Container.

Once the patient has opened their bowels, take the container to the sluice and collect two samples from different parts of the faeces (in case of false readings); smear a small amount from each on the two sample windows indicated on the card by the foldaway section. Once smeared on, close the cover and turn the card over, and then follow the instructions for administering the chemical, taking care not to spill the chemical because this can cause some hazards, e.g. a chemical might cause a skin reaction (Control of Substances Hazardous to Health [COSHH] – HMSO 1999).

The test area should be observed for a change in colour. Ouyang et al. (2005) indicated that this was a blue colour change depending whether blood was in the stool, and usually occurred within 1 minute. This can be further classified, so if pale blue it could indicate weakly positive, whereas strong blue indicates strongly positive.

 Reflection point

What hazards might you encounter with an FOB test?

Related aspects and terminology (Tortora and Derrickson 2006)

- **Jaundice:** yellow pigmentation of the skin due to build-up of bilirubin
- **Cirrhosis:** distorted or scarred liver due to chronic inflammation
- **Diabetes mellitus:** a group of disorders that lead to an elevation of glucose in the blood; as glucose (sugar) levels increase, glucose appears in the urine
- **Glycosuria:** (glucose) sugar present in the urine
- **Renal function:** kidney functioning
- **Haematuria:** presence of intact red blood cells in the urine
- **Pre-eclampsia:** condition sometimes found in pregnancy
- **Suprapubic:** above the pubes (pubic) bone
- **Meatus:** passageway or canal
- **Labia:** lip
- **Hypertension:** high blood pressure
- **Acute pancreatitis:** inflammation of the pancreas.

Common problems

Urinalysis, if not tested on a fresh sample, as noted before, can lead to false results, so always ensure that freshly passed urine is tested or that refrigerated urine has been removed for an hour before testing.

In females take care if the patient is in the childbearing age group and menstruating, because this can lead to a false reading of haematuria.

Ensure that you handle the strips correctly, when in storage and when undertaking the test, otherwise this can also affect results.

FOB testing problems may be due to poor sampling, not smearing sufficient faeces on the test areas, insufficient chemical or reading the result too quickly (before it has time to change). Please check the type of test in your area and follow the manufacturer's instructions fully. It has been suggested that false negatives or positives are related to diet and medicines; refer to advice from Kyle and Prynn (2004).

Summary

Urinalysis and FOB testing are quick and simple tests and allow for prompt results, however, they require safe and competent practice to ensure their accuracy. As discussed, there are risks with these procedures unless the healthcare assistant is aware of these and addresses them.

Case study 10.1: Urinalysis

Julie Forth is 68 years and lives in a nursing home; over the past few days she has had a couple of episodes of incontinence and is complaining of abdominal discomfort and pain on passing urine. She has been admitted with a suspected UTI.
What might you expect to find present in her urine?

Case study 10.2: FOB test

John Armour is 73 years old and has been admitted with weight loss and altered bowel habits.
Discuss why FOB will be requested, and outline how you will collect a sample of stool and test for the presence of occult blood.

 ## Self-assessment

Assessment	Aspects	Achieved ✔
Urinalysis	*Have you considered all aspects of this section?*	
	Timing of collecting	
	Specimen collection procedure	
	Observation, e.g. colour, smell	
	Performing the test	
	Recording the results	
	Reporting concerns or results	
	Problem solving	
FOB testing	*Have you considered all aspects of this section?*	
	Assessment, e.g. colour, smell and consistency	
	FOB test procedure	
	Storage and handling of equipment	
	Patient education	
	Recording the results	
	Reporting concerns or results	
	Problem solving	

Table 10.2 Competency framework: urinalysis testing

Steps		First assessment/reassessment					Date/competent signature
		Demonstration/Supervised practice					
Urinalysis testing		Date/sign	Date/sign	Date/sign	Date/sign	Date/sign	
		1	2	3	4	5	
1	Checked reagent strips are correctly stored and in date						
2	Explained procedure to the patient						
3	Washed hands, applied disposable gloves and apron						
4	Obtained fresh urine sample in clean container						
5	Dipped reagent strip fully into the urine, removed immediately, excess urine removed						
6	Held stick at an angle, to ensure no mixing						
7	Waited specified time interval for each square as noted per bottle						
8	Read and recorded findings						
9	Disposed of urine in sluice or toilet and test strip into clinical waste						
10	Washed hands, disposed of gloves and apron						
11	Reported findings and results						
12	Ensured patient is comfortable, where appropriate given results						

Supervisors/Assessor(s):

Table 10.3 Competency framework: faecal occult blood (FOB) testing

		First assessment/reassessment					Date/ competent signature
Steps		**Demonstration/Supervised practice**					
FOB testing		Date/sign	Date/sign	Date/sign	Date/sign	Date/sign	
		1	2	3	4	5	
1	Washed hands, disposable apron and gloves						
2	Collected sample from the faeces						
3	Smeared a small amount on the test card						
4	Closed test area						
5	Administered the chemical, carefully						
6	Observed the test area for change to colour						
7	Washed hands, disposed of gloves and apron						
8	Disposed of card and protective clothing						
9	Recorded and reported results						

Supervisors/Assessor(s):

References

Baillie L, Arrowsmith K (2005) Monitoring vital signs. In: Baillie L (ed.), *Developing Practical Nursing Skills*, 2nd edn. London: Hodder Education, pp. 393–436.

Cook R (1996) Urinalysis: ensuring accurate urine testing. *Nursing Standard* **10**(46): 49–52.

Dougherty L, Lister S, eds (2004) *The Royal Marsden Hospital Manual of Clinical Nursing Procedures*, 6th edn. Oxford: Blackwell Publishing.

HMSO Statutory Instrument (1999) Control of Substances Hazardous to Health. No 437. Available at: www.hmso.gov.uk/is/si1999/19990437.htm (accessed 27 January 2007).

Kyle G, Prynn P (2004) Guidelines for patients undergoing faecal occult blood testing. *Nursing Times* **100**(48): 62, 64

Ouyang DL, Chen J, Getzenberg RH, Schoen RE (2005) Noninvasive testing for colorectal cancer: a review. *American Journal of Gastroenterology* **100**: 1393–1403.

Pellatt GC (2007) Anatomy and physiology of urinary elimination. Part 1. *British Journal of Nursing* **16**: 406–410.

Rigby D, Gray K (2005) Understanding urine testing. *Nursing Times* **101**(12): 60–62.

Steggall MJ (2007) Urine samples and urinalysis. *Nursing Standard* **22**(14–16): 42–45.

Tortora GJ and Derrickson B (2006) *Principles of Anatomy and Physiology*, 11th edn. Hoboken, NJ: John Wiley & Sons Inc.

Addendum

Bristol Scoring Chart

Permission granted via Wikipedia site: http://en.wikipedia.org/wiki/Bristol_Stool_Scale (accessed 3 March 2008).

Figure A10.1 The Bristol Stool Chart or Scale is an aid for healthcare staff that classifies faeces into seven categories. It was developed by Dr SJ Lewis and Dr KW Heaton at the University of Bristol, and was first published in 1997 in the *Scandinavian Journal of Gastroenterology* **32**: 920–924.

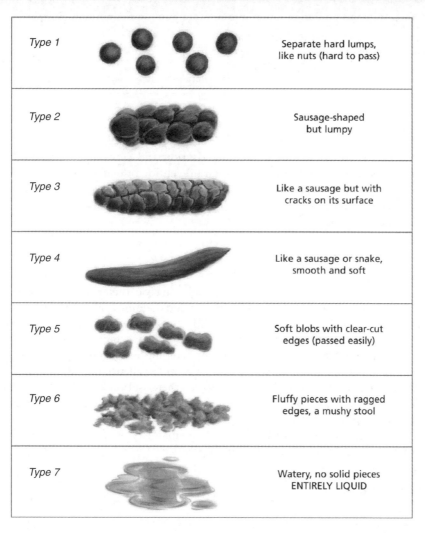

Figure A10.1   The Bristol Stool Form Scale. Source: http://en-wikipedia.org/wiki/Bristol_Stool_Scale

Chapter 11

Urinary catheterisation and catheter care

Learning objectives

- Identify the main reasons for inserting a urinary catheter
- Describe common catheters and associated equipment
- Outline how to undertake the procedure of urinary catheterisation
- Discuss catheter care and complications, and how to prevent or manage

Aim of this chapter

The aim of this chapter is to discuss urinary catheterisation and catheter care in adults and children, and to review possible complications and their prevention or management. This chapter is aimed at supporting any local training and supervision and focuses on urinary catheterisation. Intermittent self-catheterisation is also discussed, because the healthcare assistant may need to assist a patient in this process, or carry out this procedure.

Reasons for urinary catheterisation and catheter care

NHS Quality Improvement Scotland (QIS 2004) described urinary catheterisation as a procedure to enable emptying of the bladder by insertion of a catheter, and ongoing care and maintenance are considered as catheter care. The Department of Health (DH 2001) stated that the use of indwelling catheters should be considered only after alternative methods have been explored, and these include intermittent catheterisation, use of medications, voiding programmes or incontinence pads with children (National Institute for Health and Clinical Excellence or NICE 2003).

Mangnall and Watterson (2006) indicated that urinary catheterisation is one of the most common healthcare interventions with around 25% of patients in hospital requiring this procedure, so attention to infection control aspects is critical. Leaver (2007) also noted that nurses insert at least 50% of all catheters and subsequently perform the majority of catheter care, so there is a need to ensure that they are at the forefront of good practice.

Relevant anatomy and physiology

Chapter 10 should be referred to for details of the urinary system; however, a review of the relevant parts of the urinary system may be useful.

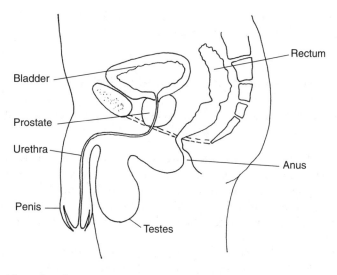

Figure 11.1   Male bladder and urethra.

The bladder is a hollow muscular organ lying in the pelvic cavity, in males directly anterior (in front) of the rectum, whereas in females it is anterior to the vagina and inferior (below) to the uterus (Tortora and Derrickson 2006). The urethra is a small tube leading from the bladder to the exterior of the body; in females it is about 4 cm (1.5 inches) long, and in males about 15–20 cm (6–8 inches) long (Tortora and Derrickson 2006) (Figures 11.1 and 11.2). This is why catheters come in different lengths and are often referred to as male and female lengths.

Elimination of urine is an essential bodily function and, normally, day- and night-time bladder control is developed by age 6 years (Pellatt 2007). Bray and Saunders (2006) suggest that children are usually toilet trained between 2 and 4½ years, and girls generally achieve dryness before boys.

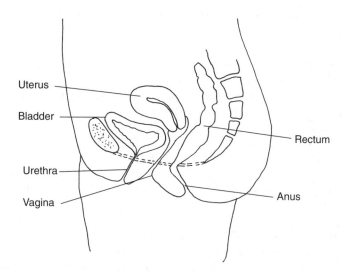

Figure 11.2   Female bladder and urethra.

In the adult the kidneys filter about 150 l/day, and concentrate this into urine of around 1.5 l/day (Pellatt 2007), while in children the output is usually 1 ml/kg body weight per hour (Bray and Saunders 2006).

How to perform urinary catheterisation and catheter care

Bray and Saunders (2006) suggested that the reasons for inserting a catheter in children are usually:

- Acute retention: with sudden onset often after surgery (after 12 hours), medication related, or after spinal or epidural anaesthesia; it can be an associated secondary complication due to acute constipation, spinal injury or obstruction at the urethral outflow.
- Postoperative urine monitoring: where a child is unwell after emergency surgery, trauma or injury, a catheter would be inserted to monitor fluid balance and measure specific gravity (see Chapter 10).
- Skin and wound integrity: a catheter is inserted after surgery to allow a wound to heal, and a catheter minimises the risk of infection, pain and discomfort for the child.

NHS QIS (2004) outlined reasons for insertion in adults due to time frames as:

- 1–7 days: postoperatively
- 7–30 days: measurement of urinary output in a critically ill patient
- Over 30 days: complications, e.g. incontinence or retention.

Baillie and Arrowsmith (2005) describe specific reasons in adults, which require urinary catheterisation, whereas Dougherty and Lister (2004) consider reasons in males and females as follows.

- Males:
  - to empty bladder contents, e.g. before surgery and some investigations
  - to accurately measure urinary output, especially if patient is acutely ill
  - to determine residual urine
  - to allow bladder irrigation or instillation
  - to bypass obstruction or where there is dysfunction
  - to relieve urinary retention
  - to introduce cytotoxic medicines (treatment in some bladder cancers)
  - to allow bladder function tests
  - to help bladder healing, e.g. after bladder, pelvic or urethral surgery
  - to relieve incontinence, if no other practical method.
- Females – all of the above and:
  - to empty bladder before childbirth
  - to avoid complications from insertion of radiotherapy.

Rees and Mawson (2007) discussed catheterisation in patients after a hip fracture and have a few additional reasons:

- If skin integrity becomes a risk, e.g. breakdown due to incontinence
- On a long journey, e.g. transfer to other hospital or care facility
- To monitor renal (kidney) or cardiac (heart) function (this patient population are often elderly and so are likely to have other illnesses too).

Types of catheterisation

This chapter focuses on indwelling catheterisation, and also discusses intermittent catheterisation by both the healthcare assistant and the patient. The other option for draining urine from the bladder is via a suprapubic catheter, where a catheter is inserted above the pubes bone; this is not a common procedure and would be carried out by trained personnel, and so is not outlined in this book.

Assessment considerations

NHS QIS (2004) suggested that intermittent catheterisation should be considered a first option, rather than inserting an indwelling catheter, and this would be done after a full patient assessment. Initial assessment would be to identify the reason for the bladder-emptying problem, which would include considering any psychological (or emotional) effects of a catheter, e.g. impact on the patient's body image or sexuality. NHS QIS (2004) also indicated that catheterisation can be a challenge with children, older, frail, confused patients, or patients with a learning disability, and they will need additional considerations, especially around communication and consent.

The decision as to the type of catheterisation could then be made, in consultation with the patient and carers or family if necessary. With older confused people or patients with a learning disability, consideration is also needed about their capacity to consent, briefly discussed in Chapters 1 and 4, as well as later in this chapter.

Let us now review the materials, gauges, balloon sizes, tip design and lengths of catheters, and drainage systems.

Materials

Dougherty and Lister (2004) suggested the need to consider how long a catheter will be *in situ*, because this will affect the choice of material (Table 11.1). Therefore, Dougherty and Lister (2004) used the following time frames:

- Short term: 1–14 days
- Short to medium term: 2–6 weeks
- Long term: 6 weeks–3 months.

Gauges (sizes)

Choose the smallest size suitable, because larger sizes can cause pain, discomfort, bypassing (urine leaks past catheter) and lead to abscess formation (Dougherty and Lister 2004; Bray and Saunders 2006).

Baillie and Arrowsmith (2005) advised that the size is the external diameter of the catheter and is measured in Charrière (Ch) or French gauge (FG) (see Table 11.2 for paediatric sizes).

NHS QIS (2004) and Baillie and Arrowsmith (2005) indicated adult sizes as:

- Females: commonly 12–14 Ch
- Males: commonly 12–16 Ch.

Bray and Saunders (2006) also described a polytetrafluorethylene (PTFE) material, which has a smooth outer surface and therefore causes less irritation and rejection. NHS Quality Improvement

Table 11.1 Catheter selection

Length *in situ*	Type of material	Discussion
Short term	PVC non-balloon for intermittent catheters or for instillation of solutions into bladder	Rigid catheter with wide lumen, so allows rapid flow rate, used mainly for intermittent catheter or postoperatively. Due to rigidity it can cause some patients discomfort or pain, or bladder spasm
	Latex	Softest material, but smooth surface tends to allow crust formation. Also risk of patient allergy with latex, so ensure that this is checked with patient
Short to medium term	Teflon or silicone Elastomer coatings	Teflon or silicone is applied to latex to prevent the risk of latex allergy and reduce urethral irritation However, NHS Quality Improvement Scotland (2004) suggested that Teflon coating is unsuitable for patients with a latex allergy, whereas silicone material is suitable
Medium term	100% silicone	Less likely to cause urethral irritation, but can still develop encrustation (inner crusting). Silicone can also allow balloon to deflate (water leaks out) and so catheter can fall out prematurely
Long term	Hydrogel coated latex	These coat the catheter and cause the least irritation and as they become rehydrated they become smoother, and so reduce friction in the urethra. This reduces the risk of becoming contaminated with bacteria or encrusted.
		NHS Quality Improvement Scotland (2004) note this type of material is unsuitable for patients with a latex allergy
	Hydrogel-coated silicone	Suitable for patients with latex allergy, however are rigid so can be uncomfortable for some patients
	Conformable catheter	Designed to conform to the shape of the female urethra and allows partial filling of the bladder. Made of latex with silicone Elastomer coating, and approximately 3 cm longer in length than usual female catheter
	Polymer hydromer (PH) (Bray and Saunders 2006)	Latex bonded with PH to create a material suitable for long-term use

PVC, polyvinylchloride.
Adapted from Dougherty and Lister (2004) and NHS QIS (2004), and Bray and Saunders (2006).

Scotland (QIS 2004) discussed studies using silver-coated (silver alloy or silver oxide) catheters compared with silicone hydrogel or Teflon latex. These catheters are designed for a maximum of 28 days and were associated with a reduced incidence of urinary infections and, are now available in the UK.

Table 11.2 Paediatric catheter sizes

Age (years)	Charrière (Ch) size
0–2	6
2–5	6–8
5–10	8–10
10–16	10–12

Reproduced from Bray and Saunders (2006) with permission.

Balloon sizes

Balloons are used to hold the indwelling catheter in place and are inflated once the catheter has been correctly inserted into the bladder (Baillie and Arrowsmith 2005). The volume in the balloon varies; in children the balloons are commonly filled with 3–5 ml of sterile water, and 5–10 ml for adults; however some balloons inflate to 30 ml, but this is used mainly after urological procedures only. Dougherty and Lister (2004) noted that too much fluid in a balloon can cause damage to the neck of the bladder or irritation to the bladder wall, often causing bypassing, or too little fluid can also cause irritation. If a Foley-type catheter (design) is inserted, always make sure that it is draining before inflating the balloon with sterile water; and this is used in case of balloon rupture and so will not cause any bladder irritation (NHS QIS 2004).

Design of catheter tip

Dougherty and Lister (2004) describe tip designs and these can affect drainage:

- Tiemann-tip is curved with one to three drainage eyes
- Whistle-tip has a lateral eye in the tip and eyes above the balloon to provide a large drainage area; helpful in drainage of debris or blood clots
- Roberts tip has an eye above and below the catheter to help drain residual urine.

Length of catheter

Authors note a variance, but all agree on three lengths (Dougherty and Lister 2004; NHS QIS 2004; Baillie and Arrowsmith 2005; Bray and Saunders 2006):

1. Paediatric: 30–31 cm
2. Female: 20–40 cm
3. Male or standard: 40–45 cm.

   However, Baillie and Arrowsmith (2005) suggested that standard length is often used for women, particularly if the patient is obese or chair bound, because it allows easier access to the connector end and the drainage bag (NHS QIS 2004).

 Reflection point

Why are there different lengths of catheters (male and female)?

Drainage systems

A drainage bag allows periodic emptying, and so reduces the number of manipulations with the catheter (Baillie and Arrowsmith 2005). Dougherty and Lister (2004) noted that the highest risk

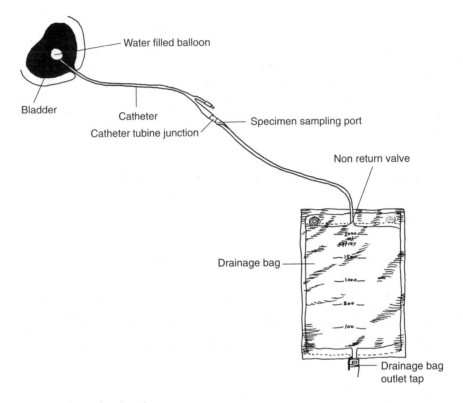

Figure 11.3 Catheter bag and outlet valve.

of infection is when emptying or changing the bag, hence NHS QIS (2004) suggested changing bags every 5–7 days.

Most drainage bags attach either to a stand on the floor or bed side, or to a patient's leg, and depend on the patient's condition and mobility, and also their preference.

Bags vary in capacity and length of inlet tube and type of outlet tap, and this may also influence choice (Baillie and Arrowsmith 2005):

- 350–750 ml in volume and up to 2 litres with overnight bags.

See Figure 11.3 for bag and outlet tap.

Baillie and Arrowsmith (2005) suggested that outlet taps are usually of a lever-type or push-across design; thus when assessing the patient, you may need to consider the mental and physical capability of patients or carers – assessing whether they can open and close the tap safely?

Reflection point

When choosing a drainage bag, what could be some factors that you should consider?

The use of a catheter valve (tap on the catheter) may provide an alternative to a bag; however, the patient needs a reasonable bladder capacity and good manual dexterity to manipulate the valve (Baillie and Arrowsmith 2005).

Bray and Saunders (2006) calculated the bladder volume in children using the formula: $30 \times$ child's age $+ 30$, so, for example, a 6 year old would have a calculated bladder volume of 210 ml. This formula is applicable until a child reaches age 12 years, and then would expect the bladder volume to be that of an adult, which ranges from 300 ml to 500 ml (Bray and Saunders 2006). Thus, for some patients a valve may offer more privacy and fewer restrictions to their mobility and lifestyle. Dougherty and Lister (2004) added that the use of a valve eliminates the need for bags and is most effective in long-term indwelling catheters, and the valve can be in place for 5–7 days.

Closed drainage systems are now considered good practice, and require effective aseptic techniques (cleansing) on insertion, emptying or removal, so care must be exercised at all times.

It is important that there is no pressure on the catheter, so ensure that the bag, if attached to a stand, is in a good position and not caught in clothing or bedclothes. The same applies to a leg bag; here the use of adjustable straps or a 'sleeve or holster' is essential to secure the bag in a suitable position, remembering patient comfort, drainage and privacy (Baillie and Arrowsmith 2005).

Reflection point

What aspects will you need to consider when assessing your patient?

Patient preparation for catheterisation

Mangnall and Watterson (2006) outlined this as:

- Explain the procedure (e.g. why catheter is being inserted, for how long)
- Educate patient, e.g. do not touch the clean area during procedure and do not play with or pull your catheter
- If possible, patients wash genital area first with unperfumed soap and water, and then men need to retract the foreskin (where possible) and clean the area thoroughly and then replace the foreskin, whereas women need to wash from front to back to prevent contamination from the rectal area.

Leaver (2007) also suggested cleansing pre-catheterisation to ensure that the area is socially clean and uncontaminated; they note that this can be carried out by staff using sodium chloride 0.9% solution, or any of the usual skin-cleansing solutions containing antiseptics.

Local anaesthetic is commonly used in male catheterisation (Dougherty and Lister 2004), and Bray and Saunders (2006) suggested that local anaesthetic gel (e.g. 2% lidocaine) be used because this also acts as a lubricant and ideally is applied 3–5 min before catheterisation. This may not, however, be achievable with younger children due to their anxiety.

Insertion technique

Catheterisation equipment: a sterile catheter pack preferably or sterile dressing pack with gallipot, sterile gloves, catheter (recommend one of assessed size and one spare plus a smaller size), sterile

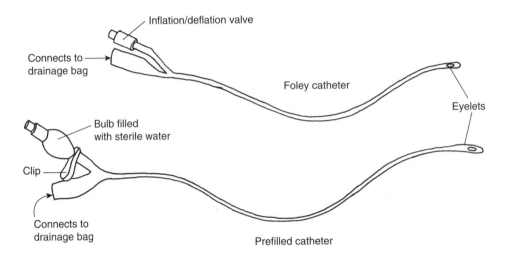

Inflation/deflation valve

Connects to
drainage bag

Foley catheter

Eyelets

Bulb filled
with sterile water

Clip

Connects to
drainage bag

Prefilled catheter

Figure 11.4 Catheter.

sodium chloride or antiseptic solution, sterile water and syringe as per age and balloon size, sterile single patient anaesthetic gel or lubricating gel, holder or leg straps, drainage bag (as appropriate), sterile receiver and waterproof protective sheet/pad (if not in catheter pack), sterile specimen container (often a sterile sample is sent to laboratory, depends on the reason for catheter insertion), apron, screens and good lighting (may require portable or angled light).

The whole procedure must follow a non-touch technique, and equipment used must be sterile and single use (Figures 11.4 and 11.5), and that all packaging is checked and intact and in date.

Table 11.3 describes the procedure for male or female catheterisation; however, in some clinical areas healthcare assistants may require additional training for male catheterisation because of technical aspects and the use of anaesthetic gel and, as this is an administration of a medicine, some clinical areas may not cover this role for healthcare assistants as usual, *please check your local policy*. (See Figures 11.1 and 11.2 re male and female anatomy for catheterisation.)

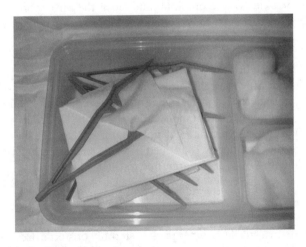

Figure 11.5 Sterile pack. (Photograph by I Lavery.)

Table 11.3 Catheterisation procedure

Step	Procedure
1	Approach the patient, explain procedure, and gain consent and cooperation
2	Help patient into a safe position, preferably flat on back, covered and screened for privacy
3	Wash hands, put on plastic apron, assemble equipment on clean trolley, take to the screened bedside/area
4	Place waterproof sheet under patient's buttocks – to protect the bed
5	Open catheter pack taking care not to touch inside – to protect sterile field
6	Open the catheter but leave in internal packing and drop onto sterile field
7	Draw up the required amount of sterile water with a sterile syringe
8	Pour sterile sodium chloride into sterile gallipot in pack, and open single use gel (lubricating or anaesthetic), set up drainage bag (on stand if being used)
9	The assistant now uncovers the patient and supports the legs, and knees bent up and apart
10	Open sterile gloves and wash hands or use alcohol rub to cleanse hands
11	Sterile gloves on, place sterile towels over patient's thighs and under buttocks
12	Males: wrap a sterile towel around the penis, and retract the foreskin to clean round the top of urethra with the sodium chloride or antiseptic solution Females: cleanse the perineal area with sodium chloride, then, using non-dominant hand, separate the inner labia (lips) and cleanse the meatus (opening)
13	Males: insert the nozzle of the anaesthetic gel into the urethra, and squeeze the gel in, remove the nozzle and discard the tube, massage the gel along the urethra (penis) and wait 5 min Females: carefully locate the urethra and insert either lubricant or anaesthetic gel and wait 5 min
14	Males: grasp the penis behind the glans (acorn-shaped rim) and raise penis until extended and maintain this grasp till procedure finished – see below Females: expose the tip of the catheter by pulling off serrated end of internal wrapper (also for male catheterisation)
15	Males: place sterile receiver between patient's legs and insert selected catheter for 15–25 cm (6–9 inches) until urine flows, pulling back internal wrapper and ensuring that catheter end is in receiver Females: place sterile receiver between patient's legs and insert selected catheter for 5–7 cm (2–3 inches) until urine flows, pulling back internal wrapper and ensuring that catheter end is in receiver
16	Males: if resistance is felt, increase the traction on the penis slightly and ask the patient to strain gently as though passing urine and apply steady gentle pressure on the catheter; this may help insertion past bladder sphincter; if not, stop and seek advice Females: Bray and Saunders (2006) noted that occasionally a catheter may enter the vagina and so no urine drains. If this happens, leave this catheter in place as a marker, and recommence with new catheter, then remove the first one once the second catheter is correctly *in situ*
17	Males: advance catheter forward to ensure safely within the bladder to bifurcation (Y section) (Figure 11.4) Females: advance the catheter a further 5 cm; never force the catheter. If resistance is met stop and seek medical advice
18	Inflate balloon with sterile water as per manufacturer's instructions, and ensure that urine is still draining
19	Withdraw catheter slightly – balloon will hold in place
20	Attach free end to drainage system and ensure secured and no drag on catheter
21	Males: ensure that penis is clean and foreskin is retracted Females: ensure that genital area is clean
22	Dispose of equipment, per local policy
23	Check that patient is comfortable and has understood catheter education
24	Document procedure, noting catheter type, size and balloon volume inserted, along with date, time and drainage, and if any specimen sent or tested

Adapted from Dougherty and Lister (2004) and Baillie and Arrowsmith (2005).

Men, particularly the older age population, may suffer from an enlarged prostate gland. Tortora and Derrickson (2006) described this as a single doughnut-shaped gland, which surrounds the urethra, so if it enlarges this can affect the flow of urine and also catheter insertion. If a male patient reports pain or discomfort during the procedure, stop and always seek advice.

Bray and Saunders (2006) noted, in children's insertion, usual aspects should be documented as for point 24 in Table 11.3, plus the catheter batch number, the inserter's name, the type of analgesia used, if any, and consent.

Intermittent catheterisation

Intermittent catheterisation can be undertaken by the patient, carer or healthcare professional, and the bladder must have sufficient capacity to store urine between catheterisations (NHS QIS 2004). Dougherty and Lister (2004) describe the procedure as the periodic removal of urine and, after the procedure, the catheter is removed, leaving the patient catheter free. The procedure is carried out (see Table 11.4 for the procedure) as often as the patient requires, usually four to five times a day.

When patients, commonly at home, carry out this procedure it is a clean procedure, whereas any healthcare assistant would carry it out as an aseptic procedure. Also, the healthcare assistant may be helping to teach the patient or carer the procedure, or assisting them in hospital, if due to an acute illness, they may not have the usual physical and manual dexterity to carry out the procedure (NHS QIS 2004).

Dougherty and Lister (2004) suggested patients who are suitable for intermittent self-catheterisation as the following:

- Those who can comprehend (understand) the technique
- Those with a reasonable degree of manual dexterity (able to use hands)
- Those who are highly motivated
- Those who have a willing partner (if suitable for both to participate)
- Those who can position themselves to attain reasonable access to the urethra, especially in females.

The benefits of intermittent catheterisation can include an improved quality of life, greater patient satisfaction, greater freedom to express sexuality and minimisation of urinary complications (Dougherty and Lister 2004).

Catheter care

NHS QIS (2004) outlined the following aspects:

- Maintain a closed system, as much as possible
- Empty drainage bags regularly (when bag two-thirds full) and always ensure positioned below level of bladder (exception: a 'belly bag' see Figure 11.6) and change every 5–7 days
- Body-worn bags, e.g. 'belly bag' (Figure 11.6): change weekly (a 'belly bag' is worn round the waist and has 1000 cm^3 capacity and can be used with Foley-type catheters)
- Bedside-type drainage bags must be supported off the floor
- A separate clean container is used for each individual; avoid contact with the drainage tap and container

Table 11.4 Intermittent self-catheterisation procedure

Step	Procedure in males	Procedure in females
1	Wash hands using bactericidal soap and water, or bactericidal alcohol hand rub and dry thoroughly	Take up a comfortable position, dependent on mobility, e.g. sitting on toilet or standing with one foot up on toilet rim (see Step 10)
2	Stand in front of toilet, or low bench with a container if easier (see Step 10)	Spread the labia (lips) and wash the genitalia from front to back with soap and water, then dry
3	Clean the glans of the penis (head) with plain water, retract foreskin, if applicable, during the procedure	
4	Hold penis with left hand (if right handed) three fingers underneath and thumb on top, holding the penis straight out. Coat the end of the catheter with the lubricating gel	Insert the catheter, use lubricant gel if wish for comfort, and a mirror to help see genitalia
5	Pass the catheter gently with the right hand (or left if left handed); it can be felt as it passes the fingers holding the penis. There will be a change in feeling as catheter passes through the prostate gland into the bladder. It may be a little painful on the first few occasions only; if any resistance is felt, stop and seek medical advice immediately	Urine will drain as soon as the catheter reaches the bladder, so have the end positioned over the toilet or the container
6	Urine will drain as soon as the catheter enters the bladder, so have end positioned over toilet or container	
7	Withdraw the catheter slowly so that all the urine is drained and it should slide out easily	Remove the catheter slowly when urine has stopped draining; it should slide out easily
8	Wash catheter through if reusable[a] and store in dry, clean container	
9	Wash hands again as Step 1	
10	If patient has a large abdomen, a mirror standing in front can assist observation and insertion	

Adapted from Dougherty and Lister (2004).

NHS Quality Improvement Scotland (QIS 2004) describe intermittent catheter cleaning (PVC reusable catheters); wash in warm soapy water, rinse thoroughly and then leave in a clean dry area to air dry, and then store in a clean dry container. These catheters can be used for up to 1 week (approximately) before being discarded, so they recommend that a patient makes note of date or day, to ensure that they remember to change the catheter.

- Wear gloves to empty drainage bags and ensure new gloves and hands washed between patients – strict aseptic technique
- Leg bags can be emptied directly into toilets
- When overnight bag is required, a new single-use 2-litre bedside bag is used and emptied and discarded in the morning
- Encourage the patient to have a daily bath or shower and wash with warm soapy water
- Frequent vigorous meatal (genital area) cleansing with antiseptic solutions is not needed, and may even increase the risk of infection.

Dougherty and Lister (2004) offer further points;

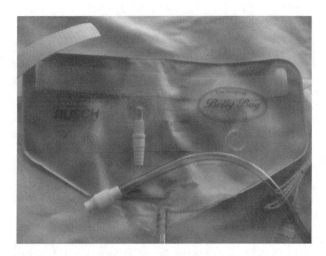

Figure 11.6   Belly bag. (Photograph by I Lavery.)

- Clean the outlet valve with 70% isopropyl alcohol-impregnated swab and allow to dry thoroughly
- Once urine drained, re-clean as above
- Record volume and document if necessary
- Always wash hands at start and finish with bactericidal soap and water.

Baillie and Arrowsmith (2005) suggested changing bags at home after 1 week, and that the bag be rinsed with water and allowed to dry between use. While in hospital, a new bag may be required every time the bag needs changing; refer to manufacturer's guidance.

Sampling

Breaking the closed system to obtain a sample increases the risk of catheter-related infection, so use of a drainage bag with a sample port (Figure 11.7) incorporated removes the need to break the closed system (NHS QIS 2004).

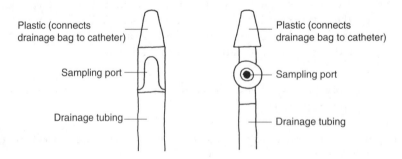

Figure 11.7   Sampling ports.

Dougherty and Lister (2004) and NHS QIS (2004) described the steps in sampling as follows:

- Only take a sample for a valid reason, e.g. suspect a urinary infection
- Wash hands, put on gloves and apron

- Cleanse port with 70% isopropyl alcohol-impregnated swab and allow to dry thoroughly
- Take the sample from the bag sample port
- Using a sterile syringe (and needle if necessary) aspirate the required amount of urine; Dougherty and Lister (2004) noted that, if no urine in tubing, it is possible to clamp the tubing below the sample port/cuff only until sufficient volume collects
- Re-clean sample port with 70% isopropyl alcohol-impregnated swab and allow to dry thoroughly
- Place specimen into sterile container and label correctly
- Wash hands again with bactericidal soap and water, and dry thoroughly
- Unclamp tubing, if necessary
- Consider recording volume, where applicable, e.g. patient is on fluid balance chart
- Send specimen and form promptly to laboratory, as per local policy.

Pellatt (2007) suggested, in young children, that placing a sterile bag over the genitalia to catch the urine may be necessary (see Chapter 10 for more information). Tables 11.6–11.9 are competency frameworks for catheterisation procedures and sampling.

Removal of catheter

NHS QIS (2004) and Baillie and Arrowsmith (2005) indicated removal as soon as possible, depending on the patient's condition and the judgement of healthcare staff. Assessment of patients should consider whether they are physically and mentally able to cope with normal micturition (passing urine).

Baillie and Arrowsmith (2005) suggested removal at 12 midnight, increasing the time before the patient would pass urine, leading to a greater initial volume and faster return to normal voiding (passing) of urine, which can decrease levels of anxiety. A Best Practice Statement from Joanna Briggs Institute (JBI 2006) discussed the time of removal and noted that this is a balance between avoiding infection (early removal) and voiding (passing urine) problems (by later removal), and midnight removal may lead to shorter hospital stays.

The urine output must be monitored after removal, to ensure that the patient is passing urine and in adequate volumes (Baillie and Arrowsmith 2005). It may be recommended that a portable bladder scan be used to measure residual volumes in the first few days, because retention can often be a problem after a catheter is removed (NHS QIS 2004). Bray and Saunders (2006) noted that careful gentle removal must be ensured in case a catheter has become encrusted (possible in medium- to long-term catheters).

Dougherty and Lister (2004) and Baillie and Arrowsmith (2005) outlined the procedure as follows:

- Explain the procedure to the patient and any possible after effects, e.g. urgency or discomfort
- Wash hands and, wearing gloves, clean the meatal/urethral area with sodium chloride, females from front to back, males around urethral opening
- Clean/change gloves, having previously checked volume of water in balloon use a syringe to withdraw the water and deflate the balloon
- Ask the patient to breathe in and out and, on an exhalation, gently but quickly remove the catheter. Advise males that they may note some discomfort as deflated balloon passes the prostate gland
- Cleanse area; dry, remove and dispose of equipment as per local policy. If urine is present in drainage bag, empty before disposal in clinical waste
- Document removal, volume in bag, and date and time; also whether any problems reported, e.g. patient discomfort

- Patient should maintain adequate fluid intake; Baillie and Arrowsmith (2005) suggested that patients should be encouraged to increase their fluid intake to 'flush' the bladder.

Baillie and Arrowsmith (2005) recommended checking that no specimens are required first; if they are collect sample and then proceed to removal.

Related aspects and terminology

Communication, consent and clinical holding

In adults this includes consideration of communication, consent and education and in children may also need to consider the issue of holding (see Chapters 3 and 4 for more information on consent).

NHS QIS (2004) discussed patient consent and gender issues, and indicated key aspects in relation to catheterisation:

- Informed consent must be obtained first and is ongoing, so patient may/can withdraw consent at any time
- Patient's capacity is crucial (e.g. in Scotland, Adults with Incapacity Act 2000 protects the interests of adults who are not capable of making a decision, e.g. learning difficulty or mental health problem)
- Ensure accurate documentation, which includes the process for consent, and indicates that the patient has understood and verbally consented to the procedure
- Patients are entitled to request the procedure be carried out by a specific gender of healthcare worker, e.g. male patient may wish a male nurse, to fit with their cultural/personal preferences.

Dingwall and McLafferty (2006) also considered patient preferences in relation to catheterisation, because the patient may be embarrassed; in addition they considered the effect that a catheter may have on body image and sexuality, and found that this was noted more in males. However, as Rees and Mawson (2007) indicated, if the reason for an indwelling catheter is because of incontinence, this in itself can cause social embarrassment and isolation and so affect their quality of life. Thus, the option of a catheter may be seen here as advantageous. Incontinence affects 6 million people worldwide and in the UK 40 in 1000 people are affected (Rees and Mawson 2007).

Bray and Saunders (2006) stated that catheterisation in children is a sensitive issue that requires effective communication, sensitivity and diplomacy skills. They further noted that a child's rights can be ambiguous where procedures such as catheterisation are to be done, as a parent or healthcare professional can override a child's wishes. Bray and Saunders (2006) therefore discussed the need for healthcare workers to understand the child's level of understanding and, as catheterisation is an unpleasant procedure, ensure that the child is involved, so that they feel they have some control over the situation.

Parents should be encouraged to be present, because they can act as chaperones and relieve their child's anxiety by being there (Bray and Saunders 2006). If the child is strongly opposed, Bray and Saunders (2006) stated that this must be fully explored with the child before the procedure is undertaken. Therefore discussions must take place with the child and their parent(s) or carer(s), including the reason for catheterisation versus other options, e.g. voiding programme or incontinence pad.

Education would include the reason for the initial catheterisation, how long the catheter might remain in place and how it will be secured and emptied, and patients can be encouraged to self-cleanse the genital area and catheter, e.g. daily bath or shower with soap and water is adequate (NHS QIS 2004; Baillie and Arrowsmith 2005). Further education would include asking the patient to drink adequate fluids; this is good practice (maintaining healthy fluid levels), and would ensure good urine drainage and output. Other aspects: advise the patient to ensure that the drainage bag (if used) is always kept below bladder level to achieve drainage and to observe that urine is draining (Baillie and Arrowsmith 2005).

Bray and Saunders (2006) talked about clinical holding – positioning a child for a medical procedure, so that it can be carried out in a safe and controlled manner, and where possible, with the consent of the child and the parent/carer. Holding must be seen as a last resort, so other options that should be considered first are use of a play specialist to help distract or guided imagery. Preparation can include acting out the procedure with a doll and playing with products that may be used (Bray and Saunders 2006). Finally, Bray and Saunders (2006) noted the use of pharmacological interventions (drugs) that may aid with relaxation and minimise discomfort, e.g. Entonox (this gas would be administered only under prescription by a registered children's nurse and/or doctor).

Terminology

- Intermittent catheterisation: catheter inserted routinely and not left in place
- Suprapubic: above the pubes bone
- Acute retention: sudden inability to pass urine (micturate)
- Epidural anaesthesia: anaesthetic drug is injected into spine to 'numb' lower body, often used in childbirth and if a patient is unable to tolerate a general anaesthetic, e.g. patient with chronic bronchitis
- Residual urine: volume left in bladder after voiding (passing urine)
- Cytotoxic: medicine therapy to destroy 'cancer' cells
- Bladder irrigation or instillation: drug therapy inserted directly into the bladder.

Common problems

The most common problem is urinary infection, hence thorough asepsis at all times is necessary (Bray and Saunders 2006). Rees and Mawson (2007) noted that a catheter increases this risk and can lead to increased temperature, bypassing of the catheter and, in an older patient, cause acute confusional states. Leaver (2007) identified rates of urinary infections at 40%, and 80% of these were associated with the use of catheters.

NHS QIS (2004) and Bray and Saunders (2006) identified other problems and these are shown in Table 11.5.

Bladder spasm: medicines would be prescribed, and can include an anticholinergic (NHS QIS 2004), and Bray and Saunders (2006) noted that, in children, the use of oxybutynin or tolterodine has been found to be successful, but care is needed because these can cause side effects and some may not be licensed for certain ages. *The administration of these would not be part of a healthcare assistant's role; check your local policy.*

Table 11.5 Problem solving

Catheter problem	Possible reason	Possible solution
Urine not draining/ blockage	Catheter in wrong position – not in bladder, maybe in vagina	Deflate balloon and gently reposition catheter forward
	Drainage bag in wrong position – above the level of the bladder	Check bag position – move to below bladder level
	Drainage tubing may be kinked	Check tubing and unkink
	Catheter blocked by debris	Prescribed flush, gently with saline preferably or sterile water
	Bladder spasm	Consider use of medication[a]
Haematuria (presence of blood in urine)	Trauma post-catheterisation	Observe output and document severity of haematuria, report to nurse in charge and/or doctor
	Infection	
	Calculi (stones)	Observe and report as above
	Cancer	
	Prostatic enlargement	Encourage fluid intake and observe and report as above
Bypassing of urine around catheter	May indicate infection	Send sterile urine specimen
	Bladder spasm/instability	Consider use of medication[a]
	Constipation	Increase fluid and dietary fibre intake: 2–3 l in adults, 1500 ml for children over 5 years and 2000 ml for teenagers
	Incorrect positioning of drainage system	Check drainage bag position
	Balloon volume incorrect	Check volume in balloon, remove if overinflated or add if less than specified volume
	Drainage bag more than two-thirds full	Regular emptying
Pain or discomfort	The eyes of the catheter may be blocked	Raise the drainage bag above the level of the bladder for 10–15 s only
	Maybe a sign of infection	Obtain sterile specimen of urine
	On removal, may indicate crusting	Ensure correct catheter size inserted in first place and the patient maintains daily cleaning of genital area and catheter
Catheter retaining balloon will not deflate	Valve port and balloon inflation channel may be compressed	Check no compression on tubing
	Faulty valve mechanism.	Aspirate balloon port slowly; if too fast can cause valve mechanism to collapse
		Can inject a small additional amount of sterile water in and then slowly aspirate again
		Do NOT cut catheter, if all fails, seek medical advice

Adapted from NHS Quality Improvement Scotland (QIS 2004), and Bray and Saunders (2006).

Table 11.6 Competency framework: indwelling catheterisation

First assessment/reassessment						
Steps	**Demonstration/Supervised practice**					**Date/competent signature**
Indwelling catheterisation	Date/sign	Date/sign	Date/sign	Date/sign	Date/sign	
Procedure stages: male and female	1	2	3	4	5	
1 Patient approached, procedure explained, consent /cooperation gained						
2 Helped patient into safe position, covered and screened						
3 Washed hands, equipment assembled on clean trolley						
4 Placed waterproof sheet/ pad under patient's buttocks						
5 Catheter pack opened protecting sterile field						
6 Catheter opened onto sterile field						
7 Appropriate volume of sterile water drawn up with sterile syringe						
8 Sterile sodium chloride prepared and single use gel opened						
9 Patient uncovered and legs supported in appropriate position						
10 Sterile gloves opened and hands washed as per policy						
11 Sterile gloves on, sterile towels placed over patient's thighs and under buttocks						
Male-specific aspects	Date/sign	Date/sign	Date/sign	Date/sign	Date/sign	
	1	2	3	4	5	
12 Sterile towel wrapped around penis, foreskin retracted, and top of urethra cleaned with sodium chloride or antiseptic solution						
13 Anaesthetic gel nozzle inserted into urethra, gel squeezed in, nozzle removed, discarded, massaged gel along penis, waited 5 min						
14 Penis grasped safely and raised until fully extended, for all procedure						
15 Sterile receiver placed between patient's legs, catheter tip exposed, then inserted smoothly and gently for 15–25 cm until urine flows						
16 Catheter advanced forward so safely within bladder, and urine is draining into receiver						

(Continued)

Table 11.6 (*Continued*)

17	Balloon inflated with sterile water and ensured urine still draining						
18	Catheter withdrawn slightly to ensure secure in bladder						
19	Free end attached correctly and securely to selected drainage system						
20	Ensured penis clean and foreskin retracted at finish						
Indwelling catheterisation: female-specific aspects		Date/sign	Date/sign	Date/sign	Date/sign	Date/sign	
		1	2	3	4	5	
12	Perineal area cleansed with sodium chloride, inner labia separated and meatus cleansed too						
13	Urethra located, lubricant or anaesthetic gel inserted, waited 5 min						
14	Tip of catheter exposed by pulling off serrated end of internal wrapper						
15	Sterile receiver placed between patient's legs, catheter inserted smoothly and gently for 5–7 cm until urine flows						
16	If no urine drained, checked if catheter in vagina, so left in place, recommenced with new catheter, then removed first once second is correctly *in situ*						
17	Advanced catheter a further 5 cm to ensure safely within the bladder and urine still draining into receiver						
18	Balloon inflated with sterile water and ensured urine still draining						
19	Catheter withdrawn slightly – to test secured in bladder						
20	Free end attached correctly and securely to drainage system and genital area is clean						
Male and female aspects		Date/sign	Date/sign	Date/sign	Date/sign	Date/sign	
		1	2	3	4	5	
21	Disposed of equipment, per local policy						
22	Checked patient is comfortable, has understood catheter education, allowed questions						
23	Procedure documented, noting catheter type, size and balloon volume inserted, along with date, time and drainage, and if any specimen sent or tested						

Supervisors/Assessor(s):

Table 11.7 Competency framework: intermittent catheterisation competency – patient/carer

Steps	First assessment/reassessment					Date/competent signature
	Demonstration/Supervised practice					
Supervised aspects for *learner* patient/carer self-catheterisation	Date/sign	Date/sign	Date/sign	Date/sign	Date/sign	
	1	**2**	**3**	**4**	**5**	
1 Patient/carer washed hands using bactericidal soap and water, or bactericidal alcohol hand rub and dried thoroughly						
2 Took up a comfortable position, e.g. sat on toilet or stood with one foot up on toilet rim (female); or stood at toilet or low bench with a container (male)						
3 Genital area cleaned correctly: **Female:** spread labia and washed from front to back with soap and water, then dried **Male:** cleaned the head of penis with water, foreskin retracted during procedure						
4 **Male:** held penis with three fingers underneath and thumb on top, straight out, coated the end of the catheter with the lubricating/anaesthetic gel **Female:** inserted catheter, used lubricant or anaesthetic gel if wished, and a mirror to help see genitalia						
5 Passed catheter gently with one hand; in males it can be felt as it passes the fingers holding the penis. Urine drained and catheter end positioned over toilet or container						
6 Withdrawn catheter slowly once all the urine is drained						
7 If container, urine disposed in toilet and container cleaned/disposed						
8 Catheter washed correctly if re-usable and stored in clean container						
9 Hands washed again post procedure						

Supervisors/Assessor(s)

Table 11.8 Competency framework: intermittent catheterisation by healthcare assistant

Steps	First assessment/reassessment					Date/competent signature
	Demonstration/Supervised practice					
Intermittent catheterisation by healthcare assistant	Date/sign	Date/sign	Date/sign	Date/sign	Date/sign	
	1	2	3	4	5	
1 Hands washed using bactericidal soap and water, or bactericidal alcohol hand rub and dried thoroughly						
2 Patient assisted into a comfortable position						
3 **Females:** perineal area cleansed with sodium chloride then inner labia separated and meatus cleansed too **Males:** sterile towel wrapped around penis, foreskin retracted and top of urethra cleaned with sodium chloride or antiseptic solution						
4 Urethra located, lubricant or anaesthetic gel inserted, waited 5 min						
5 Sterile receiver placed between patient's legs, catheter inserted smoothly and gently for required distance; Males 15–25 cm and females 5–7 cm, until urine flows						
6 Catheter withdrawn slowly once all the urine is drained						
7 Catheter washed correctly if reusable and stored in dry clean container or if single use disposed of correctly as per local policy						
8 Procedure documented and volume recorded						
9 Patient left clean and comfortable						

Supervisors/Assessor(s):

Table 11.9 Competency framework: sampling competency

	First assessment/reassessment					Date/competent signature
Steps	**Demonstration/Supervised practice**					
Sampling competency	Date/sign	Date/sign	Date/sign	Date/sign	Date/sign	
	1	2	3	4	5	
1 Checked reason for sampling valid, e.g. suspected urinary infection						
2 Washed hands, put on gloves and apron						
3 Cleansed port with isopropyl alcohol 70% swab and allowed to dry thoroughly						
4 Used sterile syringe (and needle if necessary) aspirated the required amount of urine						
5 If no urine in tubing, clamped the tubing below the sample port/cuff until sufficient volume collected						
6 Re-cleaned sample port with isopropyl alcohol 70% impregnated swab and allowed to dry thoroughly						
7 Placed specimen into sterile container and labelled correctly						
8 Washed hands again with bactericidal soap and water and dried thoroughly						
9 Unclamped tubing, if necessary						
10 Recorded volume, if patient is on fluid balance chart						
11 Sent specimen and form promptly to laboratory, per local policy						

Supervisors/Assessor(s):

Summary

This chapter has outlined the skills necessary for inserting and removing urinary catheters, discussed intermittent catheterization and sampling, as well as ongoing catheter care. All require strict aseptic technique and competent practice. Also required are effective communication and documentation

Case study 11.1

Mrs Fiona Wilson is 74 years old and lives in a nursing home; she has been unwell for a few days with urinary frequency and a fever. Yesterday she was incontinent several times, and today staff have observed that she is becoming confused and restless. On examination, you find her skin very red and sore looking around her genital area, and she is now unable to walk to the toilet, because she is very unsteady and confused.
  What actions would you recommend and why?

Case study 11.2

Brian Fredericks, aged 32 years and wheelchair bound after a road accident, is being discharged home in a few days. You are part of a team caring from him and he is being considered for intermittent self-catheterisation.
  What might be the benefits for this young male?
  How would you explain the technique?

Below there is a self-assessment checklist; however, you may also wish to review Skills for Health (2004). Competence CH88 insert and secure urethral catheters, and monitor and respond to the effects of urethral catheterisation.

 ## Self-assessment

Assessment	Aspects	Achieved ✔
Indwelling catheterisation	*Have you considered all aspects of this section?*	
	Reasons for insertion or other options explored	
	Catheter material, gauge and length considered	
	Patient assessment carried out	
	Consent, communication and patient education	
	Procedure and infection control aspects	
	Recording the procedure	
	Reporting concerns or outcome	
	Problem solving	
	Disposal of equipment	
Sampling	*Have you considered all aspects of this section?*	**Achieved ✔**
	Procedure and infection control aspects	
	Process for dealing with sample	
	If for testing refer to Chapter 10 If for laboratory purposes, is aware of local process for sending sample	

(*Continued*)

	Recording the results	
	Reporting concerns or results	
	Problem solving	
	Disposal of equipment	
Catheter care	*Have you considered all aspects of this section?*	**Achieved ✔**
	Procedure and infection control	
	Reporting concerns or results	
	Problem solving	
	Disposal of equipment	
Removal	*Have you considered all aspects of this section?*	**Achieved ✔**
	Procedure and infection control	
	Reporting concerns or results	
	Problem solving	
	Disposal of equipment	
Intermittent catheterisation	*Have you considered all aspects of this section?*	**Achieved ✔**
	Assessment – nurse or patient procedure?	
	Procedure and infection control	
	Self-catheterisation: patient education and clean technique and storage and cleaning of catheter	
	Reporting concerns or results	
	Problem solving	
	Disposal of equipment	
	Ordering of equipment	

References

Baillie L, Arrowsmith K (2005) Meeting elimination needs. In: Baillie L (ed.), *Developing Practical Nursing Skills*, 2nd edn. London: Hodder Education, pp. 278–349.

Bray L, Saunders C (2006) Nursing management of paediatric urethral catheterisation. *Nursing Standard* 20(24): 51–60.

Department of Health (2001) Guidelines for preventing infections associated with the insertion and maintenance of short-term indwelling urethral catheters in acute care. *Journal of Hospital Infection* 47(suppl) S39–46.

Dingwall L, McLafferty E (2006) Nurses' perceptions of indwelling urinary catheters in older people. *Nursing Standard* 21(14–16): 35–42.

Dougherty L, Lister S, eds (2004) *The Royal Marsden Hospital Manual of Clinical Nursing Procedures*, 6th edn. Oxford: Blackwell Publishing.

Joanna Briggs Institute (2006) *Best Practice: Removal of short term indwelling urethral catheters*, vol 10. Adelaide: Blackwell Publishing.

Leaver RB (2007) The evidence for urethral meatal cleansing. *Nursing Standard* 21(41): 39–42.

Mangnall J, Watterson L (2006) Principles of aseptic technique in urinary catheterisation. *Nursing Standard* 21(8): 49–56.

NHS Quality Improvement Scotland (2004) *Best Practice Statement: Urinary catheterisation and catheter care*. Edinburgh: NHS Quality Improvement Scotland.

National Institute for Health and Clinical Excellence (2003) *Infection Control, Prevention of Healthcare-associated Infection in Primary and Community Care*. Clinical Guideline 2. London: NICE.

Pellatt GC (2007) Anatomy and physiology of urinary elimination. Part 1. *British Journal of Nursing* 16: 406–410.

Rees J, Mawson T (2007) Guidelines on catheter use in patients with a hip fracture. *Nursing Times* 103(16): 30–31.

Skills for Health (2004) *CHS8 Insert and secure urethral catheters and monitor and respond to the effects of urethral catheterisation* www.skillsforhealth.org.uk/tools/view_framework.php?id=39 (accessed 2 September 2007).

Tortora GJ, Derrickson B (2006) *Principles of Anatomy and Physiology*, 11th edn. Hoboken, NJ: John Wiley & Sons Inc.

Chapter 12

Venepuncture

Learning objectives

- Discuss the anatomy and physiology relating to venepuncture
- Review skills and competence with regard to undertaking venepuncture
- Describe possible complications of venepuncture and how to manage them

Aim of this chapter

The aim of this chapter is to review the reasons for undertaking peripheral venepuncture (blood sampling) and the associated complications and risk prevention. *This may not, however, be a role that is expected of all healthcare assistants, so please check your local policy and access any approved training.*

Reasons for performing venepuncture

The term 'venepuncture' is used to describe the introduction of a needle into a vein to obtain a representative sample of the circulating blood for laboratory (haematological, biochemical or bacteriological) analysis, and is usually requested by a medical practitioner/doctor to diagnose or monitor a patient's condition and/or treatment.

Relevant anatomy and physiology

It is essential that the healthcare assistant undertaking the technique has a good understanding of the anatomy and physiology of arteries, veins and associated nerves.

Veins and arteries are different; both have three layers of tissues but vein walls are thinner, having less muscle and elastic tissue in the middle layer (tunica media) (Tortora and Derrickson 2006). Veins also have valves, which help blood return to the heart, and are common especially where blood return is against gravity, e.g. lower limbs. Care must be taken to avoid sites where veins meet (bifurcation) due to the presence of these valves, because these can be damaged.

Veins carry deoxygenated blood back to the heart and the pressure is significantly lower than in arteries. Arteries transport blood away from the heart under pressure and are larger vessels with more elastic tissue and muscle, although this does vary depending on the size of the vessel.

For successful venepuncture, blood is sampled from a vein in the patient's arm. As arteries, veins and nerves can be in similar locations, care must be taken during the assessment and procedure to avoid arteries and nerves.

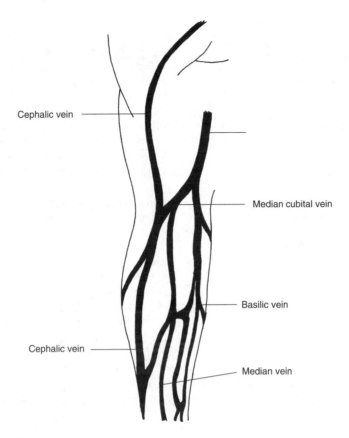

Cephalic vein

Median cubital vein

Basilic vein

Cephalic vein

Median vein

Figure 12.1 Common sites (upper arm).

Common sites for venepuncture

Usually the superficial veins of the arm are chosen for venepuncture – namely the basilic, cephalic and median cubital veins in the antecubital fossa or elbow area (Black and Hughes 1997). Preferred or first choice should be the median cubital vein (Figure 12.1).

The healthcare assistant needs to consider many aspects when selecting a vein and Table 12.1 gives some reasons for choice.

Reflection point

What are two differences between a vein and an artery?

In summary, the healthcare assistant must, as part of good assessment practice, be able to see and feel (palpate) the vein.

Infection

Venepuncture is the most common clinical practice that breaches the circulatory system, so healthcare assistants should consider their role in the prevention of infection (Box 12.1).

Table 12.1 Summary of possible considerations for vein choice

Consideration	Explanation
The vein being used is easily accessible	Makes it easier for patient comfort and ease of the procedure
Choose sizeable veins with wide inner-wall width (lumen), thick walls, not too superficial or fragile, and the vein is able to take repeated blood samples	To ensure that the vein can sustain duration of the procedure and the volume of blood required can be obtained, because this could result in further blood needing to be taken from another site
Choose sites that are less sensitive and do not bruise easily	Results in less discomfort for the patient
Do not use hard, cord-like/fibrosed (scarred), thrombosed (clotted) veins or a site of arteriovenous anastomosis (where a vein and artery have joined), e.g. for dialysis.	Could result in patient discomfort and require further sites to be needed
Do not choose veins that are next to an infected area	Area may be affected in deeper tissues and the open site vulnerable to infection
Patient has had a previous cerebral vascular accident (stroke)	Do not use the affected arm because sensation and circulation may be altered and thus, if pain or injury occurs, may not be identified at an early stage
Patient has an infusion (drip) *in situ*	Use the other arm or stop infusion for 20 minutes if medically acceptable, because otherwise this may alter blood results
Patient has lymphoedema (swelling in the tissues) or has had a mastectomy/axillary node dissection (removal of small swelling from breast or under arm)	Avoid these areas because more prone to complications, and risk of poor assessment as area swollen
Patient has rheumatoid arthritis	Joint capsule, e.g. elbow joint, may be inflamed and the tourniquet position might cause pain

Adapted with permission from NHS Lothian (2007).

Box 12.1 Predisposing infection risk factors and management

- Skin colonisation (surface bacterial spread) can allow bacteria to enter the circulatory system through the insertion of a needle, so ensure careful site selection and cleansing if evidence or concern of contamination
- Remote infection (e.g. urinary tract infection) can also lead to a risk; the patient should be educated about not tampering with the site or sterile dressing, if used, and this should reduce the risk
- Multi-use disinfectants can become colonised with bacteria very quickly, so use only single-use sachets when cleansing site
- Expired or damaged stock can be a source of infection; ensure that stock is in date and has been stored correctly, and is used for its intended purpose; single-use devices must be used (Medical Devices Agency [MDA] 2000)
- Hands of practitioners are the single most common way that bacteria are transferred onto devices (equipment), so ensure correct hand cleansing

Adapted with permission from NHS Lothian (2007).

Hand hygiene

Carry out hand hygiene before, during and after an invasive procedure such as venepuncture, e.g. after possible contact with a source of microbes (germs); wash hands with liquid soap and warm water for 10–15 seconds, dry thoroughly with paper towels then follow with alcohol hand rub. An alternative would be to use an antiseptic solution, e.g. 7.5% povidone–iodine (Betadine), 4% chlorhexidine gluconate (Hibiscrub) and warm water, and then dry thoroughly with paper towels (Royal College of Nursing [RCN] 2005b).

Aseptic (sterile) technique

This prevents microbial (bacterial) contamination of susceptible sites by ensuring that only sterile objects and fluids touch them. Aseptic technique must be used when introducing an invasive device such as a sterile needle into the circulatory system, which is a breach of the body's natural defence system (May 2000).

Wilson (2001) and Damani (2003) promoted skin cleansing with either soap and water, and drying thoroughly if visibly dirty, or cleansing proposed venepuncture site with an alcohol swab for at least 30 seconds and allowing to air dry for a further 30 seconds (Black and Hughes 1997).

Protective clothing

In venepuncture, it is appropriate for healthcare assistants to wear non-sterile disposable gloves and a disposable apron. Latex and the associated risks are now widely known and it is advisable to consider the type of glove available and ensure that it minimises exposure to harmful substances (MDA 1996; RCN 2005b). Latex and other risks can affect both patients and staff.

Environment

Good practice requires either a clean trolley or tray to assemble and hold all the necessary sterile equipment and the collection tube(s) (Dougherty and Lister 2004). Adequate lighting is recommended, to enable careful assessment of the patient and veins, as well as the patient being seated or lying on a trolley/bed, so that they are relaxed with the limb supported and are resting safely (Table 12.2).

Reflection point

Identify the common predisposing infection risk factors and describe how to prevent these risks in venepuncture practice.

Performing the skill: requirements and technique

Venepuncture equipment

For equipment using a vacuum system see Figure 12.2 and examples below.

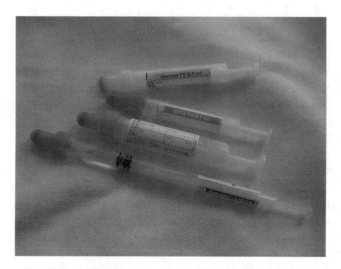

Figure 12.2   Vacuum tubes. (Photograph by I Lavery.)

Examples of venepuncture equipment

- Tourniquet: consider the quick-release type
- Non-sterile gloves
- Apron
- Alcohol wipe, e.g. 70% isopropyl alcohol
- Bactericidal alcohol hand rub, e.g. Hibisol
- Requisition forms and blood specimen bags
- Blood specimen tubes: system as used by local organisation
- Sterile needle: size (gauge) appropriate to the vein and sampling needs, using smallest where possible (RCN 2005b)
- Cotton-wool ball: non-sterile
- Tray or trolley
- Sterile hypoallergenic plaster
- Sharps disposal bin.

Patient safety must be considered in relation to the patient's position when this procedure is being performed, so ensure that the arm is supported (Figure 12.3). Where a patient has a history of fainting during venepuncture, it is advised that the patient should lie down to reduce the possibility of a fall, which could have serious consequences (Black and Hughes 1997). When performing venepuncture it is essential that the healthcare assistant taking blood is competent, because this will also help reduce the risk of avoidable complications occurring (Table 12.3). The equipment used should be considered with regard to allergies and, if the patient is allergic to either latex or plasters, then alternatives sought (Lavery and Ingram 2005).

Winged infusion device, e.g. butterfly option

The option of using a winged infusion device may not be open to all healthcare assistants; *please check local policy and confirm if this practice is taught, supported and supervised before undertaking*. Refer to Table 12.4 for specific guidance on inserting a winged device.

Table 12.2 Guide to good venepuncture practice: vacuum system

Action	Reason
1. Wash hands with liquid soap, and dry hands thoroughly followed by an alcohol hand rub, or wash with an approved antiseptic solution	To minimise the risk of healthcare-associated infection
2. Assemble the equipment required for the procedure on a trolley or a tray. Ensure that all equipment and disposables used are intact and within their expiry dates	Procedure is carried out safely, efficiently and without interruptions To maintain asepsis during the procedure
3. Identify the tests on the requisition form and select the appropriate blood collection tubes	To ensure correct sampling
4. Allow the patient time to ask questions and express concerns about the procedure	To obtain patient consent and cooperation
5. Identify the patient, check the addressograph label or written details on the requisition form and ensure that it corresponds with the details on the patient's identity wristband Check all details verbally by actively asking the patient to state their name and date of birth (DOB) Where a patient is unable to verbally state their name and DOB, good practice suggests that two staff check the identity bracelet against health records and requisition form(s)	To ensure the blood specimen is taken from the patient indicated on the request form To ensure all details are correct
6. Help the patient into a comfortable position either sitting in a chair or lying on the bed. The arm must be supported in an extended (straight) position	To enable the healthcare assistant to carry out the procedure with ease and maintain the patient's comfort
7. Prepare the area, e.g. provide adequate lighting, and heighten the bed, lower cot sides	To ensure a safe working environment

Adapted from NHS Lothian (2007).

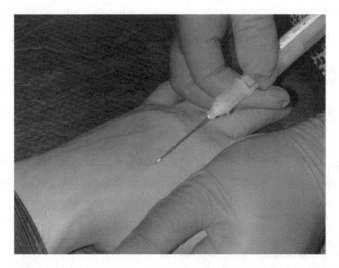

Figure 12.3 Insertion technique example. (Photograph by I Lavery.)

Table 12.3 Specific actions and observations during the procedure

Action	Reason
1. Wash hands with liquid soap, and dry hands thoroughly followed by an alcohol hand rub, or wash with an approved antiseptic solution	To minimise the risk of healthcare-associated infection
2. Identify the patient's own preferred site for the procedure based on their previous experience	To actively involve the patient in their treatment. To familiarise the healthcare assistant with the patient's medical history and factors that may influence choice of vein
3. Apply a tourniquet to the upper arm on the chosen side approx 7–10 cm (3–4 inches) above the puncture site	Increases venous pressure to help vein identification and entry. Careful attention is paid to length of time tourniquet is left on (No more than $1^1/_2$ min or can cause an adverse effect, as below)
4. Apply enough pressure to impede (slow) venous circulation but not arterial blood flow, check for arterial pulse	Prolonged pressure may lead to vein spasm, pain and haematoma (blood in the tissues)
5. To further encourage venous filling consider: • Allow their arm to hang at the patient's side • Stroke vein lightly • Ask the patient to wash their hands or place in warm/hot water • Ask patient to assist by clenching and unclenching their hand	Aid vein filling and make procedure easier *Take care because this may affect some results, so not recommended*
6. Observe and palpate (feel) the selected vein	To identify its course, depth and distinguish structures such as tendons, and to avoid nearby arteries
7. Release the tourniquet. Check that the vein has decompressed (a thrombosed vein will remain firm and palpable)	Reduce the length of time that tourniquet is *in situ* (see 3) Check for a thrombosed (clotted) vein.
8. Push the tube into the needle adaptor by twisting clock-wise	Opens the system
9. Wash hands with liquid soap, and dry hands thoroughly followed by an alcohol hand rub, or wash with an approved antiseptic solution Put on gloves	To minimise the risk of healthcare associated infection. Gloves are worn for the protection of staff against blood spillage. They will not protect against needlestick injuries
10. Ensure the patient's skin is clean. Wash with soap and water and dry thoroughly if visibly dirty Use alcohol wipe if deemed appropriate, but essential for blood cultures. *Check local policy* If using alcohol wipe, cleanse the site in a circular movement from the proposed puncture site for 30 s, then allow to air dry for 30 s	To minimise the risk of infection from the patient's own skin during this invasive procedure Recommended in hospital patients, but may not be required in a community setting
11. Reapply the tourniquet to the identified site	Encourage venous filling
12. Inspect the needle	To ensure needle is sharp with no barbs (hooks)
13. With the patient's arm in a downward position, line up the needle and collection tube with the vein from which the blood will be drawn. Using the thumb or first finger of free hand anchor the vein by applying manual traction of the skin 2–5 cm below the proposed insertion site. With the bevel of the needle upward insert the needle into the vein. A sensation of resistance will be felt followed by the needle entering the vein	To hold the vein steady and provide countertension, which will facilitate a smooth needle entry

Table 12.3 (*Continued*)

Action	Reason
14. Advance the needle a further 1–2 mm into the vein	To stabilise the needle within the vein and prevent it becoming dislodged
15. Secure the needle by holding the guide sheath firmly	To prevent movement of the needle in or out of the vein
16. Using the syringe technique for the initial specimen, fill the blood collection tube by slowly pulling back the plunger, keeping the needle in centre of the vein	To ensure appropriate filling of blood sample tube
17. Remove the tube from the needle by twisting anticlockwise (grip the needle guide sleeve firmly). The needle remains in the vein. Secure next prepared tube onto the needle by twisting clockwise	To minimise the movement of needle and prevent mechanical phlebitis (infection due to friction)
18. The second and subsequent samples may be taken either by the syringe technique or alternatively by the vacuum principle where there is good venous supply Remove the final tube from the needle	To aid blood sampling procedure To ensure system 'closed'
19. Release the tourniquet	To release venous congestion Ensure it is not left on
20. Then slip the cotton wool ball down over the puncture site and do not apply pressure until needle has been fully removed Once removed, apply firm finger pressure until bleeding stops (approximately 2 minutes). Do not allow the patient to bend the arm	Prevent bleeding and haematoma formation To prevent pain on removal Prolonged finger (digital) pressure may be required if treatment and/or medical condition interferes with clotting mechanisms Prevent shearing to vein, which causes more bleeding/bruising
21. Once venepuncture site has stopped bleeding, if required, cover site with an Elastoplast dressing, or hypoallergenic dressing if patient has an allergy	To prevent leakage of blood until healing is complete
22. Make no more than two attempts to obtain blood sample/s. If unsuccessful, obtain assistance from more experienced staff	Patient comfort Prevent trauma to vein
23. Ensure the patient is comfortable. Advise the patient to inform staff if venepuncture site starts to bleed or is tender or painful, and when to remove any dressing applied Explain to the patient that results may take some time to come back and that they will be informed when they are available	Reduce anxieties
24. Complete the labels on the blood samples you have taken prior to leaving the patient/bedside, checking details with the patient and the blood forms	Ensure that blood samples are correctly labelled

Adapted with permission from NHS Lothian (2007).

Additional requirements for winged infusion device

- Butterfly 21 or 23 gauge, size depending on patient's vein, i.e. 23 gauge for a frail elderly patient with small veins
- Adaptor: see Figure 12.4
- Tape for securing butterfly.

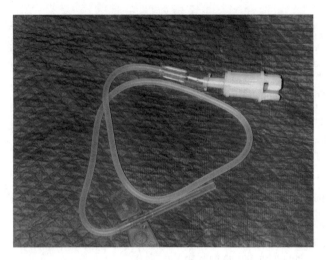

Figure 12.4   Winged device and adaptor. (Photograph by I Lavery.)

Table 12.4 Guide to good practice and winged device (butterfly) insertion

Action	Reason
1. Assess and prepare patient as 1–12 in Table 12.3	
2. Attach adaptor to the tail of the butterfly before attaching the first tube. Fold up wings of butterfly and insert needle into vein as detailed in 13–14 in Table 12.3 (Figure 12.5); bring the device level with skin and then advance along length of the needle, keeping it level and in line with the vein	To prevent blood spillage or leakage
3. Flatten the wings of the butterfly to the skin and secure with Micropore tape	To prevent dislodgement of the butterfly during specimen collection
4. Collect the first specimen using the syringe technique	
5. Complete procedure as 16–24 in Table 12.3	

Blood cultures – samples to check for blood infections

Some practice areas only use senior and experienced healthcare staff in blood culture sampling, *so again please check local policy and practice prior to undertaking this procedure, if an accepted role.*

Box 12.2 Additional requirements; (for vacuum system)

- Blood culture set (aerobic and anaerobic bottles)
- Three needles
- Two alcohol wipes
- 20 ml syringe and adaptor (Figure 12.7)

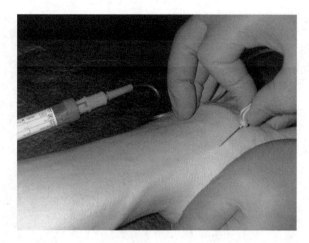

Figure 12.5   Insertion technique. (Photograph by I Lavery.)

Ernst (2001) said that the most common cause of contamination occurred when a practitioner touched the prepared site and suggested the use of mental markers, e.g. freckles, to reduce this urge.

The ideal volume for an adult is 20 ml evenly distributed between both collection bottles, and not exceeding 12 ml (Ernst 2001). Ernst (2001) also proposes that, if the yield is less than 20 ml, it is better to load (fill) 10 ml into the aerobic bottle (e.g. blue), because 98% of septicaemias are caused by aerobic (need oxygen) organisms, and most of the causative organisms can still be detected, even if the anaerobic (e.g. pink) bottle has less than the optimum volume. Overfilling can lead to false positives, so take care when filling. However, fill the anaerobic (e.g. pink) bottle first, to minimise the risk of air in the syringe getting in and altering the anaerobic (oxygen not needed) environment (Ernst 2001).

If a blood culture sample is falsely positive, due to incorrect skin cleansing or contamination from the healthcare assistant's hands, then a patient could have an increased length of hospital stay, which increases costs, with the associated risk of infection. The patient may require transfer, if thought to be septicaemic (bacteria in the blood), suffer the unnecessary use of antibiotics and the increased risks associated with this. The intravenous (IV) route would be preferred to treat septicaemia, and so would also incur increased costs and pressure on staff time. Thus the longer a patient is in hospital, the more admissions will be restricted, putting more pressure on to limited beds. Therefore extra care is needed when sampling for blood cultures (Table 12.5) (Lavery and Ingram 2005).

 Reflection point

Consider if skin surface bacteria contaminate a sample for blood culture. What might be the outcome for the patient and the service?

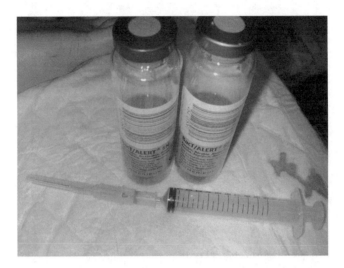

Figure 12.6   Example of blood culture set. (Photograph by I Lavery.)

Table 12.5 Blood Cultures: good practice guide

Action	Reason
1. Cleanse the proposed venepuncture site as per Table 12.3, Step 10	To prevent contamination of blood sample from microorganisms on the skin
2. Do not re-palpate the vein after the site has been cleansed	As above
3. Remove flip top cap from bottles, wipe the tops with fresh alcohol wipe, allow to dry, then insert clean needle into each	Preventing contamination of the sample
4. Withdraw 20 ml of blood (1–3 ml in neonates) from the adult patient using technique described in Table 12.3	Adequate sample for laboratory testing
5. Fill both bottles and divide blood equally, 10 ml in each	Ensure adequate sample size
6. Dispose of sharps immediately into sharps container	Reducing the possibility of a needlestick injury
7. Decontaminate (cleanse) hands	Preventing infection
8. Minimum data required on samples are surname, forename, date of birth, gender, date and time of sample, type and site of sample, location of patient	Ensuring that laboratory has correct information
9. Minimum data are also required on request form, addressographs can be used including the time and date of sampling; if high risk (e.g. HIV), any antibiotic therapy and relevant clinical details	Ensuring that laboratory has the correct and appropriate information
10. Arrange for transport to the laboratory, if not available immediately, e.g. night-time, leave cultures at room temperature	Appropriate storage of blood cultures

Adapted with permission from NHS Lothian (2007).

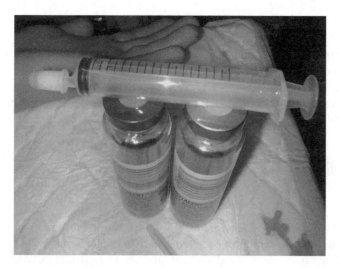

Figure 12.7 Adaptor. (Photograph by I Lavery.)

Related aspects and terminology

Consent

Lavery (2003) stated that, for consent to be valid, it must be given voluntarily and freely, e.g. without influence or undue pressure to accept or refuse treatment. With venepuncture it is sometimes thought that patients have consented when their actions demonstrate this, e.g. turning up for an appointment or simply rolling up a sleeve and presenting an arm to the healthcare assistant. Despite patients perhaps having a basic knowledge of the procedure, it is important that the healthcare assistant explore the patient's understanding relating to the need for the blood test (Lavery and Ingram 2005). For more discussion on consent refer to Chapters 1 and 4.

Anxiety

In an effort to reduce anxiety, patients should be asked whether they have had venepuncture performed previously. Attention should be paid particularly where there were any adverse (poor) outcomes or experiences, so that reassurance or further action can be taken.

With regard to the actual procedure, anxiety can be caused by a previous bad experience, a degree of 'needle phobia' (fear of a needle) or just a dislike of medical procedures. The RCN (2005a) noted the need for skilled practice that minimised pain and anxiety in relation to children or young people, but can be seen as good practice for all. Willock et al. (2004) have shown distraction to be an effective and useful coping strategy, particularly in older children, and could easily be taught to adults, e.g. asking a patient to concentrate on breathing can relax and distract.

Another method to reduce the pain of venepuncture is the use of topical (skin) creams/gels acting as local anaesthetics (Neal 1997). Despite having cost implications, they are widely used in children and could be used for anxious adults. However, for some healthcare assistants this may be out with their role, because these creams/gels must be prescribed (unless through a patient group direction/approved protocol), and administered as a medicine. *Please check your local policy.*

Common problems

Unsuccessful sampling

This may be due to poor vein assessment, incorrect choice of sampling device or poor technique. Careful review of veins and technique before starting the procedure, as well as consideration of patient comfort and position, is necessary to prevent this. Table 12.6 is a competency framework for venepuncture.

Potential complications of venepuncture

Bruising

This is caused by the infiltration (leakage) of blood into the tissues, and can be due to unskilled venepuncture technique or a patient bleeding easily, e.g. older people with friable thin veins, or patients on treatments that affect blood clotting, e.g. warfarin (RCN 2005b).

Bruising is preventable by the following:

- Accurate identification of a suitable vein
- The correct insertion technique and angle
- Ensuring that the tourniquet is not applied with excessive pressure or below previous puncture sites
- 'Fixing' the vein position by skin traction during the insertion of the needle
- Ensuring adequate pressure to the puncture site after needle removal, which will prevent further damage (Campbell 1995).

Accurate monitoring of the site and documentation of the bruise is also necessary.

Haematoma

This is caused by a collection of blood that leaks from a vein into the tissues surrounding the puncture site, and can result from poor technique, e.g. overshooting the vein (going through rear vein wall) (RCN 2005b). Other causes are inadequate pressure to the puncture site or failing to remove the tourniquet before removing the needle. It is preventable by appropriate assessment of the patient and vein, and planning of the procedure.

If a haematoma occurs during the procedure, remove the tube, release the tourniquet and then remove the needle, apply firm pressure for 2–3 min and elevate the arm (Black and Hughes 1997). Again, documentation is crucial and monitoring of the site and reassurance for the patient.

Excessive pain

This can be caused by the frequent use of a vein, or poor technique, i.e. blind plunging manoeuvres (without feeling/assessing for vein); where a nerve or valve is touched; or if the patient is anxious, fearful, or has a low pain threshold.

This is preventable by:

- ensuring that the patient is comfortable and the arm supported
- allowing the alcohol to dry at the skin site
- carrying out the procedure in a confident unhurried manner.

Consider the use of local anaesthetic cream; Black and Hughes (1997) noted that this should be prescribed individually, or under a patient group direction. *Please check your local practice and policy, because it may not be within a healthcare assistants role to apply local anaesthetic cream/gel.*

Reassurance is crucial and using diversion can also be effective, i.e. asking patients to concentrate on breathing can distract and relax them. Explanations will also aid in relaxing patients and is good practice to ensure that patients are aware and consent to the procedure (RCN 2005b). Again good practice necessitates documentation and observation, whilst, in the case of possible nerve damage, medical intervention must be sought immediately, as well as reporting this to the nurse in charge promptly.

Arterial puncture

This is caused by poor technique or inadequate assessment and the healthcare assistant would see bright red blood pulsating into the tube and needle. Prevention is by:

- thorough assessment of the site
- the use of the correct insertion technique and angle.

The management would be to immediately remove the needle and apply prolonged finger pressure for 5 minutes and then a pressure bandage for at least a further 5 minutes. The patient should be under observation, assessment and medical supervision, whilst recording the incident in the patient's case notes and following local adverse incident reporting mechanisms and reporting to nurse in charge (RCN 2005b).

Fibrosis

This is where the vein becomes hard or cord-like and may occur with prolonged use of one site. Prevent by:

- careful assessment
- rotation of sites.

Phlebitis

This is an infection caused by mechanical irritation (needle rubbing inside the vein) or poor aseptic technique, and is considered a rare complication in venepuncture. Prevention is by:

- following sound infection control practice (Franklin 1999)
- not re-palpating the vein after cleansing the site with alcohol.

Ongoing site monitoring and documentation are critical, as is investigation to identify the cause and plan the steps for future prevention.

 Reflection point

What action should be taken if an artery is punctured?
What preventive measures should have been considered?

Summary

Venepuncture is a common procedure, especially in the hospital setting, and can be carried out by a range of healthcare professionals, e.g., doctor, registered nurse, healthcare assistant or phlebotomist. Thus effective communication and prompt recording are critical for safe patient care.

Case study 12.1

Mr Robert Walls is an older man aged 90 years and requires samples for full blood count (FBC) and urea and electrolytes (U&Es).

He is frail and dehydrated after a fall, and has an intravenous infusion running into his left median cubital vein. He has a residual weakness in his right arm from a previous stroke (cerebral vascular accident). He is restless and upset at being in hospital, and slightly confused.

Outline the assessment process here and discuss the choice of venepuncture device and describe why chosen.

Below is a self-assessment checklist; however, you may also wish to review Skills for Health (2004) competence HSC376.

  ## Self-assessment

Assessment	Aspects	Achieved ✔
Patient	*Have you considered all aspects of this section?*	
	Patient assessment: veins and general condition	
	Infection control and asepsis aspects	
	Consent, communication and education	
	Problem solving	
Procedure	*Have you considered all aspects of this section?*	**Achieved ✔**
	Equipment selection and insertion technique	
	Recording and labelling	
	Reporting concerns	
	Problem solving	
	Disposal of equipment	
Winged device	*Have you considered all aspects of this section?*	**Achieved ✔**
	Selection and insertion of butterfly	
	Recording and labelling	
	Reporting concerns	
	Problem solving	
	Disposal of equipment	
Blood cultures	*Have you considered all aspects of this section?*	**Achieved ✔**
	Infection control and procedure	
	Disposal of equipment	

Table 12.6 Competency framework: venepuncture

	First assessment/reassessment				
Steps	**Demonstration/Supervised practice**				
Venepuncture	Date/sign	Date/sign	Date/sign	Date/sign	**Date/competent signature**
	1	**2**	**3**	**4**	**5**
1 Gives explanation of procedure and obtains patient's verbal consent					
2 Selects appropriate equipment and sample tubes					
3 Correctly identifies the patient against the request form					
4 Ensures patient comfort and privacy					
5 Reassures patient, and uses anxiety relieving measures (if appropriate)					
6 Hands washed, gloves and apron worn					
7 Uses appropriate methods to encourage good venous filling					
8 Identifies appropriate vein for venepuncture					
9 Prepares patient's skin as per local policy					
10 Carries out procedure successfully					
11 Removes last sample tube and tourniquet before removing needle					
12 Disposes of sharps immediately					
13 Applies pressure and seals puncture site					
14 Labels and packages samples correctly for transport					
15 Records information in patient's notes					

Supervisor/assessor(s):

References

Black F, Hughes J (1997) Venepuncture. *Nursing Standard* **11**(41): 49–55.

Campbell J (1995) Making sense of the technique of venepuncture. *Nursing Times* **91**(31): 29–31.

Damani NN (2003) *Manual of Infection Control Procedures*, 2nd edn. London: Greenwich Medical Media.

Dougherty L, Lister S, eds (2004) *The Royal Marsden Hospital Manual of Clinical Nursing Procedures*, 6th edn. Oxford: Blackwell Publishing.

Ernst DJ (2001) The right way to do blood cultures. *Nursing Journal for Registered Nurses* **64**(3): 28–32.

Franklin L (1999) Skin cleansing and infection control in peripheral venepuncture and cannulation. *Nursing Standard* **14**(4): 49–50.

Lavery I (2003) Peripheral intravenous cannulation and patient consent. *Nursing Standard* **17**(28): 40–42.

Lavery I, Ingram P (2005) Venepuncture: Best practice. *Nursing Standard* **19**(49): 55–65.

May D (2000) Infection control. *Nursing Standard* **14**(28): 51–59.

Medical Devices Agency (1996) *Sterilisation Disinfection and Cleaning of Medical Equipment: Guidance on decontamination from the Medical Advisory Committee to the DH (111)*. London: The Stationery Office.

Medical Devices Agency (2000) *Single-use Medical Devices: Implications and consequences of re-use. MDA DB2000 (04)*. London: The Stationery Office.

NHS Lothian (2007) *Adult Venepuncture and/or Peripheral IV Cannulation*. Clinical Skills Education Package. Edinburgh: NHS Lothian.

Neal M (1997) *Medical Pharmacology at a Glance*, 3rd edn. Oxford: Blackwell Science.

Royal College of Nursing (2005a) *Competencies: An education and training competency framework for capillary blood sampling and venepuncture in children and young people*. London: RCN.

Royal College of Nursing (2005b) *Standards for Infusion Therapy*. London: RCN.

Skills for Health (2004) *HSC376 Obtain Venous Blood Samples (level 3)*. Bristol: Skills for Health. Available at: www.skillsforhealth.org.uk/tools/view_framework.php?id=39 (accessed 2 September 2007).

Tortora GJ, Derrickson B (2006) *Principles of Anatomy and Physiology*, 11th edn. Hoboken, NJ: John Wiley & Sons Inc.

Willock J, Richardson J, Brazier A, Powell G, Mitchell E (2004) Peripheral venepuncture in infants and children. *Nursing Standard* **18**(27): 43–50.

Wilson J (2001) *Clinical Microbiology: An introduction for healthcare professionals*. London: Baillière Tindall.

Chapter 13

Blood glucose monitoring

Learning objectives

- Explain what causes diabetes
- Define the different types of diabetes
- List the common symptoms and risk factors
- Describe complications associated with diabetes
- Describe how to measure and record accurate blood sugar levels using appropriate equipment.

Aim of this chapter

The aim of this chapter is to understand the fundamental principles of diabetes and apply this to the skill of measuring blood glucose.

What causes diabetes?

Diabetes occurs when the hormone insulin is not functioning normally or is deficient. This results in varying degrees of failure to metabolise and store glucose and a resulting high blood glucose level. There are two main types of diabetes, type 1 and type 2, both of which are described later (Sewell 2007).

Reasons for performing blood glucose measurement

Blood glucose monitoring is performed in a number of settings: primary care, the acute hospital setting and the patient's own home. Near patient testing is a convenient and quick way to obtain blood glucose measurements without sending samples to the laboratory. To ensure that readings are accurate and reduce the number of significant risks of error, staff must have obtained competency in the skill (Department of Health [DH] 1996). Blood glucose levels are carried out for a variety of reasons and these are shown in Box 13.1.

There are benefits to patients keeping their blood glucose levels within acceptable limits and these include the patient:

- running a smaller risk of developing complications (Wallymahmed 2007) (see later)
- feeling more active and healthy
- having better clinical outcomes if they have an acute cardiovascular event, e.g. myocardial infarction (heart attack) or stroke (Malmberg et al. 1995).

Box 13.1 Reasons for taking blood glucose measurements

- Monitoring diabetic control and identifying unstable diabetic states (Dougherty and Lister 2004)
- Monitoring patients who are receiving enteral/parenteral feeding (feeding through a tube, e.g. nasogastric tube into the stomach).
- Liver disease or pancreatitis (where pancreatic tissue is destroyed) (Waugh and Grant 2001)
- Where the patient has sustained a head injury or is unconscious
- After a stroke, myocardial infarct (heart attack) or other cardiovascular event
- If the patient has alcohol or drug intoxication
- Seizures
- Due to side effects of some medication, e.g. steroid-induced diabetes (Dougherty and Lister 2004)
- Serious infection (sepsis)

Adapted from Ferguson (2005).

In order to fully understand diabetes, and the importance of blood glucose monitoring, revision of the anatomy and physiology of the pancreas is necessary.

Relevant anatomy and physiology

The pancreas

The pancreas is situated in the abdominal cavity with the head nesting in the curve of the duodenum (part of the small intestine). It is a pale grey/pink gland that consists of a broad head, body and narrow tail (Tortora and Derrickson 2006). It weighs up to 100 g and is 12–15 cm long (Thibodeau and Patton 2007). Figure 13.1 shows the position of the pancreas in relation to other organs. The adrenal glands produce steroid hormones which are essential for wellbeing and maintenance of life (Tortora and Derrickson 2006).

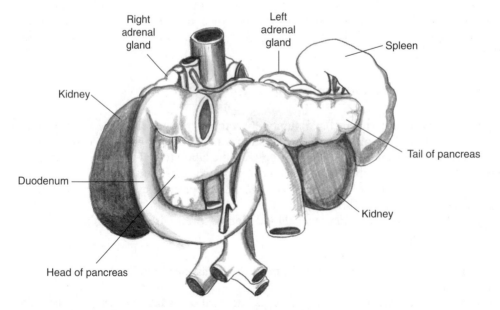

Figure 13.1   Pancreas shown in relation to the kidneys, duodenum and adrenal glands.

The pancreas has both an endocrine and an exocrine function: endocrine means excretion of substances directly into the bloodstream, in this case insulin, and exocrine means excretion via ducts and refers to digestive juices.

Only 2% of the pancreas fulfils the endocrine function and this is performed by collections of cells found in clusters irregularly distributed throughout the pancreas, known as the islets of Langerhans. Within the islets of Langerhans there are two types of cells: α (alpha) cells that produce glucagon and β (beta) cells that produce insulin. The body balances these two hormones to maintain a healthy blood glucose level and Figure 13.2 illustrates the variance in their roles.

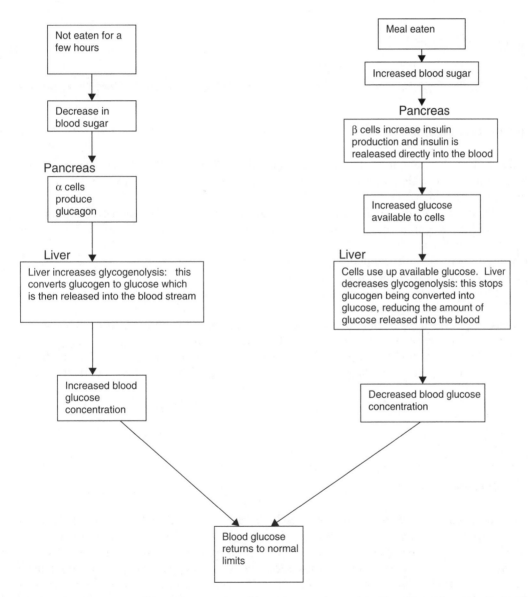

Figure 13.2 Maintenance of blood glucose. Adapted from Tortora and Derrickson (2006), Marieb and Hoehn (2007) and Thibodeau and Patton (2007).)

Related aspects and terminology

Effects of diabetes

Figure 13.2 demonstrates how the body maintains normal blood glucose levels despite periods of fasting or eating. In diabetes, the blood glucose level remains high after the intake of a carbohydrate meal due to defective glucose metabolism by body cells, thus glucose cannot cross the cell membrane and be absorbed by the body. Conversion of glucose to glycogen in the liver and muscles is diminished leading to protein being broken down instead.

Reflection point

List some signs or symptoms of diabetes

Common terminology

- *Blood glucose*: the amount of glucose (sometimes also called 'sugar') in the circulating blood.
- *Hypoglycaemia*: low blood glucose (see later). This is sometimes referred to as a 'hypo'.
- *Hyperglycaemia*: high blood glucose (see later).
- *DKA (diabetic ketoacidosis)*: dangerously high blood glucose levels (see later). This can result in the patient being in a coma, and may well be the first symptom to be noticed prior to a diagnosis of diabetes.
- *Polydipsia*: increased thirst/appetite (Tortora and Derrickson 2006).
- *Polyphagia*: excess eating (Tortora and Derrickson 2006)
- *Polyuria*: frequently needing to pass urine (micturition) due to excessive urine production, and the kidneys unable to reabsorb excess water (Tortora and Derrickson 2006).
- *Ketonuria*: ketones (a byproduct of red blood cells) present in the patient's urine. This is why people with diabetes often test their urine for both ketones and glucose.
- *HbA1c (glycated haemoglobin)*: percentage of haemoglobin bound to glucose. This is shown in a blood sample that is taken to monitor how well controlled the patient's diabetes is (see later).

Types of diabetes

Type 1 diabetes

This usually occurs as a result of the progressive destruction of β cells, within the islets of Langerhans, which leads to insulin deficiency (Sewell 2007). Type 1 diabetes is thought to be triggered by a variety of environmental factors, e.g. a prolonged period of ill-health, ingestion of certain toxins, dramatic change in life circumstances and perhaps a genetic predisposition (Currie 2007a). The presence of infection can also result in damage to some cells and the subsequent production of antibodies as part of the autoimmune response. Despite these antibodies being detectable before the symptoms of type 1 diabetes become apparent, the antibodies usually disappear within months of the diagnosis (Currie 2007a). Other symptoms of diabeties usually only appear once 80–85% of all the β cells have been destroyed. The disease is usually of sudden onset in young adults or children, with the cause being generally unknown. The only treatment option for a patient with type 1 diabetes is subcutaneous insulin replacement therapy and the condition cannot be cured, only managed.

Symptoms of type 1 diabetes

- Polydipsia
- Polyuria
- Polyphagia
- Weight loss, due to the body not being able to release insulin, which prevents glucose being released (Tortora and Derrickson 2006)
- Increased incidence of infection
- Lethargy (extreme tiredness)
- Symptoms of ketoacidosis (see below): collapse, reduced consciousness, restlessness, leading to coma and death if undetected.

Ketoacidosis

Diabetic ketoacidosis is the result of very low or zero insulin levels, and generally only occurs in type 1 diabetes, because patients with type 2 diabetes have sufficient reserves to prevent this occurring (Hand 2000). If it does occur in type 2 diabetes, this is provoked by severe illness (Wallymahmed 2007). The signs and symptoms are listed below.

Signs and symptoms of ketoacidosis (Wallymahmed 2007)

- Hyperglycaemia
- Ketonuria
- Polyuria
- Polydipsia
- Acetone: this is excreted in the patient's breath, and diagnosis would be identifying a sweet smell, often likened to the smell of 'pear drops', on the patient's breath.

Type 2 diabetes

Type 2 diabetes is related to both reduced insulin sensitivity (insulin resistance) and impaired B-cell function (Currie 2007a). It is the most common form of diabetes and occurs in around 90% of cases of diabetes in the developed world (Sewell 2007). The exact cause is unknown, but genetic factors are thought to have some role in its development, as well as age, ethnicity and lifestyle factors (Sewell 2007). The disease is usually late onset and can often be undiagnosed for many years, so in some instances the complications of diabetes will present rather than the disease. Insulin secretion may be below or above normal, but deficiency of glucose inside body cells leads to hyperglycaemia and a high insulin level. This may be due to changes in cell membranes, which block the insulin-assisted movement of glucose into cells.

Symptoms of type 2 diabetes

- Tiredness
- Blurred vision, this may be due to complications (see below) (Cradock 1996)
- Dry skin
- Increased appetite and thirst
- More frequently needing to pass urine (micturition).

Maturity-onset diabetes in the young (MODY)

This is a form of type 2 diabetes and is due to a β-cell defect that reduces the insulin secretion in response to specific blood glucose levels, rather than insulin resistance. Currie (2007a) reports that it requires strict diagnostic criteria, including: diagnosis before the age of 25 years, no requirement for insulin therapy 5 years after diagnosis and a previous familial history spanning several generations.

Gestational diabetes (during pregnancy)

Diabetes can occur for the first time during pregnancy, presenting during the third trimester (last months of pregnancy) (Bewley 2002; Sewell 2007). After delivery of the baby, glucose tolerance returns to normal. However, it is thought that, if gestational diabetes is experienced, the development of type 2 diabetes later in life is more common (Sonksen et al. 2001). Treatment involves dietary control and insulin, if required, because the use of oral diabetic medication during pregnancy is not recommended (Wallymahmed 2007).

Blood glucose levels

Blood glucose testing is used for all types of diabetes, because it is both accurate and reliable. The blood glucose level shows how well diet, insulin and exercise have been balanced. The measurement is in millimoles of glucose per litre of blood and is abbreviated to mmol/l (Sonksen et al. 2001). Long-term diabetic control can be monitored by measuring glycated haemoglobin (HbA1c). This substance can assist in reflecting blood glucose control over the past 2–3 months (Wallymahmed 2007). Depending on individual circumstances, this level is recommended to be between 6.5% and 7.5% (National Institute for Health and Clinical Excellence [NICE] 2002). This is particularly useful because, even if an individual feels well, this does not necessarily mean good blood glucose control (Sonksen et al. 2001).

In individuals without diabetes, blood glucose levels do not tend to drop >3 mmol, even if fasting, and likewise do not rise >10 mmol, despite increased food input. The desired range for patients with diabetes is shown in Box 13.2.

Box 13.2 Desired blood glucose levels for patients with diabetes

- Before meals: 4–7 mmol
- 90 minutes after meals: <10 mmol
- Bedtime: around 8 mmol

From Campbell and Song (2007).

Sites for blood glucose testing

The best site is the side of the finger, no lower down than the nailbed. The use of fleshy fingertips is discouraged due to their sensitivity, and may cause further desensitisation in some patients who are already experiencing a lack of sensation there (Ferguson 2005). The thumb and forefingers should be avoided if possible, because these are important for dexterity. Fleshy earlobes are used less commonly despite being less sensitive, and where patients are performing this procedure themselves they will require a mirror. This site can also be used by healthcare professionals undertaking this role, provided that training is given. *Check local policies and procedures for further advice on using this site.*

Rotation of the site for drawing blood ensures good health at all sites, and it is recommended that the patient or staff record the site for future reference.

Patients with diabetes will often become very skilled at taking and assessing their own blood glucose levels (Cradock 1996), so wherever possible patients should be encouraged to continue to take their own blood glucose levels while in hospital. If equipment varies from their home equipment some patient education may be required.

Equipment

Often in the acute hospital environment there is a standard meter to reduce confusion between models. However, staff in the community may be exposed to a variety of different meters because patients often purchase these themselves. There are a variety of kits available for both home and hospital use. Figure 13.3 shows an example of an Advantage meter made by Roche.

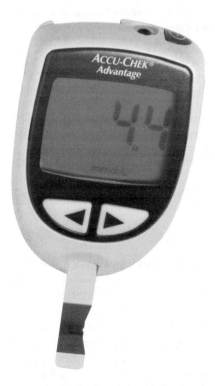

Figure 13.3   Advantage blood glucose meter by Roche. Permission kindly given by Roche.

Competency-based training and comprehensive reading of the manufacturer's instructions regarding both the meter and the associated test strips are essential to ensure safe and accurate measurement. Many meters require regular quality assurance checks to guarantee accuracy of the readings and these checks should be documented. The Department of Health (1987) has issued hazard warnings about training and quality control when measuring blood glucose, because there have been fatal errors. In addition, the Medical Devices Agency (MDA 2002) issued recommendations advising that education, training and ensuring understanding of the quality control measures are necessary for safe blood glucose monitoring.

Reflection point

Imagine that you are going to take your own blood sugar level. What anxieties would you have? If you get permission to perform a blood glucose reading on yourself, how did it feel? Consider physical, emotional and psychological aspects.

Taking a blood glucose sample

When considering taking a blood glucose level there are certain contraindications that have been identified and these are listed in Box 13.3.

Box 13.3 Contraindications to blood glucose levels

- Peripheral circulatory failure and severe dehydration, e.g. diabetic ketoacidosis, non-ketotic coma, shock and hypotension (low blood pressure). In these situations capillary blood glucose readings can be artificially low due to peripheral shut down (reduced blood to peripheral areas)
- Haematocrit (red blood cells) values >55% may lead to inaccurate results if the blood glucose level is >11 mmol/l
- Intravenous infusion of ascorbic acid
- Pre-eclampsia: a condition in pregnancy where the placenta is low lying
- Some treatments for renal dialysis
- Hyperlipidaemia (increased fat levels): cholesterol levels >13 mmol/l may lead to artificially raised capillary blood glucose readings.

It would not be expected that a healthcare assistant would identify these contraindications, but it may assist in explaining the treatment plans for some patients. Blood samples for glucose measurement can be capillary, venous or arterial (Dougherty and Lister 2004). Capillary blood is the blood obtained by using a lancing device and is described later. To obtain venous blood the patient would require blood to be taken from their veins (see Chapter 12), which would involve an invasive procedure. An arterial sample would be obtained if the patient has either a central line or similar in place, e.g. in an intensive care unit (ICU). Table 13.1 describes the procedure for taking a capillary blood sample to measure blood glucose.

Usually the role of the healthcare assistant will be to carry out the procedure following guidance from either nursing or medical staff. This will be based on many factors, some of which are detailed in Box 13.4.

Reflection point

A patient with type 1 diabetes is having hip replacement surgery tomorrow. What factors do you think should be considered for this patient with regard to their diabetic control?

Documentation

Results may be recorded in the patient's case notes, the patient's own documents or, if an inpatient, on a specific blood glucose chart.

Hypoglycaemia

This is when the blood glucose level is <4.0 mmol/l, occurring with or without symptoms (Table 13.2). If it is not possible to test the blood glucose, but symptoms are experienced, immediate action (treatment) should be considered. It is sometimes abbreviated to 'hypo'.

Symptoms

The symptoms of hypoglycaemia occur when glucose levels drop, which triggers hormones that result in early onset symptoms; if left untreated it leads to severe symptoms (see Table 13.2).

The causes of hypoglycaemia can be varied and are shown in Box 13.5. These causes should be taught to patients because taking preventive steps could prevent hypoglycaemia occurring.

To ensure patient safety and prevention of late symptoms, where possible treatment should be prompt. Table 13.3 gives the series of actions that should be undertaken, *but check local policy for any variations*.

Reflection point

If a patient is hypoglycaemic, explain why a diet drink would not be effective.

Table 13.1 Procedure for taking blood glucose measurements using a capillary blood sample

Action	Rationale
Before the procedure Collect the required equipment:	
• Blood glucose monitor – check that it is clean, has been calibrated for use with the test strips and has had the quality control test performed and documented (Dougherty and Lister 2004)	A clean meter will prevent cross-infection; follow local policy if it requires cleaning
	Calibration will ensure the meter is fit for purpose and gives accurate readings
• Test strips, ensure that they are in date and have not been exposed to air (Dougherty and Lister 2004)	To ensure accurate readings
	To prevent cross-infection
• Single-use disposable finger-pricking device or lancets (DH 1990; Dougherty and Lister 2004)	To stop bleeding at site
• Cotton wool or sterile gauze (Ferguson 2005)	To prevent needlestick injury
• Sharps container	To prevent cross-infection
• Gloves/apron (Ferguson 2005)	
The procedure	
1. Describe the procedure to the patient and gain consent Explain that some patients want to look away at the sight of a lancing device (Dougherty and Lister 2004)	To get cooperation from the patient, ensure that they understand the procedure fully
	Patient comfort and safety; some patients may faint when blood is taken (Dougherty and Lister 2004)
2. Ask the patient to wash and dry their hands with soap and water (Dougherty and Lister 2004)	Prevention of cross-infection (Dougherty and Lister 2004; Wallymahmed 2007)
3. Position the patient comfortably – either lying down or sitting up	For patient comfort
4. Wash own hands and put on protective gloves and an apron (Ferguson 2005; Wallymahmed 2007)	Prevention of infection
5. Massage the finger from its base to its tip to increase its perfusion (blood flow (Burton and Birdi 2006).	
6. Take blood from the side of the finger, using a site that has not been used recently, if possible (Fig. 13.4)	As there are comparatively fewer nerve endings in the side rather than the tip of a finger it is less painful (Burton and Birdi 2006)
The finger may bleed without assistance (Fig. 13.5) or may need to be milked to form a droplet of blood large enough to cover the test pad (Dougherty and Lister 2004; Wallymahmed 2007)	
7. Some strips 'suck' blood up automatically, stopping when the correct volume is obtained whilst others may still require blood to be dropped onto the strip (Wallymahmed 2007)	
8. Read the blood glucose level from the machine, using it as per manufacturer's recommendation.	To provide an accurate reading
9. If there is not enough blood, prick the finger again with a new lancet ensuring the patient is fully informed and offer sympathy to the patient (Burton and Birdi 2006)	To ensure accurate results by using disposables as intended by the manufacturer
After the procedure Immediately dispose of the lancet in the sharps box (Dougherty and Lister 2004; Ferguson 2005; Wallymahmed 2007)	To prevent sharps injury and cross-infection
Apply cotton wool or gauze, with pressure applied	To stop bleeding at the site
When the result is available document into patient's notes/blood glucose chart or patient records, informing the patient	Accurate recording of the results The patient may self-manage their condition and make adjustments themselves to the regimen (Wallymahmed 2007)
Inform the nurse in charge of any abnormal or unusual results (Ferguson 2005)	To allow further intervention if required
Assess the patient clinically, repeating the procedure if they do not appear to correlate (agree) with the results and report to nurse in charge	Incorrect reading, could result in inappropriate management
Dispose of waste as per local policy.	Prevent cross-infection
Observe site for further bleeding, applying further pressure to stop bleeding if necessary	To allow management of any further bleeding
Ensure the patient is comfortable and reassure if necessary	Patient comfort
Wash and dry hands.	Prevent cross-infection

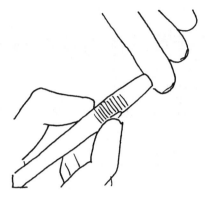

Figure 13.4   Site for blood glucose sampling.

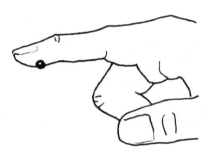

Figure 13.5   Blood specimen for blood glucose testing.

Box 13.4 Factors that influence how often blood glucose should be tested

- Whether the patient has type 1 or type 2 diabetes: patients with type 1 diabetes generally test more often and are advised to test between one and four times per day, but more often on diagnosis or if the patient is unwell (Cradock 1996)
- The quantity and frequency of the patient's medication
- The variance of the blood glucose level during the day, increasing if the variance is abnormal
- If the patient is ill or under stress; this often results in patients who are in hospital requiring more frequent testing (Wallymahmed 2007)
- If dietary intake is altered or eating is prevented, e.g. fasting before a surgical procedure
- If more exercise is taken than is normal for the patient
- If medication has been altered

Table 13.2 Symptoms of hypoglycaemia

Early onset	Severe symptoms
Tremor (Tortora and Derrickson 2006)	Mental disorientation/confusion
Nervousness/shaking (Tortora and Derrickson 2006)	Convulsions
Sweating (Tortora and Derrickson 2006)	Unconsciousness
Increased heart rate (tachycardia) (Tortora and Derrickson 2006)	Shock
Hunger (Tortora and Derrickson 2006)	
Drowsiness	
Abnormal speech (Waugh and Grant 2001)	

Box 13.5 Causes of hypoglycaemia

- Too much insulin or oral medication
- More than the usual amount of exercise or activity
- Changing the patient's insulin injection site (it is important to rotate sites regularly as overuse of an area may result in the site losing the ability to absorb insulin effectively). Increase uptake of glucose can also occur at a new site
- Change of insulin schedule
- Missing or postponing regular meals or eating less than normal
- Liver failure (Dougherty and Lister 2004)
- Infection (Dougherty and Lister 2004)
- Insulin-secreting tumours (Dougherty and Lister 2004)
- Consuming alcohol

Table 13.3 Treatment for hypoglycaemia

Action	Rationale
1. Report to registered staff and/or medical staff	To alert other personnel of patient's condition
2. Assist in giving the patient fast acting glucose, or give on instruction from a registered nurse, without delay. Possible examples include three to six dextrose tables, a sweet soft drink (not diet), or three to five sugar lumps. Glucose gels are also now available (Wallymahmed 2007)	To increase patient's blood glucose
3. Test the patient's blood glucose level both immediately, and after 15 min	To assess if the glucose has entered the patient's bloodstream
If the patient's blood glucose has increased, and it is over an hour and a half until the patient's next meal, a sandwich, some fruit or biscuits, etc. may be given.	If the patient eats too soon after the first dose of glucose it will delay the absorption of glucose into the bloodstream
4. If the level has not increased seek further advice	To decide on patient management that may include further glucose
5. Monitor the patient as directed	To ensure that the patient makes a full recovery

Hyperglycaemia

Hyperglycaemia is when blood glucose level is too high, usually >10 mmol/l of glucose. The symptoms are shown in Box 13.6.

Box 13.6 Symptoms of hyperglycaemia

- Increased urination
- Ketones in urine
- Increased thirst
- Lethargy
- Dehydration
- Weight loss
- Blurred vision
- Cramps/weakness caused by excessive urination
- Increased likelihood of infection

As with hypoglycaemia the symptoms and causes of hyperglycaemia should be taught to the patient with a view to the patient taking preventive action. The possible causes of hyperglycaemia are shown in Box 13.7. Hyperglycaemia can affect the patient's wellbeing and should be treated promptly. Table 13.4 gives the actions required for patients who are hyperglycaemic.

Box 13.7 Possible causes of hyperglycaemia

- Untreated diabetes
- Decreased mobility/reduction of physical activity
- Infections/illness
- Stress
- Too much food
- Insufficient medication
- Overuse of injection sites/poor injection technique
- Increase in weight
- Insufficient insulin
- The wrong type of food

Reflection point

Go through the possible causes of hypo- and hyperglycaemia and give examples of how this may apply to patients in hospital.

Common problems

Complications of diabetes

It is of vital importance for the patient with diabetes to have well-controlled blood glucose, because uncontrolled diabetes can lead to either short or long-term complications. Chronic

Table 13.4 Treatment for hyperglycaemia

Action	Rationale
1. Report to registered staff and/or medical staff	To alert other personnel of patient's condition
2. Insulin will be reviewed by medical staff and if prescribed will be administered. The healthcare assistant may assist with this	To reduce blood glucose levels
3. Test the patient's blood glucose level both immediately, and after 15 min	To determine blood glucose level
4. Encourage the patient to drink fluids	Prevent dehydration
5. Monitor the patient as directed	To ensure the patient makes a full recovery

complications can be divided into macrovascular and microvascular disease (Currie 2007b). Macrovascular applies to atherosclerotic plaques ('hardening'), which can build up in arteries (and lead to blockages), whereas microvascular applies to the narrowing of the inside of the blood vessels. Table 13.5 summarises some of the common complications.

Table 13.5 Complications of diabetes

Complication	Effect on the body
Cardiovascular disease (Currie 2007b)	This leads to an increased risk of heart attack and cardiovascular accidents (stroke)
Nephropathy (reduced renal function)	Changes in the small blood vessels can damage the kidneys, leading to renal failure (Sewell 2007)
Retinopathy (ophthalmic [eye] problems)	Damage to the small vessels in the eyes (Sewell 2007) which can lead to blindness or the formation of cataracts (Currie 2007b)
Neuropathy – nerve damage	This can cause sensory deficits, particularly in the feet (Currie 2007b, Sewell 2007) and can increase the incidence of injury, ulcers and infections, resulting in poor circulation
Erectile dysfunction (problems with getting or maintaining an erection) (Currie 2007b)	Changes in the blood vessels reduces the blood flow to the penis

Common problems in obtaining a blood glucose measurement

The problems associated with taking a blood glucose measurement can be divided into three areas: the patient, the equipment and technique.

The patient

If the patient has poor circulation obtaining a sample can be more challenging. Keeping the hand warm can improve circulation and, if the fingers are massaged, this can increase blood flow (perfusion) to the site, allowing the capillaries to bleed more easily (Cradock 1996; Dougherty and Lister 2004; Burton and Birdi 2006). Where the skin has become hardened the patient should be discouraged from using alcohol gel to wash hands (this can also affect the blood glucose reading) (Dougherty and Lister 2004). If the patient is uncooperative with regard to the procedure, despite a full explanation, seek assistance because this may be the first signs of hypoglycaemia.

The equipment

As mentioned earlier it is essential that the machine be serviced and calibrated as per local policy to ensure that accurate results are obtained. If the machine displays an error code or is malfunctioning another machine should be used. Regular quality control checks are required with both the machine and the strips and these need to be documented (Dougherty and Lister 2004). The strips should be in date, have not been exposed to the air and calibrated for use with the specific machine being used (Dougherty and Lister 2004). The lancets (finger-pricking devices) should be for single patient use to prevent infection (DH 1990; Dougherty and Lister 2004). Competency-based training with the machine should have been completed as per local policy.

Technique

The site for obtaining a sample (as mentioned earlier) should be the side of the finger and, where possible, a site that has not been used recently to prevent damage. Due to the fact that there are comparatively fewer nerve endings in the side than the tip of the finger, this site is less painful (Burton and Birdi 2006). If the finger does not bleed it should be milked but not squeezed because this can give inaccurate results (Blake 1999; Dougherty and Lister 2004; Wallymahmed 2007). It is essential that all staff performing this procedure should have had competency-based training on the specific machine and accessories being used. When recording the blood glucose level, best practice is also to assess the patient's other observations to ensure that the result appears correct, reporting any concerns immediately. This is highly significant because inaccurate results can lead to mismanagement of patients and can be potentially life threatening.

Summary

Taking blood glucose levels provides important information, which affects patient management. It is essential that quality control and good technique be mastered to ensure best practice. Where possible, if patients have previously been active in this procedure, they should be encouraged to preserve self-care, especially for management of diabetes at home. As with all abnormal or unusual results, the healthcare assistant should report these immediately to the nurse in charge or medical staff. An example of competency framework for blood glucose measurement is shown in Table 13.6.

Case study 13.1

The blood glucose level of an acutely ill patient is taken. Instead of taking the current reading, a value from the previous patient is retrieved from the history function of the machine.
What do you think are the implications of this error?

Table 13.6 Competency – blood glucose monitoring

Steps	First assessment/Reassessment					Date/competent/signature
	Demonstration					
	Date/sign	Date/sign	Date/sign	Date/sign	Date/sign	
	1	2	3	4	5	
Blood glucose monitoring						
1 Define the types of diabetes						
2 Describe the effect of insulin on the body						
3 Discuss conditions where a patient's blood glucose may require careful monitoring						
4 Identify the contraindications to blood glucose measurement						
5 State the normal range for blood glucose readings						
6 Identify signs and symptoms of hypoglycaemia						
7 Identify signs and symptoms of hyperglycaemia						
8 Discuss the equipment required to undertake this task						
9 Demonstrate an understanding of using appropriate calibration and quality control techniques and what checks should be made on the monitor before use						
10 Demonstrate the proper use of the equipment as laid down by the operating instructions and specifications and discuss the consequences of improper use						

No.		Date/competent/signature
11	Demonstrate that, before taking device to patient, the monitor is checked for the following: That one pack of strips is open and are in date, ensure that the monitor and the test strips have been calibrated together. Discuss the actions that would be taken if there was doubt about the quality of the strips	
12	Check that the quality control test has been carried out that day, when the batteries require changing, when opening new strips and any unusual, unpredicted result	
13	Confirm that the quality control check has been recorded in the record book and signed	

Blood glucose monitoring procedure	Demonstration					Date/competent/signature
	1	2	3	4	5	
1 Demonstrate satisfactory explanations of the procedure to the patient						
2 Show awareness of preparation of site before blood sampling						
3 Demonstrate appropriate positioning of patient						
4 Demonstrate safe hand washing according to infection control policy						
5 Demonstrate procedure for safe practice in obtaining a blood sample from the patient to apply to the test pad						
6 Demonstrate safe disposal of lancet						
7 Demonstrate the proper use of the monitor as per individual manual and local policy						
8 Demonstrate the procedure for recording and reporting the result						
9 Show awareness of appropriate disposal of waste						
10 Demonstrate knowledge of care for the patient following the procedure						

Supervisors/Assessors:

Case study 13.2

Ben is a 17-year-old boy who has taken his own blood glucose level. The level recorded is very high but he appears asymptomatic (he has no symptoms). You notice a bag of sweets on his locker. *What explanation do you think may be applicable to this patient and what would be your planned actions?*

 ## Self-assessment

Assessment	Aspects	Achieved ✔
Patient/Disease	*Have you considered all aspects of this section?*	
	Types of diabetes and the role of the pancreas	
	Signs and symptoms of diabetes	
	Complications that can occur due to diabetes	
Procedure	*Have you considered all aspects of this section?*	**Achieved ✔**
	Selecting equipment and reasons for blood glucose measurement	
	Technique required	
	Normal values	
	Recording and reporting concerns	
	Safe disposal of sharps	

References

Bewley C (2002) Diabetes in pregnancy. *Nursing Standard* **16**(25): 47–52, 54–55.

Blake J (1999) An insight into blood glucose sampling. *Practice Nursing* **12**(2): 73–74.

Burton NL, Birdi K, eds (2006) *Clinical Skills for OSCEs*, 2nd edn. London: Informa Healthcare.

Campbell IW, Song S (2007) Blood glucose levels. Available at: www.netdoctor.co.uk/health_advice/facts/diabetesbloodsugar.htm (accessed May 2007).

Cradock S (1996) Diabetes mellitus at diagnosis. *Nursing Standard* **10**(30): 41–48.

Currie J (2007a) Types of diabetes. *Scottish Nurse* **10**(10): 40–41.

Currie J (2007b) Diabetic complications. *Scottish Nurse* **10**(11): 28–29.

Department of Health (1987) *Blood Glucose Measurements: Reliability of results produced in extra-laboratory areas*. DHSS Hazard Notice 15 October. NHS Procurement Directorate DHSS Blood Glucose Measurement. London: Department of Health and Social Security.

Department of Health (1990) *Lancing Devices for Multi-patient Capillary Sampling: Avoidance of cross infection by correct selection and use*. DEF 41/00/10003. London: Medical Services Directorate.

Department of Health (1996) *Extra laboratory use of blood glucose meters and test strips: contraindications, training and advice to users*. Medical Devices Agency Incident Safety Notice. SN 9616. London: DH

Dougherty L, Lister S, eds (2004) *The Royal Marsden Hospital Manual of Clinical Nursing Procedures*, 6th edn. Oxford: Blackwell Publishing.

Ferguson A (2005) Blood glucose monitoring.*Nursing Times* **101**(38): 28–29.

Hand H (2000) The development of diabetic ketoacidosis. *Nursing Standard* **15**(8): 47–55.

Jeffrey A (2003) Insulin resistance. *Nursing Standard* **17**(32): 47–55.

Malmberg K, Ryden L, Efendic S, et al. (1995) Randomized trial of insulin-glucose infusion followed by subcutaneous insulin treatment in diabetic patients with acute myocardial infarction (DIGAMI study): effects on mortality at 1 year. *Journal of the American College of Cardiology* **26**: 57–65.

Marieb EN, Hoehn K (2007) *Human Anatomy and Physiology*, 7th edn. San Francisco, CA: Pearson Benjamin Cummings.

Medical Devices Agency (2002) *Management and Use of IVD Point of Care Test Devices*. London: The Stationery Office.

National Institute for Health and Clinical Excellence (2002) *Management of Type 2 Diabetes. Management of blood glucose*. London: NICE.

Sewell J (2007) Diabetes: causes, complications and management. *British Journal of Healthcare Assistants* **1**(1): 6–9.

Sonksen P, Fox C, Judd S (2001) *Diabetes at Your Fingertips*, 4th edn. London: Class Publishing.

Thibodeau GA, Patton KT (2007) *Anatomy and Physiology*, 6th edn. Elsevier, MO: Mosby.

Tortora GJ, Derrickson B (2006) *Principles of Anatomy and Physiology*, 11th edn. Hoboken, NJ: John Wiley & Sons Inc.

Wallymahmed M (2007) Capillary blood glucose monitoring. *Nursing Standard* **21**(38): 35–38.

Waugh A, Grant A (2001) *Ross and Wilson Anatomy and Physiology in Health and Illness*, 9th edn. London: Churchill Livingstone.

Chapter 14

Fluid balance and intravenous maintenance

Learning objectives

- Define the importance of fluid balance in the body
- Discuss the body's response to an increased/decreased fluid balance
- List the instances when intravenous (IV) fluids are necessary
- Describe how to prime (run through) an IV line
- Describe how to discontinue an IV line
- Identify the common problems with IV administration via gravity infusion sets

Aim of this chapter

The aim of this chapter is for the reader to understand the importance of fluid balance and the need for intravenous (IV) fluids via a cannula.

This chapter discusses fluid balance and IV maintenance; to revise the anatomy and physiology of the placement of a cannula please refer to Chapter 16. Fluids administered by the subcutaneous route are not covered.

Reasons for monitoring fluid balance

Fluid and electrolyte balance within the body is necessary to maintain health and function in all body systems, and for transportation of nutrients, gases and waste products (Tortora and Grabowski 2003).

Related anatomy and physiology

The total body water for adults is about 60% of the body weight, with a higher percentage in young people and adults of below-average weight (Waugh and Grant 2001; Tortora and Derrickson 2006). Older people have a reduced amount of water, whereas in infants it is around 75% (Thibodeau and Patton 2007). Women also tend to have slightly lower water content than men due to a higher percentage of fat (Thibodeau and Patton 2007).

Dougherty and Coote (2006) describe a number of regulators that work together to maintain fluid balance (Table 14.1).

Table 14.1 Regulator of fluid balance

Organ	Role in fluid balance
Kidneys	If the kidneys reabsorb more water, fluid will remain in the body and prevent loss. This would result in the patient passing concentrated urine
Hypothalamus/Pituitary gland	If there is a reduction in blood volume, e.g. haemorrhage (blood loss) the body will respond by trying to restore normal fluid levels. It does this by releasing the hormone antidiuretic hormone (ADH), which, after being made in the hypothalamus, is released from the posterior pituitary gland. ADH increases the reabsorption of water and therefore increases the circulating blood volume
Adrenal cortex	Reabsorption of sodium is an important part of fluid balance and aldosterone is a hormone secreted to regulate both the reabsorption of sodium and water.

Adapted from Dougherty and Coote (2006.)

The body's required input can be maintained by the patient drinking or eating (as some foods contain fluids) or, after medical intervention and insertion of a cannula, subcutaneous or IV fluids. Output is maintained mostly by urine output but sweating and body functioning also contribute to small losses.

The body is in balance when the required amounts of water and solutes (dissolved substances) are present and are correctly proportioned among the various compartments (Tortora and Derrickson 2006). The body keeps fluid levels constant when water loss equals water gain (Tortora and Derrickson 2006). Imbalances will cause discomfort to patients and is associated with some diseases, e.g. renal (kidney) problems. The body has a process for regulating fluid balance called homoeostasis; this means that, when the body notices a shift from normal values, it takes steps to regulate it back to normal limits. Figure 14.1 shows how the body reacts to a stimulus that caused a decreased volume of fluid in the body. If the patient is very unwell a central venous pressure (CVP) line may be placed in the right atrium (top chamber) of the heart to determine the amount of fluid contained within the body but currently this would be the role of a registered nurse (Mooney 2007).

Body fluids are distributed within two compartments in the body known as extracellular and intracellular. Extracellular is fluid outside the cells, consisting of fluids in the blood, lymphatic system (a system that fights infection), spinal fluid (cerebrospinal [CSF]) and fluid that bathes body cells. Intracellular or interstitial fluid both bathes the cells of the body and is contained within cells (Waugh and Grant 2001). Intracellular and extracellular compartments are separated by a plasma membrane (Tortora and Derrickson 2006).

Electrolytes

These are particles that have a positive or negative charge attached to them, and they play an essential role in the body because they control the movement of water between body fluid compartments (Thibodeau and Patton 2007). Patients who have an imbalance in the blood's electrolytes can develop fluid imbalance (Mooney 2007). Examples of some common electrolytes are shown in Box 14.1.

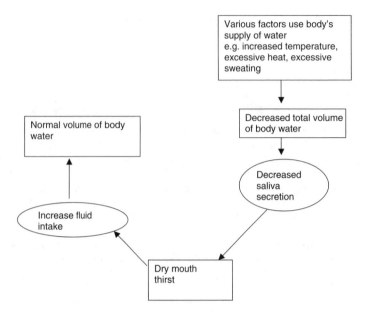

Figure 14.1 Temperature regulation in the body. (Adapted from Thibodeau and Patton 2007.)

Box 14.1 Common electrolytes in the body

Na^+: sodium
Cl^-: chloride
K^+: potassium
Ca^{2+}: calcium
Mg^{2+}: magnesium

Reflection point

Ask to view a patient's blood results and analyse the levels of the electrolytes contained in the blood. Most wards will also have a list of the 'normal' values with which you can compare the results.

Related aspects and terminology

- *Hypovolaemia*: loss of fluid (Mooney 2007)
- *Hypervolaemia*: fluid overload (Mooney 2007)
- *Electrolytes*: negatively or positively charged particles within the body
- *Extracellular*: fluid outside cells
- *Intracellular*: fluid contained in or around cells.

Hypovolaemia/Dehydration

The term 'dehydration' is used to describe the condition that results from excessive loss of body water and electrolytes (Thibodeau and Patton 2007).

Causes of dehydration

- Gastrointestinal problems that cause fluid loss are commonly vomiting and diarrhoea (Tortora and Derrickson 2006; Mooney 2007). This can be of sudden onset and have rapid effects on fluid loss, particularly in vulnerable patient groups such as babies and older people. Some chronic diseases can also cause these symptoms, e.g. ulcerative colitis (inflammation of the bowel) or irritable bowel syndrome.
- Where there is a reduced oral input, this can be due to altered mental state, e.g. dementia, depression or the patient being unconscious (Tortora and Derrickson 2006). In such instances the role of the healthcare assistant may be to ensure that the patient is given regular drinks. Where patients have poor or reduced mobility it is essential to ensure that fluids are within easy reach. Localised problems in the mouth may also affect the patient's desire to drink because it may cause further discomfort and this should be reported to the nurse in charge.
- Environment can also contribute to a reduced oral input, e.g. lack of water in a hot climate (Thibodeau and Patton 2007).
- Excessive urination (passing urine) may be due to diuretic medication (encourages increased urine output) with less absorption occurring in the kidneys (Mooney 2007). If fluid balance is being monitored, giving the patient a jug to measure urine output can be successful in recording an accurate output. If the patient has mobility problems, ensuring that they are near a toilet after the diuretic medication can reduce any anxiety and prevent incidents of incontinence.
- Any disease or condition that alters fluid loss can cause dehydration, e.g. haemorrhage, severe burns, diabetes, vomiting/diarrhoea (Marieb and Hoehn 2007).

Signs and symptoms of dehydration

- Dizziness/light-headedness, leading to mental confusion (Marieb and Hoehn 2007)
- Muscle weakness (Thibodeau and Patton 2007)
- Poor skin 'firmness', sometimes referred to as 'turgor' (Thibodeau and Patton 2007)
- Dry flushed skin (Marieb and Hoehn 2007)
- Decreased urine output; will also be very concentrated (Marieb and Hoehn 2007)
- Increased pulse (tachycardia)
- Thirst (Thibodeau and Patton 2007).

Treatment

Medical and nursing staff need to find out and then treat the symptoms or cause, e.g. if the patient is vomiting they can be give an antiemetic (anti-sickness medication) to try to rectify the problem.

Fluids require to be replaced either orally or intravenously if necessary (e.g. patient unable to tolerate oral fluids). Monitoring the patient's fluid balance is essential to promote recovery.

Hypervolaemia (excess fluid)

This is an expansion of fluid in the body.

Cause

- Over-infusion of intravenous fluids
- Congestive cardiac failure, renal (kidney) failure, cirrhosis of the liver due to the kidneys retaining large amounts of sodium and water (Mooney 2007; Thibodeau and Patton 2007).

Signs and symptoms of excess fluid

- Weight gain
- Oedema (excess fluid in tissues)
- Breathlessness
- Increased pulse rate
- Lung problems – congestion.

Treatment

- Once medical and nursing staff identify the underlying cause, treat it, e.g. if the patient has had too much IV fluid the regimen should be reviewed by medical staff and nursing staff, and ensuring that the drip is closely monitored is essential.
- If prescribed, assist in giving diuretic medication that will promote excretion of fluid in the kidneys, resulting in increased urine output.

If a person steadily consumes more water than the kidneys can excrete, water intoxication can occur, which results in the cells within the body swelling dangerously; this can result in death (Tortora and Derrickson 2006).

Fluid balance charts

Fluid balance charts are used to monitor the patient's input and output, and are an important aspect of care, particularly with critically ill patients, because failure to maintain fluid balance can have serious consequences for the patient, e.g. severe dehydration (Reid et al. 2004). Figure 14.2 shows an example of a fluid balance chart. In some areas 'insensible loss' which is loss of fluid due to evaporation from the body is also calculated (see Chapter 7).

If the role of the healthcare assistant involves completing the fluid balance chart, some training should be undertaken to ensure that the correct information is recorded, given the importance of the information in patient management. Reid et al. (2004) suggest that mandatory education for fluid balance should be incorporated within local training programmes for all staff, to overcome the problems of incomplete charts. Involving patients in completion can be very useful to promote accuracy and can reduce workload for the nursing team (Chung et al. 2002). Box 14.2 shows the potential problems in fluid balance chart completion.

To reduce some of these variables, education of both staff and patients in the importance and completion of the charts would prove beneficial. A sign can be put at the bed space too, which can raise the awareness of fluid balance in general, and give specific instructions for individual patients (Reid et al. 2004).

The intravenous route

When IV fluids would be commenced

- Patient is nil by mouth, e.g. before or after surgery
- Medication only available in this form
- Where the patient is feeling nauseous and not taking oral fluids
- Where the patient is vomiting, so medication not able to be absorbed in the gut
- To assist in fluid balance maintenance or correct dehydration
- To correct electrolyte imbalance.

IV fluids are delivered by a cannula inserted into a vein (Figure 14.3; see Chapter 16). Cannulation involves direct entry into the circulatory system and is a route for infection (Lavery and Ingram 2006). Great care must therefore be taken to prevent infection, and this would involve only touching the cannula/IV line when necessary. Preventing equipment coming into contact with potentially harmful organisms can be maximised by taking great care not to touch the equipment where possible, a technique known as aseptic or non-touch technique (Rowley 2001). If the healthcare assistants role involves manipulation of IV lines training and competency in this skill are recommended.

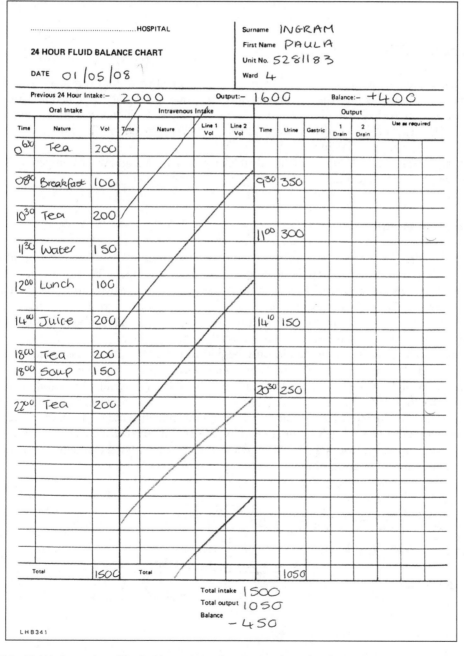

Figure 14.2 Fluid balance chart. (Used with permission from NHS Lothian 2008.)

Box 14.2 Potential problems in fluid balance chart completion

- Chart not completed at all
- Inaccurate volumes entered, e.g. sips/??? or wet pad/used toilet (Reid et al. 2004)
- Staff unaware of the volumes in cups/glasses, etc. and estimate wrongly
- Patient forgets to measure output
- Patient cannot remember input
- Patient may be unable to give a history due to previous cerebrovascular accident (stroke) or dementia
- Domestic staff remove cups without alerting staff to volume consumed

Priming an IV line

To administer fluid via an IV line the line must first be filled with fluid (primed). This involves running the fluid through the line to prevent air remaining in the line, which could cause an air embolus (air entering the circulatory system) (Higgins 2004). The line, sometimes also referred to as an IV set, comes packed in a sterile pack to prevent infection. Table 14.2 describes the procedure for priming an IV line.

Priming the line should be undertaken only if local policy allows, and when competency training in both aseptic technique and the actual task has been undertaken.

Flushing an IV line

If an IV cannula is in place but is being used only intermittently, often fluid (e.g. sodium chloride or 'saline') will be introduced to keep the line patent (free from blockages). This is known as 'flushing the line'. The administration of IV medication is currently a post-registration role and therefore flushing before, between and after medicine – also seen as good practice – is performed by the registered nurse (National Institute for Health and Clinical Excellence [NICE] 2003; Infusion Nurses' Society 2000). However, it is anticipated that this may change in the future. Where this role is permitted in the future it should only be performed by healthcare assistants under local protocols and after competency-based training, including aseptic technique (see earlier).

As mentioned, the medicine used for flushing peripheral lines is usually 0.9% sodium chloride, provided that this does not react with other medications being administered via this route. The volume should be equal to twice the volume of the cannula plus any additional devices, e.g. needle-free connectors (Royal College of Nursing [RCN] 2005). The recognised technique is a pulsated push–pause (stop–start, stop–start), which creates turbulence with the cannula, removing debris from its internal wall (Gabriel et al. 2005).

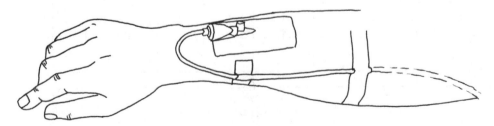

Figure 14.3 Cannula with intravenous line attached.

Table 14.2 The procedure for priming an intravenous (IV) line

Action	Rationale
1. Ensure that the registered nurse has checked that IV fluid has been prescribed, and not already given. Two practitioners should have checked this, because it is by the IV route	Administration of medicines is the role of the registered nurse (Nursing and Midwifery Council [NMC] 2008)
Check the IV fluid, ensuring that it is clear, so has no contamination or debris and that in date	IV fluid fit for purpose and within expiry date
2. Collect all other equipment: administration set, gloves/apron, receptacle for any discarded fluid, drip stand, air inlet if the container is glass or rigid, alcohol swab	To ensure that the process can be done timely
3. Wash hands, put on gloves and apron. Where possible undertake procedure in sterile environment, e.g. clinical treatment room in the hospital	Prevent cross-contamination
4. Read the instructions on the IV line packaging, including expiry date if applicable	
Remove the line from outer packaging and close the roller clamp. Remove the IV fluid from outer bag if applicable	All outward packaging removed
5. Remove the seal on the IV bag where the trocar (spike) will be inserted	
Insert the trocar into the bag taking care not to spike and puncture the bag (Figure 14.4)	Mis-spiking the bag will allow entry for microorganisms and potentially could cause sharps injury
6. Squeeze the drip chamber at the top to fill around half to two-thirds full (check manufacturer's recommendation) (Figure 14.5)	Some manufacturers' sets may have specific instructions
7. Slowly open the roller clamp allowing the fluid to flow down the IV line	Slow priming of the line will reduce the amount of air in the line
8. Close the roller clamp when the fluid has filled the line completely and come out the end (Figure 14.6)	To expel all air from the line
9. The line is now filled with fluid and ready for connection to the patient. Place a sterile cap over the end ready for connection to the patient	Sterile cap prevents contamination of the line before it is connected to the patient

Care of the cannula

Refer to Chapter 16; however, a summary of care is as follows:

- The cannula site should be inspected regularly to identify potential problems promptly. Phlebitis refers to the inflammation of a vein and there are phlebitis scales to assist in reviewing the cannula (Jackson 1998). This would not be expected from an healthcare assistant but you may be the first person to whom the patient reports symptoms or who visually views the site. It is also beneficial to teach the patient the signs and symptoms of infection so that they can detect any problems early or even once discharged home (Lammon et al. 1995).
- If the dressing becomes wet or bloodstained, or is no longer secure it will need to be changed (Nicol et al. 2005).
- A bandage should only be used when absolutely necessary because this obscures the view of the cannula site. It should also be applied carefully to ensure that it does not compress the vein (Nicol et al. 2005).

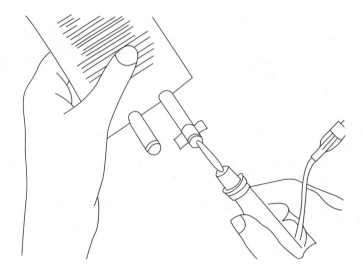

Figure 14.4　Spiking an IV bag.

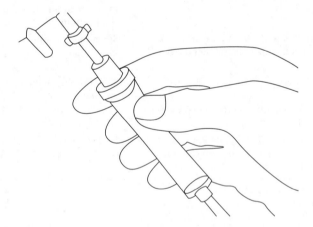

Figure 14.5　Filling the drip chamber.

Discontinuing an IV infusion

Discontinuing an infusion if a line is attached requires the line to be clamped off (by closing off the roller clamp and then removing it (Figure 14.7)). Disconnection at the cannula requires competency in aseptic technique (discussed earlier), and a sterile cap to be applied where the line previously entered the cannula. The reason for the infusion is important, because this may affect the care of the patient after removal (Lammon et al. 1995). An example of this would be if the infusion had been in place to keep the patient hydrated; the patient may then need advice and assistance in drinking fluids regularly. Table 14.3 details the procedure for discontinuing an intravenous infusion (IVI).

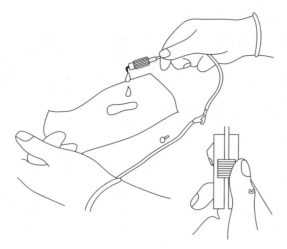

Figure 14.6   Priming the IV line.

Common problems

Despite IV administration being a qualified nursing role, the role of the healthcare assistant could be in ensuring that the infusion is running and there are no complications, if competent to do so. As mentioned earlier patients may well report symptoms of pain, discomfort, swelling or leakage to the healthcare assistant first.

IV infusions can be delivered via infusion devices or by a gravity infusion set (as seen previously). Infusion devices should be used only by individuals who have had competency-based training on their use, with local policy dictating which staff are permitted. When an infusion device is being used, the role of the healthcare assistant may be to alert staff to infusion problems, which may have resulted from either the patient reporting problems or the alarm on the pump being activated.

A standard gravity set is used for fluid administration, with specialised blood sets for blood and blood products. Table 14.4 details the common problems, presentation and actions that should be taken in relation to gravity infusion sets.

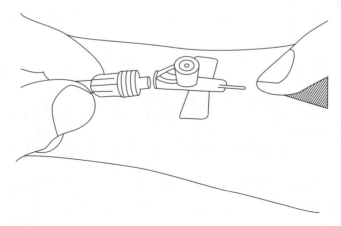

Figure 14.7   Discontinuing an IV line.

Table 14.3 Procedure to discontinue an intravenous infusion

Action	Rationale
1. Explain the procedure to the patient and obtain verbal consent	To ensure that patient understands and cooperates. Consent for legal purposes
2. Gather all necessary equipment, which includes: gloves, sterile cap, clinical waste bag and sharps bin	To promote safe and efficient removal
3. Close roller clamp on IV line Put on gloves and apron	To prevent spillage of fluid Gloves prevent cross infection
4. Open sterile cap and place carefully ensuring aseptic technique. Ensure that within easy reach	Prevents contamination
5. Remove IV line carefully (Figure 14.7) asking the patient to elevate the arm upwards if the cannula is in the back of the hand. Application of some light pressure over the cannula (where the cannula enters the vein) can also prevent bleeding (Figure 14.7)	To prevent blood spillage
6. Attach sterile cap	Ensures line is capped off securely
7. Wash hands, dispose of all equipment as per policy	Prevents infection
8. Observe site	To identify any problems with the site
9. Document removal in the patient's notes	Provides a legal record

In some instances, the registered nurse may delegate the task to close the roller clamp on the infusion line to a healthcare assistant, but this should only be done when instructed to do so and under local protocol or policy.

Summary

Fluid balance is an important aspect of patient care with serious clinical problems where there is an imbalance. The healthcare assistants role may involve encouraging and recording oral fluids and the reporting of potential problems where the patient is receiving fluids by the IV route. The healthcare assistant can also assist in monitoring the output either by recording when the patient goes to the toilet or in the care of indwelling catheters. The healthcare assistant is often the first person who may witness or deal with problems regarding IV infusions, but any interaction must be underpinned by a strong knowledge base and competency-based training in accordance with local policies and procedures.

Tables 14.5 and 14.6 are competency frameworks for recording fluid balance and IV maintenance.

Case study 14.1

Mrs Jones, who is 88 years old, has been admitted to correct dehydration. Her IV infusion has now been discontinued. What is the role of the healthcare assistant in ensuring that a correct fluid balance is both maintained and recorded?

Case study 14.2

Mr Bob Mills is a 49 year old who has had prostate surgery. He has an intravenous infusion running and is complaining of pain at the site. Describe the actions that you would take.

Table 14.4 Common problems with gravity infusion sets

Problem	Presentation	Action
The infusion has stopped dripping Causes: • Cannula may be blocked • The infusion bag needs to be elevated • The infusion is switched off	No drips evident in the chamber	Inform nurse in charge
The infusion is not running to time Causes: • The patient may have interfered with the infusion • The cannula may allow only intermittent flow depending on the position of the patient's arm • The rate has been set incorrectly.	The infusion bag appears to have a volume that is not consistent with the planned infusion duration	Inform nurse in charge
The dressing is not clean, dry and secure Causes: • The infusion may have leaked • The patient has caused contamination of the dressing • The patient may have interfered with the infusion	Dressing visually contaminated or dislodged	Change dressing if competent to do so; report
The patient reports pain or wetness at the cannula site (see also Chapter 16) Causes: • The IV may have leaked • An acute inflammation of the vein has occurred due to the presence of the cannula, known as phlebitis (Jackson 1998) • Infiltration or extravasation has occurred. This involves leakage of medication into the surrounding tissues. • The classification is linked to the type of medication that has caused the leakage (Ingram and Lavery 2005)	Dressing is wet. Site is painful	Report to nurse in charge. Stop infusion

✔ Self-assessment

Assessment	Aspects	Achieved ✔
Patient	*Have you considered all aspects of this section?*	
	Describe the regulators that maintain fluid balance in the body	
	The role of electrolytes in the body	
	The symptoms of dehydration/over hydration	
Procedure(s)	*Have you considered all aspects of this section?*	**Achieved ✔**
	Maintaining and recording on fluid balance charts	
	Priming an IV line	
	Common problems with gravity infusion lines	
	Discontinuing an IV line	

Table 14.5 Competency framework: record clinical observations (fluid balance)

Steps	First assessment/Reassessment					
		Demonstration				Date/competent/signature
	Date/sign	Date/sign	Date/sign	Date/sign	Date/sign	
	1	2	3	4	5	
Fluid balance						
1 List the two fluid compartments in the body						
2 Describe how the body controls fluid balance						
3 Discuss the symptoms of dehydration/ hypervolaemia (excess) fluid						
4 Demonstrate how to complete a fluid balance chart						

Table 14.6 Competency framework: record clinical observations (intravenous [IV] maintenance, including priming and discontinuing an infusion [IVI])

Steps	First assessment/Reassessment					Date/competent/signature
	Demonstration					
	Date/sign	Date/sign	Date/sign	Date/sign	Date/sign	
	1	2	3	4	5	
IV maintenance						
1 Describe the instances where the IV route is required						
2 Explain why aseptic technique is important when dealing with the IV route						
3 Demonstrate the correct procedure for priming (running through) an IV line						
4 Demonstrate the correct procedure for discontinuing an IV line						
5 Discuss the common problems associated with the IV route, giving the actions expected from a healthcare assistant						

References

Chung LH, Chong S, French P (2002) The efficiency of fluid balance charting: an evidence based management project. *Journal of Nursing Management* **10**(2): 103–113.

Dougherty B, Coote S (2006) Fluid balance monitoring as part of track and trigger. *Nursing Times* 102(45): 28–29.

Gabriel J, Bravery K, Doughert, L, Kayley J, Malster M, Scales K (2005) Vascular access: indications and implications for patient care. *Nursing Standard* **149**(26): 45–54.

Higgins (2004) Priming an IV infusion set. *Nursing Times* 100(47): 32–33.

Ingram P, Lavery I (2005) Peripheral intravenous therapy: key risks and implications for practice. *Nursing Standard* 19(46): 55–64.

Infusion Nurses' Society (2000) Infusion nursing standards of practice. *Journal of Intravenous Nursing* **23** (6 suppl): S56–S569.

Jackson A (1998) Infection control: a battle in vein; infusion phlebitis. *Nursing Times* **94**(4): 68–71.

Lammon CB, Foote AW, Leli PG, Ingle J, Adams MH (1995) *Clinical Nursing Skills*. London: WB Saunders.

Lavery I, Ingram, P (2006) Prevention of infection in peripheral intravenous devices. *Nursing Standard* **20**(49): 49–58

Marieb EN, Hoehn K (2007) *Human Anatomy and Physiology*, 7th edn. San Francisco, CA: Pearson Benjamin Cummings.

Mooney GP (2007) Fluid balance. *Nursing Times*. Available at: www.nursingtimes.net/ntclinical/ Fluid_balance.html (accessed 16 October 2008).

National Institute for Health and Clinical Excellence (2003) *Infection Control: Prevention of healthcare-associated infection in primary and community care*. Clinical Guidelines 2. London: NICE.

NHS Lothian (2008) *Fluid Balance Chart*. Edinburgh: NHS Lothian.

Nicol M, Bavin C, Bedford-Turner S, Cronin P, Rawlings-Anderson K (2005) *Essential Nursing Skills*, 2nd edn. Edinburgh: Mosby.

Nursing and Midwifery Council (NMC) (2008) *Standards for Medicines Management*. London: NMC.

Royal College of Nursing (RCN) (2005) *Standards for Infusion Therapy*, 2nd edn. London: RCN.

Reid J, Robb E, Stone D, et al. (2004) Improving the monitoring and assessment of fluid balance. *Nursing Times* **100**(20): 36–39.

Rowley S (2001) Aseptic non-touch technique. *Nursing Times* **97**(7): 6.

Sheppard M (2001) Assessing fluid balance. *Nursing Times* **97**(6): 11.

Thibodeau GA, Patton KT (2007) *Anatomy and Physiology*, 6th edn. St Louis, MO: Mosby.

Tortora GJ, Derrickson B (2006) *Principles of Anatomy and Physiology*, 11th edn. Hoboken, NJ: Wiley & Sons.

Tortora GJ, Grabowski SR (2003) *Principles of Anatomy and Physiology*, 10th edn. Chichester: John Wiley & Sons.

Waugh A, Grant A (2001) *Ross and Wilson Anatomy and Physiology in Health and Illness*, 9th edn. London: Churchill Livingstone.

Section 3
Complex clinical skills

Chapter 15

Medicines

Learning objectives

- Clearly identify the role and accountability of healthcare assistants in administration of medicines
- Identify the main components of the Medicine Act that have an impact on the role of the healthcare assistant
- Identify the circumstances where nurses can prescribe medication
- Identify the common routes and considerations for administration of medicines with which healthcare assistants may assist
- Discuss the circumstances where the healthcare assistant may check medications

Aim of this chapter

The aim of this chapter is for healthcare assistants to understand the law and the role of the healthcare assistant in administration of medicines.

Healthcare assistants role within medicine administration

The role of the healthcare assistant in medicines administration is currently under the delegation of a registered nurse who will take accountability for this task (see Chapter 1). This is identified in the Nursing and Midwifery Council (NMC) summary of standards relating to medicine administration (2008a), which will be referred to throughout the chapter.

Where possible, any duties associated with medicine administration should be clearly stated in the healthcare assistant's job description and, in addition, local policies, procedures or protocols should be in place to support this role. It is anticipated that a very small number will participate in this task currently, but that this is an area that will develop in the future. Healthcare assistants who undertake administering medication despite not having competency to do so are potentially endangering patients (McKenna et al. 2004).

This chapter focuses on some of the issues surrounding medicine administration, but local policies will dictate accepted local practice. It is also acknowledged that when the healthcare assistant role becomes regulated (see the chapter on accountability), then this role may well expand and develop further.

Types of medicines

Different classification of medicines are defined by the Medicines Act 1968, including the three classification categories given overleaf.

Prescription-only medicines (POMs)

These are medicinal products that may be supplied, including sold, to a patient on the instruction of a doctor/dentist supplementary prescriber or nurse/pharmacist as an independent prescriber. (see later)

Pharmacy-only medicines (Ps)

These are medications that do not require a prescription but can be purchased only from a registered pharmacy, with the sale being supervised by a pharmacist, e.g. cough medicines.

General sales list medicines (GSLs)

These include all medications that can be bought by the public, e.g. in supermarkets, and do not require either supervision of a pharmacist or a prescription, e.g. paracetamol. However, in a hospital setting there is control over these mediations and patients cannot take these without prior consultation with medical and nursing staff.

Reflection point

Think of an example of each of the categories of medicine. If you are unsure, you could take a trip to a supermarket with a pharmacy department and view what is out on the shelves (thus not requiring a pharmacist to be present), and the medications that are behind the counter (requiring a pharmacist to be present). For a prescription-only medication this needs to be prescribed by an approved person either in the community or hospital setting and could be medication for yourself, a family member or a patient.

Medication prescribing and legal aspects

Any qualified and registered independent prescriber may prescribe all prescription-only medicines for all medical conditions, with some nurse independent prescribers also able to prescribe some controlled drugs (Nursing and Midwifery Council [NMC] 2008a).

Supplementary prescribers can prescribe where there is a management plan for the patient, provided that an arrangement with the doctor or dentist and the patient has been formulated (NMC 2008a).

Nurses and midwives who have recorded their medication qualification on the NMC register fall into two categories (NMC 2008a): practitioner nurse prescribers, where they can prescribe from the community *Practitioner Nurse Prescribers' Formulary*, which includes dressings and some POMs; and independent or supplementary nurse and midwife prescribers who are trained both to make a diagnosis and to prescribe (independent prescribing) (NMC 2008a). These practitioners can also review and change medication as part of a clinical management plan; this is known as supplementary prescribing (NMC 2008a).

It is essential to check local policies and procedures about both prescribing and administration of medicines because local policy will dictate current practice.

The law

Two pieces of legislation have been identified as important in medicines management: the Medicines Act 1968 and the Misuse of Drugs Act 1971 (Corben 2005; Dougherty and Lister 2004).

Medicines Act 1968

This provides a legal framework for manufacture, licensing, prescription, supply and administration of medicines that must be adhered to (NMC 2008a). POMs are covered by the Human use order 1997 (SI no. 1830), which gives information and legislation on medicines that require a prescription to be written by specific personnel (NMC 2008a).

In the NHS, hospitals adhere to this act by ensuring that a pharmacist supervises the purchasing and supply of medicines, and that supply or administration to a patient is only by personnel authorised to prescribe (Dougherty and Lister 2004).

Within a community setting, doctors, dentists, pharmacists and nurses are exempt from this restriction, allowing them to supply and use medication in the practice of their respective professions without pharmacy supervision (Dougherty and Lister 2004).

Misuse of Drugs Act 1971

This prohibits the possession, supply and manufacture of medicinal and other products unless legal (NMC 2008a). It is mostly concerned with 'controlled' drugs, which are medications that are potentially addictive or habit forming, e.g. morphine substances (Dougherty and Lister 2004).

The role of the healthcare assistant in controlled drug administration can exist in the community through local policy, but this is usually advised only where no other registered nurse is available. In this instance, the accountability of the preparation and administration of the medicine still lies with the registered nurse (see below under 'Delegation').

Reflection point

You are asked to assist in the preparation and checking of diamorphine for use in an MS26 syringe driver. Do you think this is an appropriate task to be delegated to you? (Think about your knowledge, skills, training and competence.)

In relation to controlled drugs, healthcare assistants may be required, through local policy, to witness the preparation and administration of controlled medicines including in a syringe driver. This is a portable device that is often used for palliative care and delivers medication via a syringe, which is placed in the syringe driver. Where controlled medicines are used, if the unregistered practitioner is assisting with the ingestion or application, the unregistered practitioner must remain under direct supervision at all times (NMC 2008a). Competency-based training should have been undertaken for all registered nurses undertaking this role to ensure patient safety. Local policies should be in place if an healthcare assistant is to assist with this method of administration, and education about palliative care (management of symptoms where there is no cure) and the device should be undertaken.

Related aspects and terminology

Registered nurses' role

All nurses who administer medication must have undertaken a programme of education and demonstrated competence under supervision (Ferguson 2005). Medicine management is described by the Medicines and Healthcare products Regulatory Agency (MHRA) as:

> the clinical, cost effective and safe use of medicines to ensure patients get the maximum benefit from the medicines they need, while at the same time minimising potential harm. (MHRA 2004)

This highlights the fact that, with changes in legal, professional and cultural boundaries in healthcare, the role of the nurse has broadened to encompass medicine management rather than just administration (Dougherty and Lister 2004).

The NMC (2008b) have set out principles that must be considered by registered nurses before the administration of medicines; these are detailed in Box 15.1.

Box 15.1 Standards for practice of administration of medicines (NMC 2008b)

Standard 2

As a registrant, before you administer a medicinal product you must always check that the prescription or other direction to administer is:

- Not for a substance to which the patient is know to be allergic or otherwise unable to tolerate
- Based, whenever possible, on the patient's informed consent and awareness of the purpose of the treatment
- Clearly written, typed or computer generated and indelible (cannot be rubbed out)
- Specifies the substance to be administered, using its generic or brand name where appropriate and its stated form, together with the strength, dosage, timing, frequency of administration, start and finish dates, and route of administration
- Signed and dated by the authorised prescriber
- In the case of controlled drugs, specifies the dosage and number of dosage units or total course, and is signed and dated by the prescriber using relevant documentation as introduced, e.g. patient drug record cards

And that you have:

- Clearly identified the patient for whom the medication is intended
- Recorded the weight of the patient on the prescription sheet for all children, and where the dosage of medication is related to weight or surface area (e.g. cytotoxics – cancer medication) or where clinical condition dictates the patient's weight to be recorded

---

Once the 'direction to supply or administer' principles above have been adhered to the registered nurse would follow the principles for administration, detailed in Box 15.2.

These principles aim to improve and standardise practice, which in turn can reduce errors.

Delegation

The NMC guidelines (2008a) state that nurses who delegate the responsibility of administration must ensure that the patient, carer or healthcare assistant is competent to carry out the task. This needs education, training and assessment of the patient, carer or healthcare assistant, including further support if necessary. This is in the best interests of both the registered nurse, and the healthcare assistant and patient, with the ultimate responsibility for ensuring the correct patient, dose, drug, time and route lying with the registered nurse who delegated the task (Ferguson 2005).

Box 15.2 Standards for practice of administration of medicines (NMC 2008b)

Standard 8

As a registrant, in exercising your professional accountability in the best interests of your patients:

- You must be certain of the identity of the patient to whom the medicine is to be administered
- You must check that the patient is not allergic to the medicine before administering it
- You must know the therapeutic uses of the medicine to be administered, its normal dosage, side effects, precautions and contraindications
- You must be aware of the patient's plan of care (care plan/pathway)
- You must check that the prescription or the label on medicine dispensed is clearly written and unambiguous
- You must check the expiry date (where it exists) of the medicine to be administered
- You must have considered the dosage, weight where appropriate, method of administration, route and timing
- You must administer or withhold in the context of the patient's condition (e.g. medication to be given prior to physiotherapy)
- You must contact the prescriber or another authorised prescriber without delay where contraindications to the prescribed medicine are discovered, where the patient develops a reaction to the medicine or where assessment of the patient indicates that the medicine is no longer suitable
- You must make a clear, accurate and immediate record of all medicine administered, intentionally withheld or refused by the patient, ensuring the signature is clear and legible; it is also your responsibility to ensure that a record is made when delegating the task of administering medicine

In addition:

- Where medication is not given the reason for not doing so must be recorded
- You may administer with a single signature any prescription-only medicine (POM), general sales list (GSL) or pharmacy (P) medication

---

It is also recommended that the competence of the person to whom the task has been delegated should be reviewed periodically (NMC 2008a).

Consent

Patients should give consent for medication and unless they are incapable, and proved not to have the mental capacity to consent, no medication should be given without their agreement (NMC 2008a) (see Chapter 1). In cases such as the unconscious patient, when the patient recovers consent should be sought at the earliest opportunity (NMC 2006). Children are generally considered to lack capacity, and the right to refuse treatment, including medication, usually lies with their parents, unless the child is considered to have significant understanding where an exception may occur (NMC 2006).

Giving medications to patients by hiding it in foods must be carried out only where this is in the best interests of the patient and the registered nurse is accountable for this decision (NMC 2008a). Therefore, if medication is being given to a patient by disguising it, there should be local policies and clear guidelines advising staff, because failure to adhere to these principles could potentially result in court action (NMC 2006).

Patient group directions or group protocols

A patient group direction is a specific written instruction for the supply and administration of a named medicine or vaccine in an identified clinical situation (NMC 2008a). A pharmacist and a doctor or dentist should have been involved in the development, and then approval must be obtained from the appropriate Health Board, Trust or Division. The role of the healthcare assistant may well be in giving a medicine within specific guidelines, but further training and assessment is essential.

Reflection point

Does your clinical area have any patient group directions? If so, identify which medications and patients they cover.

One-stop dispensing

Following the publication of *A Spoonful of Sugar* in England and Wales (Audit Commission 2002) and *The Right Medicine* (Scottish Executive 2002) in Scotland, one-stop dispensing has been encouraged within the hospital setting. This is a system of administering and dispensing medicinal products involving the use of patients' own medications while in hospital (NMC 2008a). In some instances this may also involve patients administering their own medication via a locked locker at the bedside.

Self-administration

In the hospital setting, self-administration is useful when preparing patients for discharge (Dougherty and Lister 2004). Indeed, self-administration is not merely the process of patients taking their own drugs, but can also help patients retain or regain control over their health. The NMC (2008a) both 'welcomes' and 'supports' self-administration of medicines by both patients and carers.

Some patients will require assistance in order to be able to take their medication safely and the use of a compliance aid or monitored dosage system allows each day's medication to be stored in a box with dividers for each day. It is recommended that they should be dispensed, labelled and sealed by a pharmacist and, if a pharmacist is not available and another personnel performs this task, it must be to the same standard (NMC 2008a). An example is shown in Figure 15.1.

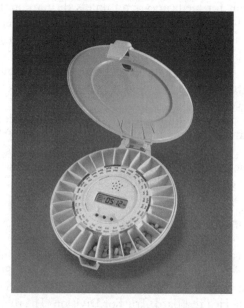

Figure 15.1   Compliance aid for medication delivery. Used with kind permission from Pivotell.

Clarification about the role of the healthcare assistant in the community is required at a local level if healthcare assistants are assisting patients to open these containers, which may be due to reduced dexterity, poor eyesight or loss of memory.

Record keeping

Accurate records detailing medication given or omitted are essential parts of medicine administration (see Chapter 4 for further information).

Common medications

There are multiple routes and preparations available, often for the same medication. The choice of route or preparation may be a result of a patient's symptoms, e.g. if a patient is vomiting oral medication may have to be changed to an alternative route, e.g. rectal administration. Healthcare assistants involved in medicine administration will be following local policies and procedure, and this will determine the level of knowledge required about the medicine and the side effects that may present.

Qualified personnel must prescribe all medications and the role of the healthcare assistant must be clearly defined. There are many different routes of administration and the most common are discussed below. Before and after all medicine administration, hands should be washed to prevent infection.

Reflection point

Think of some other medication routes and why these may be used instead of oral.

Oral route

This can take the form of either tablets (e.g. paracetamol tablets) or liquids (e.g. amoxicillin preparation for children). Consider if the patient has difficulty swallowing and, if so, report to the nurse in charge, where the medicine may need to be changed from tablets to a liquid, e.g. a patient who has had a cardiovascular accident (CVA or stroke) may have dysphagia (problems swallowing), especially if the tablets are large.

When administering tablets, their placement can vary, but this will be clearly indicated on the medicine bottle and the accompanying leaflet. Examples of different oral placement include buccal (which is placement between the gum and the inside of the mouth) or sublingual, which is under the tongue (Dougherty and Lister 2004).

Tablets should not be crushed or opened to release the medication unless the manufacturer states that this is acceptable, because this can alter the chemical properties of the medication (Morris 2005; NMC 2006). The advice on the label or leaflet will show if the medication needs to be administered depending on digestion, e.g. medication to be taken with/after meals. Tablets can be broken with a file if scored, or a tablet cutter can be used where appropriate, provided that the manufacturer's instructions are consulted.

Accurate measurement of liquid preparations is essential to prevent medication errors, and in some instances, this may require a drug calculation to be performed. Local policy dictates if a healthcare assistant can measure liquids.

In the case of mixtures, many have a relatively short shelf-life, and some need to be kept in the fridge, e.g. antibiotics. Tablets and capsules may be susceptible to moisture and need to be kept in a cool dry place (Dougherty and Lister 2004).

Topical creams

This refers to the application of cream, ointments or gels that have been prescribed to relieve symptoms experienced by the patient, e.g. hydrocortisone (steroid) cream or E45 cream for dermatological (skin) complaints.

As the cream/liquid is the active ingredient and is applied by direct contact, gloves should be worn. This prevents the person applying the cream or ointment receiving a dose of the medication, or a reaction on their skin. Where the application site includes broken skin, an aseptic technique (a technique that involves using sterile gloves and minimal touch to prevent infection) is required.

After application, the site should be observed for a local reaction or worsening of the condition, and reported to the nurse in charge. Patients may require assistance to apply topical creams due to difficulty in the patient reaching the site, e.g. if the area for application of the medication is on the patient's back.

Storage should be in conjunction with the manufacturer's recommendations, but extremes of temperature should be avoided because deterioration may occur (Dougherty and Lister 2004). Creams and ointments containing a medicine should have a date recorded, preferably on the medication, because many should only be used for a specific time after opening, e.g. 4 weeks after opening.

In some instances topical creams can be applied in preparation for a further procedure in either children or anxious patients (Spiers et al. 2001), e.g. venepuncture (taking blood; see Chapters 12 and 16). In such instances local protocols or patient group directions (see earlier) may be in place to allow administration (Ingram and Lavery 2007).

Ear

Administration via the ear canal is to relieve the symptoms of local symptoms, e.g. eardrops to soften wax.

Correct positioning of the patient both before and after administration is essential to ensure that the medication has the desired local effect and does not run out of the ear. This involves the patient tilting the head to the opposite side, which allows access to the ear canal and prevents the medication running out of the ear. The use of cotton wool can prevent this.

Local training and competency are needed to undertake this task.

Eyes

Administration into the eyes is to relieve local symptoms, e.g. due to infection, or postoperatively (after surgery), e.g. after cataract surgery.

Correct positioning of the patient both before and after administration is essential to ensure that the medication has the desired local effect. The patient will need to tilt the head back and look upwards. Care should also be taken to ensure that the medication does not run out of the eye before absorption. Local training and competency are needed to undertake this task.

Eyedrops and ointment may become contaminated with microorganisms during use and then pose a danger to the recipient. Therefore, in the hospital environment they are discarded 7 days after they are first opened, but this may be extended to 28 days in the community (Dougherty and Lister 2004). Some products need to be kept in the fridge; ensure that this is checked and guidance followed.

Subcutaneous

This involves a needle administering medication into the subcutaneous tissue (under the skin), e.g. insulin for a patient with diabetes (see Chapter 13). It is essential that correct disposal of the needle occurs to prevent needlestick injury.

It may be the patient who usually administers this medicine, but due to illness or lack of dexterity has become unable to do so.

Again, training and supervision are essential to ensure competence.

Some injections may need to be kept in the fridge and manufacturer's recommendations should be followed, e.g. insulin needs to be kept in the fridge.

Suppositories

These are solid wax pellets for rectal administration which may melt at body temperature or dissolve in the mucous secretions of the rectum (Dougherty and Lister 2004). Examples include glycerine suppositories to relieve constipation (local action) or some pain-relieving medications that have a systemic (widespread) effect, e.g. Voltarol (diclofenac) suppositories for pain relief.

The patient needs to lie on the left side if possible and draw the knees upward for best results and to be put at ease because they may find the procedure embarrassing.

Storage instructions may involve storage in the fridge and, again, manufacturer's instructions should be followed.

Administration by this route should only be undertaken after training and supervision, and in accordance with local policy.

Inhalation

This can include short-term symptomatic relief, e.g. inhalation of menthol crystals for a blocked nose, or inhalation of medication to treat a long-term condition, e.g. a Ventolin inhaler for asthma.

Inhalers can be adapted for use by children or those with poor dexterity – sometimes referred to as a 'spacer' (Figure 15.2).

Correct positioning: an upright position may need to be adopted to allow full lung expansion and allow correct medication delivery.

A good inhaler technique is essential with this route of administration and, where healthcare assistants are involved in patient education and assessment of inhaler technique, further training and assessment must be undertaken.

Aerosol containers should not be stored in direct sunlight or over radiators, because there is a risk of explosion if they are heated (Dougherty and Lister 2004).

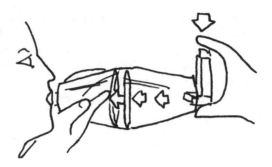

Figure 15.2   A 'spacer' inhaler.

Oxygen

Oxygen is a medication and requires a prescription to allow administration to patients. It is delivered in varying concentrations and is measured in percentages, e.g. 24%, 28%, 35% or 40%, depending on the patient's clinical symptoms (Baillie et al. 2005).

Different masks exist that include simple masks with no special features, a non-rebreathing mask, and a Venturi mask, where different coloured fittings dictate the oxygen percentage and flow rate that is required, depending on the prescription (Baillie et al. 2005). Masks are disposable and for single-patient use. They should be changed regularly to prevent infection.

Nasal cannulae can be used (Figure 15.3), which make it possible for the patient to eat, drink and talk while receiving oxygen (Moore 2007).

In the hospital setting oxygen is often 'piped', i.e. available at the bedside with a meter on the wall to apply tubing. In the community or in an ambulance this would involve an oxygen cylinder.

Wound dressings

If the healthcare assistant is performing simple dressings, which include applying a dressing to a wound, a prescription for the dressing will be required. The district nurse, who has undergone additional training, or the GP may prescribe this.

Best practice would be for the same person to carry out the dressing to monitor improvement or problems at the wound and always report to the nurse in charge. Further training and competence should be undertaken in line with local policy with regard to this skill.

Intravenous (medication administered directly into a vein)

This route should be performed only under strict local policies/procedures and competency-based training. It may include administration of fluids or medications. See Chapters 16 and 14 for further information about an intravenous flush (administration of 0.9% sodium chloride via a cannula to keep it patent, i.e. prevent blockage).

The NMC (2008a) state that, where a registered nurse delegates the task of giving a patient medication, this may be drawn up in advance after a full risk assessment and delegating the task to a 'named individual' (NMC 2008a).

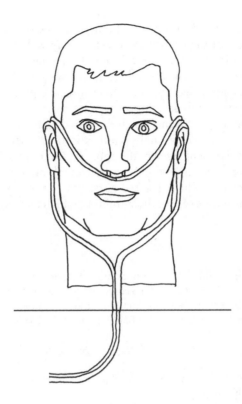

Figure 15.3   Nasal cannula.

Errors in administration and adverse reactions

As a registered nurse, if an error is made in medicines administration, there is a duty to take action to prevent harm to the patient (NMC 2008a). If the healthcare assistant is involved in medication administration under the delegation of the registered nurse and an error is made, it is essential that this is reported immediately to safeguard the patient.

In the case of an adverse incident occurring where actual harm has occured, it may be the healthcare assistant who is the first to notice the patient becoming unwell, and reporting this to the nurse in charge is essential. The duty of the registered nurse is to take action to remedy the harm, record it in the patient's notes, notify the prescriber and use a 'Yellow Card reporting system' if applicable (NMC 2008a). The Yellow Cards are at the back of the *British National Formulary* and online, and provide an important role in collecting evidence of adverse drug reactions. Where errors occur it is important to report as per local policy. In many cases these incidents will be anonymised and analysed either locally and/or nationally to allow lessons to be learnt and prevention of the same errors occurring again.

Summary

The evolving role of the healthcare assistant and imminent regulation means that medicine administration will probably play a key role in the future. In addition, the changes in healthcare result in more care being delivered in patients' homes and away from the hospital setting. To meet patients' needs, the role of the healthcare assistant may well develop as clinical team roles and responsibilities change (Scottish Executive 2005; Department of Health 2006).

However, before taking on any task involving medication, the healthcare assistant must be equipped with the relevant knowledge and skills to ensure safe patient care, and the role should ideally be incorporated into their job description.

Education in preparation for this role may include formal education, e.g. NVQ/SVQ (National Vocational Qualification/Scottish Vocational Qualification) as discussed in Chapter 1, or local training. This ensures that the patient receives the appropriate standard of care and the healthcare assistant is also safe to perform the task, with the employer taking responsibility for the healthcare assistants actions (see Chapter 1). The registered nurse who delegates this task should check this with the healthcare assistant and be sure of their abilities, which include reassessment periodically.

References

Audit Commission (2002) *A Spoonful of Sugar*. London: Audit Commission.

Baillie L, Corben V, Higham S (2005) Respiratory care: assessment and interventions. In: Baillie L (ed.), *Developing Practical Nursing Skills*, 2nd edn. London: Hodder Arnold, Chapter 11.

Corben V (2005) Administration of medicines. In: Baillie L (ed.), *Developing Practical Nursing Skills*, 2nd edn. London: Hodder Arnold, Chapter 4.

Department of Health (2006) *Our Health, Our Care, Our Say: A new direction for community services*. White paper London: DH.

Dougherty L, Lister S, eds (2004) *The Royal Marsden Hospital Manual of Clinical Nursing Procedures*, 6th edn. Oxford: Blackwell Publishing.

Ferguson A (2005) Administration of oral medication. *Nursing Times* 101(45): 24–25.

Ingram P, Lavery, I (2007) Peripheral intravenous cannulation: safe insertion and removal technique. *Nursing Standard* 22: 1 44–48.

McKenna H, Hasson F, Keeney S (2004) Patient safety and quality of care; the role of the health care assistant. *Journal of Nursing Management* 12: 452–459.

Medicines and Healthcare products Regulatory Agency (MHRA) (2004) Cited in Nursing and Midwifery Council (2008a).

Moore T (2007) Respiratory assessment in adults. *Nursing Standard* 21(49): 48–56.

Morris H (2005) Administering drugs to patients with swallowing difficulties. *Nursing Times* 101(39): 28–29

Nursing and Midwifery Council (NMC) (2006) *A–Z Advice Sheet*. London: NMC.

Nursing and Midwifery Council (2008a) *Standards for Medicines Management*. London: NMC.

Nursing and Midwifery Council (2008b) *The NMC Code of Professional Conduct: Standards for conduct, performance and ethics*. London: NMC.

Scottish Executive (2002) *The Right Medicine*. Edinburgh: Scottish Executive.

Scottish Executive (2005) *Delivering for Health*. Edinburgh: Scottish Executive.

Speirs AF, Taylor KH, Joanes DN, Girdler, NM (2001) A randomised, double-blind, placebo-controlled, comparative study of topical skin analgesics and the anxiety and discomfort associated with venous cannulation. *British Dental Journal* 190: 444–449.

Chapter 16

Peripheral intravenous cannulation

Learning objectives

- Review the anatomy and physiology relating to peripheral intravenous (IV) cannulation (see Chapter 12 for the anatomy and physiology of the arm)
- Review the skills and competence with regard to undertaking peripheral IV cannulation
- Describe possible complications of peripheral IV cannulation and how to manage them

Aim of this chapter

The aim of this chapter is to review the reasons and procedure for undertaking peripheral intravenous (IV) cannulation in the arm, and discuss the possible complications and risk prevention. *This may, however, not be a role that is expected of all healthcare assistants; check your local policy and access any approved training via your manager/charge nurse.* Also insertion of a cannula requires a saline flush to confirm patent (working); again many healthcare assistants may not be covered or allowed to administer this because classed as a medicine and many clinical areas do not allow healthcare assistants to administer any medicines (see Chapter 15); *again check your local policy for guidance.*

Reasons for cannulation

Peripheral IV cannulation is the introduction of a cannula into a peripheral vein as a means of gaining direct access into the venous circulation. Davies (1998) observed that cannulation is not just a technical skill, but also one that requires specialist knowledge, as well as good communication skills, time and patience. Parker (2002) noted that the risk of colonisation (presence of bacteria) of intravenous lines and cannulae was higher when inserted and maintained by inexperienced staff. *Please ensure that you are given local training and support, to make sure that you are competent in this role before commencing this skill.*

Why perform peripheral IV cannulation

The following list gives some indication of why a patient may require insertion of a cannula; however, many of these are not within the scope of the healthcare assistant to carry out:

- To administer intravenous fluids for the maintenance of fluid and electrolyte balance (elements carried in the blood)

- To administer intravenous medicines (bolus, intermittently or continuously)
- To transfuse blood and blood products
- Just in case, e.g. a professional judgement, in case patient collapses
- Venesection (bleeding a volume of blood from patient, similar to blood donation)
- To provide access for nutritional support
- To aid in monitoring of a patient's condition.

The decision to insert a cannula will usually be made by a doctor or registered nurse; however, in some practice settings this may also be made based on a care pathway or protocol. *Be aware of your local policy and adhere to local guidance.*

Relevant anatomy and physiology

See Chapter 12 for the anatomy and physiology of the arm. Figures 16.1 and 16.2 are a review of the anatomy and physiology of the arm and hand relating to the veins commonly used in peripheral IV cannulation, and Figure 16.3 shows a cross-section of a vein. It is essential that

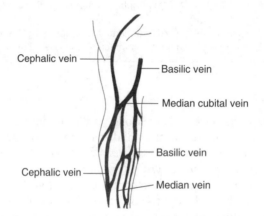

Figure 16.1   Venous anatomy of upper arm.

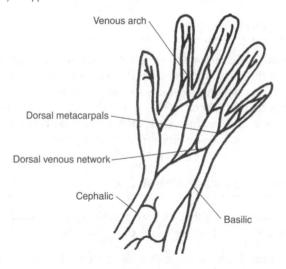

Figure 16.2   Hand Veins.

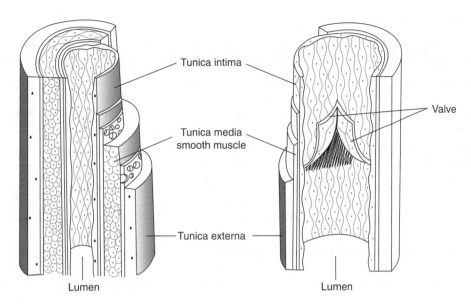

Figure 16.3   Cross-section of vein.

the healthcare assistant undertaking peripheral IV cannulation has a good understanding of the anatomy and physiology of arteries, veins and associated nerves.

How to insert and remove a peripheral IV cannula

Assessment of the patient and their veins

The healthcare assistant must take time to observe and assess patients and their veins. This is essential because the healthcare assistant must be able to see and feel the vein, so ensure that they choose the most appropriate site (Ingram and Lavery 2007; Dougherty and Lister 2004).

Use veins that feel soft and resilient, and refill when depressed, often described by practitioners as 'juicy' or 'bouncy'. Also consider the length of the cannula, so ensure that a straight vein suitable for the length of the cannula is selected with large veins being preferable to small veins. Patient involvement is essential, so ensure that the procedure is discussed with the patient, to gain consent and identify any site preference, e.g. the patient's non-dominant arm (Lavery 2003; Dougherty and Lister 2004).

Tagalakis et al. (2002) indicated risk factors relating to the cannula, the patient and other aspects that should be considered when proceeding in this role (Table 16.1).

Common sites (see Figure 16.1)

- Dorsal venous arch on hand
- Forearm vein
- Cephalic vein on thumb side of wrist
- Basilic vein on pinkie side of arm.

Take care because the most prominent vein is not necessarily the most suitable.

Table 16.1 Risk factors

Catheter specific	Patient specific	Other
How long it will be in; over 72 h increases risk, e.g. infection	Poor quality peripheral veins	Experience of inserter, e.g. how skilled
Cannula material	Site of cannula insertion	Insertion in an emergency
Cannula size (gauge)	Gender, e.g. females higher risk	Daily gauze dressing changes
Type of fluids/medicines infusing/transfusing	Underlying medical disease or history, e.g. diabetes	
Cannula-related infection, e.g. existing infection	Patient age, e.g. very young or very old	

Adapted from Tagalakis et al. (2002) and Hadaway and Millam (2005).

Criteria for selecting a site for cannulation

Hadaway and Millam (2005) note many crucial factors in selecting an appropriate vein and the device:

1. The patient's medical history
2. Age, body size, weight, general condition and level of physical activity
3. Condition of the patient's veins
4. Type of fluid or medication to be infused/transfused
5. Expected duration of IV therapy
6. The skill of the individual inserting the device.

Hadaway and Millam (2005) suggested, for adults, starting with veins in the hand, but Millam (2003) recommended avoiding hand veins in the older person, because they lose subcutaneous tissue surrounding the veins, so the veins are more likely to 'roll', resulting in an unsuccessful insertion. The healthcare assistant can observe this when palpating (feeling), because the vein tends to move easily under the skin. Moreau (2004) and Rosenthal (2005) also suggested caution in the older patient, because they lose skin tone and elasticity, which results in their skin being more fragile and prone to bruising, and the vein 'blowing' (rupturing).

Areas to avoid (Rosenthal 2005)

- Areas of joint flexion, e.g. wrist/elbow, because can cause cannula to kink
- Veins in legs, because they can increase risk of deep vein thrombosis
- Veins close to an artery, in case of accidental arterial puncture
- Previously cannulated veins, due to scarring or possible infection
- Veins on the palm side of the wrist because of risk of pain from the radial nerve
- Veins that feel hard or 'cord like' because scarring will prevent successful cannulation
- Limbs with fractures due to local pain and possible limited access
- Median cubital veins (elbow area): reserved for venous blood sampling
- Sites with infection or active skin conditions, e.g. psoriasis
- Black and Hughes (1997) also noted care when applying the tourniquet if a patient has rheumatoid arthritis, especially over the elbow joint, because the joint capsule may be inflamed and so cause pain.

Choosing the appropriate cannula

There is a range of cannula sizes (gauges), and the healthcare assistant must be aware of the reason for the cannula being inserted, because this should help in selection of the correct gauge and site. A cannula should be the smallest possible to prevent any internal vein damage and allow any medicines being administered to 'mix' with the blood in the vein (Hadaway and Millam 2005). A small cannula will also cause the patient the least discomfort and this is an important factor. Table 16.2 gives guidance; seek local guidance when necessary.

Table 16.2 Cannula choice guidance

Cannula size	Care situation
14 gauge	Emergency, e.g. cardiac arrest
16 gauge	Major trauma or surgery, massive fluid replacement
18 gauge	Routine blood transfusions, rapid infusion, surgical or trauma patient
20 gauge	Routine infusions, bolus drug administration, medical, post op patient
22 gauge	Small fragile veins, short-term access
24 gauge	Small or fragile veins, children, older patient

Adapted with permission from NHS Lothian (2007).

Reflection point

Why is the patient's age a factor that you need to think about when assessing for a site?

Infection

Peripheral IV cannulation breaches the circulatory system, so healthcare assistants should consider their role in the prevention of infection (Box 16.1).

Box 16.1 Predisposing infection risk factors and management

- Skin colonisation (surface bacterial spread) can allow bacteria to enter the circulatory system through the insertion of the needle and cannula, so ensure careful site selection and cleansing
- Remote infection (e.g. urinary tract infection) can also lead to a risk; the patient should be educated about not tampering with the site, cannula or sterile dressing, and this should reduce the risk of transferring bacteria
- Multi-use disinfectants can become colonised with bacteria very quickly, so use only single-use sachets when cleansing the site
- Expired or damaged stock can be a source of infection; ensure stock is in date and has been stored correctly, and is used for its intended purpose; single-use devices must be used (Medicines Devices Agency [MDA] 2000)
- Hands of practitioners are the single most common way in which bacteria are transferred onto devices (equipment), so ensure correct hand cleansing

(NHS Lothian 2007 with permission.)

Hand hygiene

Before, during and after an invasive procedure such as peripheral IV cannulation, e.g. after contact with a source of microbes (germs): wash hands with liquid soap and warm water for 10–15 seconds, dry thoroughly with paper towels then follow with alcohol hand rub. Alternatives are discussed in Chapter 12.

Aseptic (sterile) technique

This prevents microbial (bacterial) contamination of susceptible sites by ensuring that only sterile objects and fluids touch them. An aseptic technique must be used when introducing an invasive device such as a cannula into the circulatory system, which is a breach of the body's natural defence system (May 2000). Wilson (2001) and Damani (2003) promoted skin cleansing with soap and water and drying thoroughly if the site is visibly dirty, then cleansing proposed cannulation site with an alcohol swab for at least 30 s, and allowing to air dry for a further 30 s.

Protective clothing

Healthcare assistants should wear non-sterile disposable gloves and a disposable apron. Latex and the associated risks are now widely known and so it is advisable to consider the type of glove available and ensure it minimises exposure to harmful substances (RCN 2005).

Environment

Good practice requires either a clean trolley or tray to assemble and hold all the necessary sterile equipment (Dougherty and Lister 2004). Adequate lighting is essential to ensure careful assessment of the patient and their veins, as is the patient being relaxed, so should be sitting or resting on a trolley/bed with the arm supported on the bed or with a pillow. The safety of the healthcare assistant is also important, so ensure comfort by adjusting bed height and sitting, if suitable, and have a sharps bin in position.

Discussion point

When using a tourniquet ensure it is either cleaned between patients or use single patient disposable tourniquets.

Performing peripheral IV cannula: requirements and technique

Please refer to Box 16.2 for the equipment required for a cannulation insertion and Table 16.3 for preparation.

Table 16.4 outlines the specific actions and observations required throughout the procedure.

Box 16.2 Equipment required for cannulation procedure

Tourniquet – consider quick release, latex free
Non-sterile gloves and apron
Alcohol swab (70% isopropyl)
Appropriate size cannula
Closed system*(recommended)*, e.g. Smartsite
Sterile dressing (e.g. Tegaderm or IV3000)
Pad to protect from spillage
Clean tray/trolley
10 ml syringe
5 ml ampoule sterile 0.9% NaCl flush
Sterile green or blue needle or sharps-less needle
Appropriate IV fluid for administration[a]
Medical device (if required)[a]
Sharps bin/container

[a]As mentioned at the start of the chapter, some healthcare assistants may not be covered to administer either flush or intravenous fluids; check local policy. If this is the case, the healthcare assistant may require a registered nurse or doctor to flush the device once they have inserted the cannula (Figure 16.4).

Table 16.3 Preparation for procedure

Action	Reason
1. Wash hands with liquid soap, and dry hands thoroughly, followed by an alcohol hand rub, or wash with an approved antiseptic solution	To minimise the risk of healthcare-associated infection (HAI)
2. Assemble all the equipment required for the procedure on a clean trolley or a tray	In order that the procedure is carried out smoothly, efficiently and without interruptions
3. Ensure that all the equipment used is intact and within expiry dates	To maintain asepsis
4. Approach the patient and explain the procedure in a confident manner	To obtain patient consent and cooperation
Allow the patient time to ask questions and express concerns about the procedure, if any	
5. Help the patient into a comfortable position, e.g. sitting in a chair or lying on bed and support arm with a pillow	To maintain the patient's comfort
	To enable the operator to carry out the procedure with ease
Ask patient if they have ever had problems with procedure, e.g. previous fainting episode; if so lay the patient on a bed, to prevent a vasovagal (faint) episode	
6. Prepare the area, e.g. provide adequate lighting, privacy and heighten the bed, lower cot sides, check positioning	Safe working environment
7. Verbally check the identity of the patient – name, date of birth (DOB) against identification (e.g. patient ID bracelet) and documentation, e.g. care pathway.	Identify the need for the procedure
	To ensure that the peripheral IV cannula is being inserted into the right patient

Adapted with permission from NHS Lothian (2007).

Table 16.4 Specific actions and observations during the procedure

Action	Reason
1. Wash hands with liquid soap, and dry hands thoroughly followed by an alcohol hand rub, or wash with an approved antiseptic solution	To minimise the risk of healthcare-associated infection (HAI)
2. Consult with the patient with regard to preferences for cannulation site, based on previous experiences	To actively involve the patient in own treatment. To be aware of the patient's history and factors that may influence choice of vein
3. Apply tourniquet to the arm on the chosen side approximately 7–10 cm (3–4 inches) above selected site for cannulation	Increases venous pressure, aiding vein identification and entry
Apply enough pressure to impede (restrict) venous circulation	Check radial pulse to ensure that arterial flow is not affected
Consider the use of a disposable tourniquet, if available	Reduce risks of cross-contamination
3. To further encourage venous filling try one of the following;	Helps make vein more prominent and so easier to assess and cannulate
(a) Stroke the vein gently (b) Allow the arm to hang by patient's side (gravity) (c) Immerse limb in warm/hot water for 5–10 min (d) Ask patient to clench fist and then relax, several times	
4. Palpate (feel) the selected vein	To identify its course, depth and structures, i.e. tendons, and to avoid nearby arteries or nerves
5. Release the tourniquet and check vein decompresses (returns to normal)	To prevent cell damage due to decreased oxygen (O_2) supply
6. Choose and prepare the smallest practical cannula size (gauge)	Ensure appropriate size
7. Hand antisepsis; use either an alcohol hand rub or wash with an approved antiseptic solution	To minimise the risk of healthcare-associated infection (HAI)
8. Reapply tourniquet to the chosen site	
9. Cleanse the proposed cannulation site with alcohol skin prep, using a firm circular motion from centre to the periphery, for 30 s and at least a 5–7 cm (2–3 inches) area – size of dressing area	To minimise the risk of HAI
Allow the alcohol to air dry, for a minimum of 30 s	Prevent stinging as cannula pierces the skin
DO NOT re-palpate the vein after the site has been cleansed; use a mental marker, if necessary, e.g. freckle	Increases risk of infection
DO NOT shave the skin at the insertion point	Can cause microscopic damage to skin
10. Put on gloves	Gloves will give some protection from blood spillage
11. Fold down the wings of the cannula	This grip reduces the risk of contaminating the cannula
12. With the patient's arm in a supported downward position, anchor the vein by applying tension to the skin below and to side of the cannulation site	Prevents vein from rolling or moving Prevents risk of injury to nurse inserting
13. Insert the device into the vein at an angle (depending on device used) holding the cannula firmly with a three-point grip and bevel (cut) up	Ensures correct positioning between needle and catheter tip, and stabilises cannula within the needle
Fragile veins usually require a lower angle of insertion	Reduce overshooting
Watch for the presence of blood in the flashback chamber	This flashback indicates that the needle has successfully entered the vein (Figure 16.5)

Table 16.4 (*Continue*)

Action	Reason
14. Lower the angle of the cannula to almost skin level. Advance the cannula a few millimetres into the vein and avoid contamination by holding at the wings or protection cap	To prevent puncture of the rear wall of the vessel
	This ensures that the cannula tip also enters the vein
No resistance should be felt as cannula advances into vein	If resistance felt, consider if pierced rear of vein due to angle, or cannula not in vein initially. Remove cannula
15. Withdraw the introducer needle partially (approx. 2–5 mm)	To avoid exit through the rear of vein wall and provide stability to cannula
16. First hold the flashback chamber immobilising the needle. Then advance the cannula forward off the needle into the vein with the other hand; this should be in a smooth single movement	The plastic cannula advances only into the vein
	Consider point 14 as cannula should advance easily; if not may require removal and new cannula insertion in different vein and site
17. Release the tourniquet	Release venous pressure
18. The needle must never be reinserted while cannula is in the vein (some devices now prevent this, e.g. Vasofix)	To avoid risk of needle severing the cannula and cause plastic embolus
Apply pressure over the vein distal to the cannula tip (beyond the end of cannula)	To avoid spillage of blood when needle is removed (raising the patient's arm also reduces risk of spillage)
19a. Remove the introducer needle completely, and dispose of immediately into sharps bin, e.g. Vasofix needle cap flips over as it is withdrawn and a slight resistance might occur	Reduces risk of needlestick injury
	Ensure firm grasp of device while withdrawing needle to prevent accidental removal or dislodging of cannula
19b. Close the cannula with a closed system, e.g. Smartsite, or device cap if closed system not used	Reduce number of times cannula is reconnected to reduce infection rate and mechanical irritation
20. Flush the cannula with 5 ml 0.9% NaCl (physiological saline) or flush volume of twice the length of the cannula, plus any device, e.g. closed system, using push–pause method and positive pressure via the intermittent port or closed system connector[a]	To confirm correct placement of the cannula, the push–pause method helps create turbulence and so maintains flow, and positive pressure means that no blood can backflow into the cannula
21. Secure the cannula in position with sterile dressing, e.g. IV 2000 or Tegaderm IV (Figure 16.6)	Good fixation is essential to prevent poor position, rolling or other movements of the cannula, because can cause irritation of the vein
Skin may be clipped adjacent to, but not at insertion site, to secure the dressing	Reducing the risk of HAI
22. Make no more than two attempts to insert cannula. If unsuccessful, obtain assistance from more experienced staff	Patient comfort
	Prevent trauma to vein
23. Ensure that patient is given appropriate education once cannula is in place	Ensure cannula safety and sustain for duration required or 72–96 hours
24. Enter date and time of insertion, site, cannula size and reason for insertion in patient notes, and record signature of operator	Good record keeping and legal requirement
	Some areas may record date and time on dressing too, to aid monitoring

Adapted with permission from NHS Lothian (2007).

[a] Push–pause and positive pressure stage 20 – holding plunger with thumb, insert small volume then pause, then repeat, till all the saline is flushed in, then maintain pressure on plunger as syringe is removed.

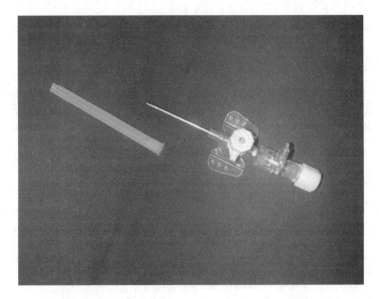

Figure 16.4 Example of cannula. (Photograph by I Lavery.)

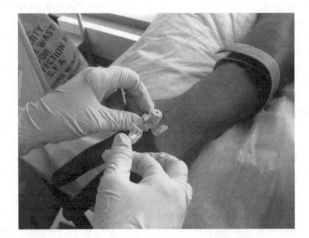

Figure 16.5 Inserting the cannula. (Photograph by I Lavery.)

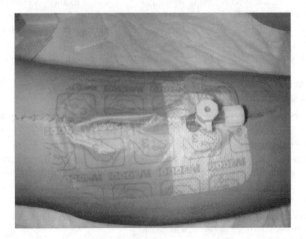

Figure 16.6 Device in place. (Photograph by I Lavery.)

Patient education for peripheral IV cannulation

Before and during insertion take care to use language that will not distress the patient. Rosenthal (2005) suggested avoiding the use of words such as 'needle' and 'stick', and use 'plastic tube' and 'insert' instead, and explain to the patient that it is the 'plastic' cannula that is inserted not the needle.

Ensure that the patient has also understood the reason for the cannula, and keep them informed about ongoing treatments (Lundgren et al. 1998).

Advise the patient to report any concerns, including if the site becomes painful, swollen, hot or tender, if there is any leakage or the dressing becomes loose. Also advise patients to take care when dressing and undressing because this can dislodge the cannula. Ask them not to tamper or touch the dressing and to try to minimise movement in the arm, especially if near an area of flexion, e.g. wrist or elbow. All these should ensure a safe cannula for the duration and help the patient comply with the procedure (Ingram and Lavery 2007).

Refer to Table 16.5 for information on the maintenance and care of a cannula after insertion.

Table 16.5 Maintenance and care of the intravenous (IV) cannula after insertion

Action	Reason
1a. Inspect the cannula each shift or more frequently depending on patient's clinical condition and type of therapy	To ensure cannula is in correct position and observe for potential complications, e.g. phlebitis
1b. Flush cannula with 5 ml 0.9% NaCl or the flush volume is twice the length of the cannula plus any device, e.g. closed system	To maintain patency of cannula and ensure flush volume adequate *Not all healthcare assistants are allowed to administer medicines – check your local policy*
1c. The cannula site should also be monitored each shift or at least daily Recommendations for resiting are after a period of 72–96 h However, cannula may be left in for longer and reason documented, e.g. 　– when initial cannulation was difficult 　– when therapy will be completed shortly afterwards	To reduce complications including healthcare-associated infection and to ensure that length of time cannula is in place reflects individual management of each patient and needs To provide reason and justify decisions
2. Use a rigorous aseptic technique when handling the cannula/lines: 　– reduce manipulations of the system to a minimum 　– keep number of stopcocks and taps to a minimum 　– injection sites and bungs cleaned with an alcohol swab and allowed to dry	Any connection in an IV system is a potential point of entry for microorganisms Recommend use of closed system to minimise infection from port
3. Maintain appropriate level of hand hygiene antisepsis before handling the cannula/lines at any time	To minimise risk of infection
4. Document in care plan/notes: 　– date and time of insertion 　– gauge (size) of catheter 　– site of insertion 　– signature 　– flush and amount (volume)	Good record keeping and legal requirement

Adapted with permission from NHS Lothian (2007).

Reflection point

While inserting a cannula you encounter resistance. What would you do?

Re-siting of a peripheral IV cannula (*once discussed and agreed locally*)

- Follow the same procedure as for initial insertion
- After 72–96 hours, if still required, check with senior/charge nurse or notes
- If inserted in an emergency re-site after 24 hours (e.g. emergency insertion may not have had time to include appropriate skin cleansing)
- If site becomes infected, cannula is blocked or leaking, or infiltrates the surrounding area (see under problems)
- Select another vein, alternating between arms if possible, for the new cannula, but proximal (above) to the previously cannulated site
- Choice of cannulation site will depend on the patient's local anatomy, patient mobility and the required flow rates; however, rotation of sites is essential
- Continue to use the distal veins of the arms if possible
- Document reason for removal, including any signs and symptoms of infection or problems and record (see point 4 in Table 16.5).

Related aspects and terminology

Consent

Consent requires the patient to understand what the procedure is and why a cannula is required (Lavery 2003). Therefore, a careful explanation is essential not only to help the patient agree to the procedure, but also to help relax the patient. The communication should also include patient education, which was discussed earlier; however, see Chapters 4 and 12 for more on consent.

Anxiety

As already discussed in Chapter 12, patients may experience anxiety, so they should be asked if they have had a cannula inserted previously, because anxiety may be due to a previous bad experience, a degree of 'needle phobia' (fear of a needle) or just a dislike of medical procedures. See Chapter 12 for suggestions on reducing or managing anxiety.

Reflection point

What options might you consider if your patient were very anxious about the procedure?

Terminology

- Vasovagal episode: blood pressure drops and patient may feel faint
- Erythema: redness
- Cerebrovascular accident (CVA): commonly known as a stroke
- Phlebitis: inflammation/infection of the vein.
- Rigors: shivering associated with high temperature
- Hypotension: low blood pressure
- Malaise: tiredness, weakness
- Venesection: blood is taken from the patient, e.g. to reduce haemoglobin level, and commonly this technique is used in patients with chronic bronchitis.

Common problems/potential complications of peripheral IV cannulation

Unsuccessful cannulation

This may be due to the healthcare assistants inexperience or the condition of the patient and their veins (Ingram and Lavery 2007). Careful assessment and appropriate supervision of the healthcare assistant while 'learning' this skill are essential. *Ensure that you have followed local policy to achieve competent and safe practice.*

Management

Pull firmly downwards on the skin to straighten and stabilise the vein during insertion. If the vein is mobile, especially in older patients, the needle can pass along the outside of the vessel and fail to enter the lumen (inner layer of vein) (Dougherty 1996).

Damaged device

Hamilton (2006) suggested that re-sheathing the needle into the cannula would cause damage to the interior of the cannula. Or, if excessive pressure is exerted within the cannula, often due to flushing with a syringe smaller than 10 ml, this causes internal pressures that can rupture the device (Hamilton 2006).

Prevention

- Never re-sheath needle; where possible use a safety device, e.g. Vasofix
- Flush using a 10 ml syringe and a pulsated gentle push–pause technique.

Haematoma

Dougherty and Lister (2004) defined this as a collection of blood that leaks from a vein into the tissues surrounding the insertion site; it is often caused by poor technique during insertion, which may cause a hard painful lump. The presence of haematomas may limit the use of the vein for future cannulation (or venepuncture).

Prevention

- Correct insertion technique
- Firm pressure on cannula site after removal.

Management

If a haematoma occurs during the procedure, release the tourniquet, remove the cannula and apply firm pressure for 2–3 min and elevate the arm. Apply a sterile dressing and ensure that this is documented; also ensure regular monitoring of the site.

Bruising

Ingram and Lavery (2007) noted this common risk, caused by leakage of blood into the tissues, e.g. poor technique during cannulation, or in patients who bleed easily, such as older patient with friable veins, or on treatments that thin the blood/affect clotting.

Prevention

- Accurate identification of a suitable vein
- Use of a blood pressure cuff instead of a tourniquet in the older patient (Hadaway 1991; Rosenthal 2005)
- In an older patient apply a tourniquet over a thin layer of clothing (Dougherty and Lamb 1999)
- Select the appropriate cannula after your patient assessment
- Correct insertion technique, including angle of entry (Dougherty 1996)
- Firm pressure on the puncture site on removal of the cannula.

Infiltration and extravasation

Infiltration (often referred to as 'tissueing') occurs when the cannula pulls out of the vein and the infusion fluid accumulates in the tissue around the cannula site (Workman 1999; Hadaway 2004). Workman (1999) proposed careful monitoring of the site in an older patient, who may not report discomfort as quickly, because loss of skin tone and elasticity means that tissues around the site have a greater capacity to expand with the leaking fluid.

Extravasation is the infiltration of a vesicant (irritating agent) medicine from an IV line into the surrounding tissue, and can cause severe tissue injury or destruction (Hadaway 2004).

Prevention

- Secure the cannula firmly with a sterile dressing while in place
- Ensure that appropriate gauge of cannula is selected
- Replace cannula after 72–96 h (Ingram and Lavery 2007)
- Secure lines and extensions to the limb to prevent accidental pulling (Workman 1999).

Signs

- Swelling
- Discomfort

- 'Tightness' at the site
- Pain
- Burning sensation – associated with extravasation
- Blanching and coolness of the skin.

Management (Workman 1999)

1. Immediately stop the infusion and disconnect the tubing; alert medical staff.
2. If a cannula is needed, re-site in the other arm to allow swelling to subside.
3. Where infiltration has occurred, elevate the arm and apply a warm compress.
4. Intervene rapidly to any suspected extravasation injury, e.g. either apply an ice pack or warm compress depending on vesicant (agent), elevate the arm and administer antidote; *this would be the role of registered nurse or doctor only, and would require a local policy.*
5. Reassure the patient that the swelling will subside in a few days.
6. Document and monitor the patient and site to prevent permanent damage.

Phlebitis

This is inflammation of the vein and can be caused by mechanical damage, chemical irritation or infection (Ingram and Lavery 2005).

- Mechanical damage is caused by the rubbing of the cannula against the inner (intima) wall of the vein if a cannula is not secured with a sterile dressing.
- Chemical irritation is caused by the infusion of irritant medicines/fluids or a reaction to the cannula material.
- Infection is caused by the contamination of the cannula by microorganisms.

Prevention (Lavery and Ingram 2007)

- Remove the cannula as soon as it is no longer clinically indicated
- Change the IV cannula every 72–96 h
- Regularly inspect the IV site (at least daily)
- Remove the cannula at the first sign of phlebitis
- Use strict aseptic technique during insertion and manipulation of cannula
- Secure the device with a sterile dressing.

Signs

- Erythema
- Pain at the insertion site
- Localised skin temperature
- Swelling
- Leakage
- In extreme cases, pus at the insertion site on removal of cannula.

Management

It is recommended to use a phlebitis scale to monitor (Jackson 1997; Davies 1998; Rosenthal 2004).

- Mechanical and chemical phlebitis: remove cannula and apply warm moist compress
- Bacterial phlebitis: remove cannula, take blood cultures, then apply warm compress
- Post-infusion phlebitis: this can occur 24–96 h after the cannula is removed; apply a warm moist compress (Macklin 2003).

Thrombophlebitis

Tortora and Derrickson (2006) defined this as inflammation of the vein and clot formation. Thromboembolism occurs when a blood clot on the cannulated vein wall becomes detached, and could pass by venous flow to the heart and pulmonary (lung) circulation.

Prevention

- Use a small gauge cannula, allowing continuous blood flow around it
- If an infusion stops as a result of clot formation, do **not** flush the cannula because it may dislodge the clot into the circulation; remove the cannula
- Ensure correct insertion technique.

Air embolism

This is a possible hazard during IV therapy; *however, few healthcare assistants would be involved in administering IV fluids,* and it is caused if lines and connections are not secure, and any attachment, e.g. closed system, is not flushed first before connection.

Prevention

- Air must be removed from all extension lines, stopcocks and administration sets during the priming of the system
- Ensure that Luer locks are tight fitting
- Clamp the infusion line before the bag empties completely.

Arterial cannulation

This is identified by bright red blood pulsating into the flashback chamber and is caused by inappropriate assessment and insertion angle.

Prevention

- Plan procedure carefully
- Apply sound knowledge of venous and arterial structures in the arm
- Insert cannula at the appropriate angle; consult manufacturer's guide.

Action

- Remove the cannula immediately and apply firm pressure for 5 min, until bleeding stops
- Apply a pressure bandage for 10–15 min
- Elevate the arm
- Check the patient's radial pulse, to ensure that pressure bandage is not too tight
- Inform medical staff; once they are satisfied that bleeding has stopped the pressure bandage is removed and the site covered with a sterile dressing
- Do not use that site for a further 24 hours
- Monitor the site over 24 hours and document the incident in patient's notes.

Nerve damage

This is a rare complication caused by poor assessment and inappropriate angle of insertion. The patient may report pain, numbness or tingling in the arm (Dougherty and Lister 2004).

Management

1. Remove the needle/cannula immediately
2. Apply pressure to stop the bleeding
3. Inform the doctor
4. Record the incident in the patient's notes
5. Observe and advise the patient to report if symptoms worsen
6. Treatment is symptomatic, so analgesia may be prescribed for pain
7. Reassure the patient
8. Physiotherapy may be necessary (Dougherty and Lister 2004).

Delay

In the situation where a patient has collapsed, ensure that help is on the way using the normal emergency procedures. Stay with the patient. It is essential that peripheral IV cannulation be undertaken as soon as possible, as the patient's worsening clinical condition is likely to make cannulation more difficult. **Do not delay** in gaining access (Ingram and Lavery 2007).

Reflection point

Consider, if an emergency and a patient had collapsed, whether the insertion of a cannula would be your priority. What is your local policy?

Other complications of peripheral IV cannulation

- Use of inappropriate sites
- Circulatory overload: too rapid IV rate, wrongly prescribed, wrongly set rate; *this would not be an aspect in which the healthcare assistant would be involved*

- Kinking of cannula; common if sited in an area of flexion, e.g. elbow
- Plastic embolism: this risk is reduced with safety cannula, e.g. Vasofix, because it is now not possible to reinsert the needle back into the cannula
- Tourniquet left in place
- Septicaemia: result of bacteria entering the bloodstream; patient presents with general malaise, temperature, rigors and hypotension.

Table 16.7 is a competency framework for peripheral IV cannulation.

Reflection point

While removing a cannula, you observe some redness around the site. What might be the cause and what actions will you take?

Removal of peripheral IV cannula

Once a decision has been made to remove the cannula, explain the procedure to the patient, and obtain patient consent and cooperation (see Table 16.6 for the procedure).

Table 16.6 Specific nursing actions during procedure-removal

Action	Reason
1. Close the flow clamp to discontinue the infusion of fluid (if necessary and if an accepted part of a healthcare assistant's role)	Prevent fluid leakage
2. Decontaminate (wash) hands, put on gloves	Prevention of infection and of healthcare assistant's hands being contaminated with blood
3. Expose the cannula site and, using aseptic technique, remove the dressing. Do not use scissors	May inadvertently cut the cannula resulting in fragments that can cause embolus (clot)
4. Apply gentle pressure with a swab/cotton ball above the cannulation site while withdrawing the cannula On removal, apply firm pressure for approximately 2–3 min until bleeding stops	Excessive pressure applied to a cannula that is blocked could result in thrombus (fixed clot) being expelled into the blood stream causing an embolus
5. Check patient has no allergy, then cover the site with a plaster/sterile dressing, until the puncture site has healed Continue to observe the site	To prevent bacteria from entering the puncture site Cotton ball may adhere and when removed bleeding restarts
6. Check that cannula removed is undamaged and intact. Discard immediately into a sharps bin However, if there are signs of infection present, report this to a senior nurse and it may be necessary to obtain a swab from the insertion site and the tip of cannula, and send to the laboratory for culture	Ensure no trauma to vein Microbiological investigations
7. Document the date and time of cannula removal and any problems encountered or not	Good record keeping and legal requirement

Adapted with permission from NHS Lothian (2007).

Equipment required: as well as a clinical waste bag and sharps bin:

- Gloves and apron
- Tray or clean receptacle
- Cotton ball/gauze swab
- Pad for spillage
- Sterile dressing/plaster
- Tape to secure dressing, if used.

Summary

Peripheral IV canulation requires specialist knowledge and skill (Davies 1988), and effective communication to ensure the patient is aware of the procedure and risks so they can consent and cooperate fully. Allied with these skills are the need for aseptic technique, monitoring and prompt recording to ensure the patient is not open to risks of infection or a neglected canula.

Case study 16.1

Miss Winifred Allsop, aged 72 years, has had a stroke (CVA) affecting her right arm and has rheumatoid arthritis. What assessment factors do you need to consider?

Below, the reader will find a self-assessment checklist; however, the reader may also wish to review Skills for Health (2004) competence HSC72.

 ## Self-assessment

Assessment	Aspects	Achieved ✔
Patient	*Have you considered all aspects of this section?*	
	Patient assessment: veins and general condition	
	Infection control and asepsis aspects	
	Consent, communication and education	
	Problem solving	
Procedure	*Have you considered all aspects of this section?*	**Achieved ✔**
	Selecting equipment and insertion technique	
	Problem solving	
	Recording	
	Monitoring, maintenance and reporting concerns	
	Removal	

Table 16.7 Practical assessment form: competency – peripheral IV cannulation

Steps	First assessment/Reassessment					Date/competent/signature
	Demonstration					
	Date/sign	Date/sign	Date/sign	Date/sign	Date/sign	
	1	2	3	4	5	
1 Washed hands and apron worn						
2 Assembled all equipment required on clean tray or trolley and equipment in date and intact						
3 Procedure explained, verbal consent gained						
4 Patient's comfort considered and positioning appropriate for safe practice						
5 Environment prepared – lighting, bed height, privacy if required, and sharps bin ready						
6 Patient's identity confirmed per local policy						
7 Considers with patient; vein of choice by assessing sites and patient comfort						
8 Prepares cannula – depending on patient's condition and reason for cannula						
9 Tourniquet applied 7–10 cm above chosen site, and vein assessed as suitable						
10 Tourniquet released and vein checked decompressed						
11 Hands washed or bactericidal hand rub used						
12 Tourniquet re-applied to chosen site						
13 Site cleansed for at least 30 s and allowed to air dry for minimum of 30 s						

14	Gloves put on		
15	Vein cannulated successfully following approved local procedure and policy		
16	Tourniquet released		
17	Pressure applied distally to vein, needle is removed, while cannula supported to prevent dislodging		
18	Needle disposed of as per local policy immediately		
19	Considers closed system, e.g. Smartsite, to minimise trauma and infection from port site		
20	Cannula flushed at appropriate rate to confirm patency and position		
21	Secures cannula using appropriate dressing		
22	Patient education given and aware of need for prompt communication if any concerns		
23	Identification of cannula site by recording in appropriate documentation, noting gauge, site, reason for insertion, date, time and signature of operator		

Supervisors/Assessor(s):

References

Black F, Hughes J (1997) Venepuncture. *Nursing Standard* **11**(41): 49–55.

Damani NN (2003) *Manual of Infection Control Procedures*, 2nd edn. London: Greenwich Medical Media.

Davies S (1998) The role of nurses in intravenous cannulation. *Nursing Standard* **12**(17): 43–46.

Dougherty L (1996) Intravenous cannulation. *Nursing Standard* **11**(2): 47–54.

Dougherty L, Lamb J, eds (1999) *Intravenous Therapy in Nursing Practice*. London: Churchill Livingstone.

Dougherty L, Lister S, eds (2004) *The Royal Marsden Hospital Manual of Clinical Nursing Procedures*, 6th edn. Oxford: Blackwell Publishing.

Hadaway L (1991) IV tips: venepuncture in the elderly. *Geriatric Nursing* **12**(2): 78–81.

Hadaway L (2004) Preventing and managing peripheral extravasation. *Nursing* **34**(5): 66–67.

Hadaway L, Millam D (2005) On the road to successful I.V. starts. *Nursing* **35**: 1–14.

Hamilton H (2006) Complications associated with venous access devices: part two. *Nursing Standard* **20**(27): 59–65.

Ingram P, Lavery I (2005) Peripheral intravenous therapy: key risk and implications for practice. *Nursing Standard* **19**(46): 55–64.

Ingram P, Lavery I (2007) Peripheral intravenous cannulation: safe insertion and removal technique. *Nursing Standard* **22**(1): 44–48.

Jackson A (1997) Performing peripheral intravenous cannulation. *Professional Nurse* **13**(1): 21–25.

Lavery I (2003) Peripheral intravenous cannulation and patient consent. *Nursing Standard* **17**(28): 40–42.

Lavery I, Ingram P (2006) The prevention of infection in peripheral intravenous devices *Nursing Standard* **20**(49): 49–56.

Lundgren A, Ek AC, Wahren L (1998) Handling and control of peripheral intravenous lines. *Journal of Advanced Nursing* **27**: 897–904.

Macklin D (2003) Phlebitis: A painful complication of peripheral IV catheterization that may be prevented. *American Journal of Nursing* **103**(2): 55–60.

May D (2000) Infection control. *Nursing Standard* **14**(28): 51–59.

Medical Devices Agency (MDA) (2000) *Single-use Medical Devices: Implications and Consequences of Re-use. MDA DB2000 (04)*. London: The Stationery Office.

Millam D (2003) On the road to successful I.V. starts. *Nursing* **33**(suppl): 1–7.

Moureau N (2004) Tips for inserting an I.V. in an older patient. *Nursing* 34 (7) 18–20

NHS Lothian (2007) *Adult Venepuncture and/or Peripheral IV Cannulation: Clinical Skills Education Package*. Edinburgh: NHS Lothian.

Parker L (2002) Management of intravascular devices to prevent infection. *British Journal of Nursing* **11**(1): 240–246.

Rosenthal K (2004) Phlebitis: An irritating complication. *Nursing Made Incredibly Easy* **2**(1): 62–63

Rosenthal K (2005) Tailor your I.V. insertion techniques special populations. *Nursing* **35**(5): 36–41

Royal College of Nursing (2005) *Standards for Infusion Therapy*. London: RCN.

Skills for Health (2004) *HSC72 Cannulation*. Bristol: Skills for Health. Available at: www.skillsforhealth.org.uk/tools/view_framework.php?id=39 (accessed 2 September 2007).

Tagalakis V, Kahn SR, Libman M, Blostein M (2002) The epidemiology of peripheral vein infusion thrombophlebitis: A critical review. *American Journal of Medicine* **113**: 146–151.

Tortora GJ, Derrickson B (2006) *Principles of Anatomy and Physiology*, 11th edn. Hoboken, NJ: John Wiley & Sons Inc.

Wilson J (2001) *Clinical Microbiology: An introduction for healthcare professionals*. London: Baillière Tindall.

Workman B (1999) Peripheral intravenous therapy management. *Nursing Standard* **14**(4): 53–60.

Chapter 17

Recording a 12-lead ECG

Learning objectives

- Review the anatomy and physiology of the heart and its conduction system
- Review the technique for recording a 12-lead ECG and its related equipment
- Discuss potential problems of the procedure, and actions to prevent or reduce these

Aim of this chapter

The aim of this chapter is to review briefly how the heart's electrical conduction works, and to describe the process of recording a standard 12-lead ECG (electrocardiograph). This chapter does **not** discuss how to interpret the recording; *its focus is on the procedure only*. However, Tough (2004) suggested that a doctor must review any 12-lead ECG recording within 10 min, so you must be aware of to whom to report results and within what time frame.

Please note that this is a specialised role and *requires specialised training*, so this role *may be limited to healthcare assistants working in specific practice areas only*, e.g. cardiology ward/clinic. *Check your local policy.*

Relevant anatomy and physiology

Some aspects of the heart have been covered in Chapters 5 and 6; however, as Tough (2004) reminded us, the heart lies in the thoracic (chest) cavity and consists of four chambers divided by the vertical septum (partition). (See Chapter 6 for a diagram of the heart and its chambers.) The upper chambers are known as the left and right atria and the lower chambers as the left and right ventricles.

However, Hampton (2006) suggested that, although the heart *has* four chambers, from the electrical point of view it can be thought of as having only two, because both atria contract together and then both ventricles contract together.

The two main functions of the heart are (Hand 2002):

1. To circulate oxygenated blood to the tissues via the high-pressure arterial system
2. To pump deoxygenated blood to the lungs through the low-pressure venous circulation.

The heart is a small muscular organ, roughly the size of an adult's fist, and is found in the thoracic cavity, immediately above the diaphragm and between the lungs (Hand 2002). The heart beats roughly 70 beats/min (bpm) throughout a person's life and pumps more than 6500 litres of blood a day. Cardiac output (the volume of blood that reaches the tissues each minute) is the most important index of cardiovascular performance, and in adults with a heart rate of 70 bpm gives a cardiac output of 4900 ml/min (Hand 2002).

The heart's conduction system

The heart uses an electrical conduction system to pump blood through the circulation and comprises the sinoatrial (SA) node, atrioventricular (AV) node, bundle of His, left and right Bundle branches and Purkinje fibres (Hand 2002) (Figure 17.1).

Each cardiac (heart muscle) contraction produces a distinctive wave on ECG paper, with each component of the wave being assigned a letter (Henderson 1997). Henderson (1997) and Palatnik and Faran (2007) described the ECG complex (an electrical recording of the events occurring in

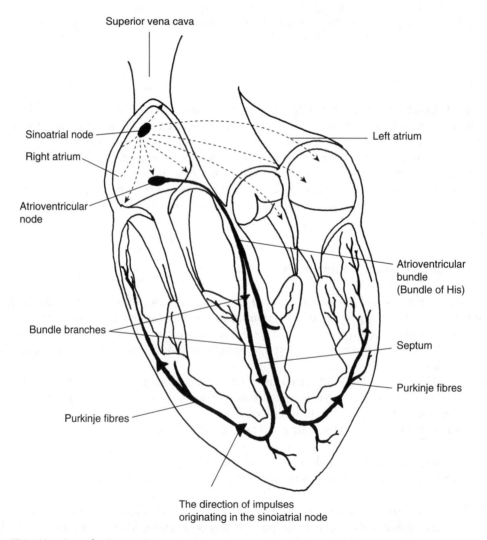

Figure 17.1 Heart's conduction system.

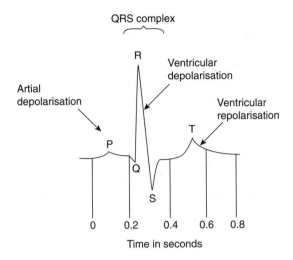

Figure 17.2   The QRS complex.

one cardiac cycle) and this consists of a P wave, a QRS complex and a T wave (see Figure 17.2 for the QRS complex).

- P wave: atrial contraction (known as depolarisation)
- P–R interval: the time required for the impulse to pass the AV node and Bundle of His, and cause ventricular contraction
- QRS complex: represents ventricular contraction
- T wave: represents the resting stage (called repolarisation).

In a healthy heart the size and rhythm of these waves tends to remain constant.

Electricity of the heart

The contraction of any muscle is associated with electrical charges known as depolarisation, and these changes are detected by electrodes attached to the surface of the body (Hampton 2006). Dougherty and Lister (2004) noted that body fluids are good conductors of electricity, so it is possible, through the use of an ECG, to observe how the currents generated are transmitted through the heart. Henderson (1997) indicated that the production of these electrical impulses can be detected on the skin surface, but the currents involved are relatively weak and so the use of an amplification device is required, an ECG machine.

Hampton (2006) added that all muscular contraction will be detected, so the electrical changes associated with the contraction of heart muscle will be clear only if the patient is fully relaxed and no skeletal (bone) muscles are contracting.

Reasons for recording a 12-lead ECG

Dougherty and Lister (2004) noted that the ECG provides a graphic representation and record of the electrical activity as the heart beats, and can pick up changes in the pattern or timing to indicate problems with the heart's conduction, e.g. myocardial infarction (heart attack). While Hampton (2006) describes an ECG as a tool to aid diagnosis, in some cases it is crucial for patient management. The ECG can best identify rhythm abnormalities; however, where a patient is breathless, it may be of value in indicating if there is any underlying heart disease present (Hampton 2003).

Tortora and Derrickson (2006) state that the standard ECG produces views from different combinations of chest and limb leads. By comparing these tracings with each other and normal records, it is possible to determine three things:

1. If the heart's conduction pathway is abnormal
2. If the heart is enlarged
3. If certain regions of the heart have been damaged, e.g. from a heart attack.

How to perform a 12-lead ECG

The ECG test is inexpensive, uses portable equipment, which is easy to operate, and can be undertaken anywhere, including at a patient's bedside, giving a prompt result and allowing rapid treatment decisions and actions to be made by the doctor(s).

Indications for performing an ECG (NHS Lothian 2004)

- After a cardiac arrest
- If the patient complains of chest pain (either recurring or persistent)
- If the patient has a history of collapse or syncope (sudden loss of consciousness)
- In a medicine overdose – if known or suspected
- In confusion of an older patient
- Preoperatively, as a screening process
- Routinely as screening for heart disease
- Routine screening in certain occupations, e.g. pilot
- If the patient has hypertension (high blood pressure)
- If the patient has acute and/or chronic heart failure
- If the patient has valvular heart disease
- Any cardiac arrhythmias (abnormal heart rhythm) – recurring or sustained.

How to record a 12-lead ECG

NHS Lothian (2004) noted that this varies from the standard 12-lead ECG to continuous monitoring (likely in intensive or high dependency units) or even over a 24-hour period (set up as an outpatient). This chapter focuses only on a standard 12-lead ECG where electrodes are placed at strategic points of the chest area and limbs as a diagnostic tool (Henderson 1997).

Preparation for the procedure

Henderson (1997) suggested that many patients will be anxious, so careful explanation and reassurance are essential, e.g. the monitoring device will not affect their cardiac function, and recording is not painful because it is non-invasive. Also reassurance can be offered that there is no danger with electrical impulses or of connection to an ECG machine causing electrocution (Henderson 1997). In fact, Henderson (1997) noted that many patients found machines reassuring; however, this is more likely with constant monitoring, so still need to ensure good communication at all times.

Language and cultural aspects may also be worth considering, so take care to check that the patient understands, and therefore consents to and cooperates with the procedure. As part of the explanation, the healthcare assistant would be asking the patient to remain still throughout the recording because movement can affect results. Allow the patient to ask questions; this helps check their understanding and, if they do not speak English, whether there is a need to use an interpreter (Henderson 1997).

Also consider cultures, as some patients, especially females, may find the need to undress and have electrodes placed around the chest area upsetting. Time taken to reassure and explain is therefore important, as is the offer of privacy and a chaperone if so desired. Some females may prefer a chaperone, especially if the healthcare assistant is male, but a male patient may equally find a female operator embarrassing, so offer all patients the option of a chaperone.

Reflection point

Mrs Wang, aged 82 years, is to be prepared for a standard 12-lead ECG. What might you need to consider if you were going to carry out this procedure?

Recording a 12-lead ECG

This section looks at the equipment required for the procedure the patient preparation and the actual procedure. It also reviews the care of the equipment, before moving on to discuss potential problems and the means of addressing these.

Equipment

The equipment for a standard 12-lead ECG is an ECG machine (with tracing paper), a patient lead cable (with limb and chest leads labelled accordingly), disposable electrodes and paper towel/tissues (Dougherty and Lister 2004). If the patient has a hairy chest, it will be necessary to use a razor to shave the chest area and ensure good skin contact (Henderson 1997).

Care of equipment

Please ensure that the ECG machine is checked regularly, under some maintenance regimen (e.g. annual check), and restocked with the equipment and stored correctly after each use. If battery operated, ensure that it is always plugged into the mains electricity when not in use, so that the battery remains charged (NHS Lothian 2004).

Electrodes

NHS Lothian (2004) described electrodes as sensors, which are placed on specific designated (more later) areas of the patient's skin surface of their chest and limbs. These sensors are usually disposable and self-adhesive, prepared with an inner moist conductive gel and kept stored in the manufacturer's foil packing. This prevents the conductive gel on each electrode from drying out and also protects the sensor from any damage or contamination (NHS Lothian 2004).

Reflection point

You have been asked to carry out a standard 12-lead ECG. What checks of the equipment must you make before proceeding?

Skin preparation

This is essential to ensure good skin contact, otherwise the results may be affected or distorted. Henderson (1997) suggested that, if a patient has body hair, this will impair the connection and so it may be helpful to shave the patient. Please ensure that this is carefully explained to the patient before shaving, to get his cooperation and understanding of the reason for shaving. Henderson (1997) and Hand (2002) also noted that skin sweat can cause adherence problems, so paper towel or dry gauze swab should be used to rub area gently until skin reddens, to remove any dry skin.

Placement of electrodes

NHS Lothian (2004) requested that the expiry date on the foil pack of electrodes be checked to ensure in date and stored correctly, and that all are the same product (electrodes not mixed from different packs). When ready, remove the protective electrode backing to expose the gel-covered disc and ensure that gel is still moist and enough covers the disc.

Hampton (2006) stressed the importance of correct positioning and attachment, because all 10 positions provide a whole record and, if electrodes are wrongly attached, the ECG recording becomes uninterpretable (unable to be read).

Placement of the four limb electrodes: right arm, right leg, left arm and left leg
The electrodes are usually placed on the outer aspect 3–4 cm above the forearm (wrist) and medial (inner) aspect 3–4 cm above the foreleg (ankle) (Figure 17.3a gives the placement). However, if required these electrodes can be placed on another area, e.g. if the patient had a right arm amputation, the electrode can be placed on the right shoulder and this is noted on the record (NHS Lothian 2004). Hampton (2006) indicated that should check and confirm electrode before placing, e.g. LA = left arm, RA = right arm, LL = left leg and RL = right leg (see Table 17.1 for the procedure).

Placement of the six chest leads V1, V2, V3, V4, V5, V6
The electrodes are placed on the chest wall at the designated positions (see Figure 17.3 for placement). NHS Lothian (2004) discussed placement of chest leads in women and noted that electrodes must not be placed on breast tissue, but positioned under the breast from V4 to V6. Hampton (2006) noted that these six chest leads record from six places along the chest wall, overlying (on top of) the fourth and fifth rib spaces (Figure 17.3b). This allows the heart to be looked at from the front left side, as V1 and V2 are over right ventricle, V3 and V4 over the septum (partition) between the ventricles, and V5 and V6 over the anterior (front) walls and lateral (side) walls of the left ventricle (Hampton 2006).

Thus accurate placement is crucial, and is why this role may be restricted to healthcare assistants working in specialist cardiac areas only.

(a)

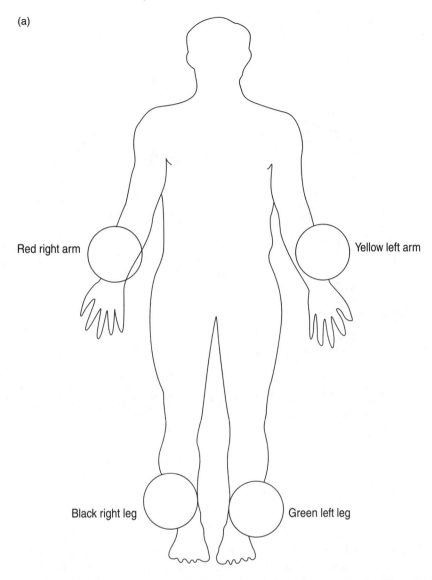

Red right arm

Yellow left arm

Black right leg

Green left leg

Figure 17.3 Electrode and lead placement for standard 12-lead ECG: (a) Limb electrode placement and (b) electrode placement on the chest.

NHS Lothian (2004) offered practical guidance on attaching electrodes for patient comfort and accuracy of reading:

- Chest lead wires should be attached to electrodes first (if snap button type), so avoiding having to press down on patient's chest and causing discomfort and problems with sticking.
- Press down on the adhesive area with a circular motion; do not press directly on centre area, as this can displace the gel and reduce conduction (tracing reading).

Times and calibration of ECG

Hampton (2006) noted that all ECG machines run at a standard rate and use paper with standard-sized squares.

(b)

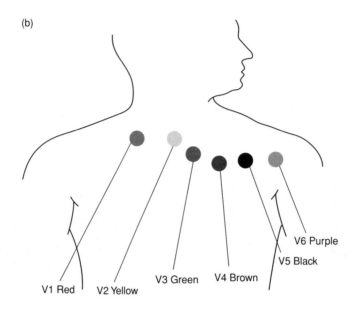

V6 Purple

V5 Black

V3 Green   V4 Brown

V1 Red   V2 Yellow

Figure 17.3   (*Continued*)

▷Delayed

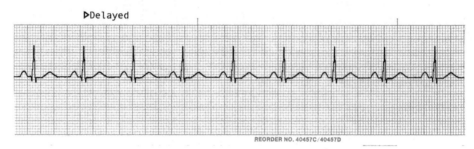

REORDER NO. 40457C/40457D

Figure 17.4   Example of sinus rhythm. Reproduced from NHS Lothian.

For information only
Each large square = 5 mm and this represents 0.2 s, so there are five large squares per second and 300 for 1 min. The standard signal of 1 millivolt (mV) moves the stylus (recording needle) vertically 1 cm (two large squares).

Related aspects and terminology

Even though this chapter does *not cover how to interpret an ECG recording*, it is useful to have an understanding of some terminology relating to the procedure, especially what a normal ECG recording is.

- *Sinus rhythm*: normal rhythm and usually 60–100 bpm; it is regular and complexes (PQRST wave) are identical. The word sinus indicates that the heartbeat originated in the SA node (Hand 2002) (Figure 17.4). Hampton (2003) noted that in a child up to 1 year of age, the rate is 140–160 bpm, falling slowly to 80 bpm by puberty (approximately 10 years old).

Table 17.1 Procedure for recording a standard 12-lead ECG

Action	Reason
Position ECG machine close to patient	Minimise risk of leads, cables, etc. becoming disconnected during the procedure
Check that power cable and patient lead fitted correctly to machine, and route power cable away from patient	Working correctly and minimise any electrical interference
Press power on; multi-lead machine will do self-test, then check machine set at:	To ensure that machine set and working correctly
1 mV or 10 small squares (two large squares)	
Paper speed is 25 mm/s Filter is on; check local policy	
Introduce self and patient provides name and date of birth (DOB); this is checked against identification, e.g. ID bracelet	Ensure correct patient
Patient explanation given to reassure and inform, to allow questions and gain consent	Understand reason for procedure and how it is done, so relaxed and cooperative
Offer patient chaperone, if appropriate	If female patient and male operator this is good practice
Ensure privacy, screens or close door	To protect patient and ensure privacy
Patient resting comfortably, lying if able (semi-recumbent or supine), with limbs supported, arms at sides	To ensure best recording and patient safety and comfort
Ask or assist the patient to undress exposing forearms, chest and forelegs. Ensure modesty; also the patient may need to remove jewellery	To prepare patient for the procedure and ensure no contact with leads from jewellery, e.g. watch
Wash hands or use alcohol gel	To prevent infection
Check that patient has understood that, once the electrodes are in place and test starts, must keep still and breathe normally	Reduce electrical noise (Henderson (1997)
Clean limbs and chest area as outlined earlier: select flat fleshy areas, avoid bony or muscular areas	To ensure that skin has good contact for electrodes and good placement
Place the 10 electrodes, as per Figure 17.3; first ensure electrodes are in date, in foil pack and gel is still moist, e.g. RA = right arm	To ensure accurate reading, and check the patient has no allergy with the adhesive on the electrodes
Attach leads to electrodes correctly (follow colour coding and labelling), e.g. LA = left arm and yellow (refer to Figure 17.3)	Correct monitoring (Henderson 1997). NHS Lothian (2004) noted that manufacturers use different colour schemes so follow UK colour code
Extend patient cable along the side of patient or centre of body from feet to chest	To ensure that all cables fully supported and prevent pulling on the electrodes
Also ensure that the leads are not pulling on the electrodes or lying over each other	To reduce electrical noise from movement and so get good reading
Make sure that patient is ready and relaxed, remind him or her not to talk or cough and allow 10 s for the patient to settle and relax	Procedure proceeds safely

(Continued)

Table 17.1 (*Continued*)

Action	Reason
Commence the 12-lead ECG recording by pushing auto-button	Allow machine to automatically run rhythm strip and leads one at a time to obtain ECG recording
Observe that paper strip is moving and recording	Ensure connected and recording correctly
Observe recording; do not alarm the patient; however, if anxious about the recording, seek advice or support, e.g. ask a colleague to get a senior nurse or doctor, and reassure the patient	It is not the role of the healthcare assistant to interpret; however ,if any irregularity is observed in the rate or rhythm, it may be prudent to get a doctor or experienced nurse to come and check immediately
During procedure reassure patient and explain what's happening	So patient informed and relaxed
If poor tracing (noise – muscle movement), check electrodes, connections and leads, then redo (repeat) recording	Ensure best recording
Before finishing ECG, check first that the recording is free from artefact (noise) and confirm settings: paper speed 25 mm, standard setting 1 mV, 10 mm	Recording technically accurate, so ready for interpretation by doctor
Let the patient know that procedure is finished, what you will do with recording, and then remove the electrodes. Offer to help wipe off the gel and redress, if necessary	Ensure that patient comfortable and aware of next steps
Document as local policy, suggested that ECG has full patient name, DOB, date and time of recording, relevant clinical details, e.g. chest pain during test, ward/department, operator signs (on the reverse of the ECG recording strip) and before leaving patient	Record maintained and accurate details Avoid errors and risk of ECG being filed in the wrong patient's notes
Turn off machine	Save power
Inform a doctor or senior nurse and ensure that doctor sees recording at earliest or agree time frame, e.g. 10 min (Tough 2004)	To ensure that results acted upon and procedure documented
Remove machine and restock; remember to plug into mains if battery operated	Good practice

Adapted from Dougherty and Lister (2004) and NHS Lothian (2004), with permission from G Brady Education Coordinator Cardiology, NHS Lothian (2004).

- *Sinus bradycardia*: regular rate originating from SA node but less than 60 bpm. Hampton (2003) indicated that this can be due to physical fitness or caused by, for example, hypothermia (low temperature) or some medicines, e.g. digoxin
- *Sinus tachycardia*: regular rate also from SA node but 100–180 bpm; this can be in response to stressors, e.g. fever, anxiety, pain, exercise (Hampton 2003). Some stimulants, e.g. caffeine, alcohol, also can cause tachycardia; check the patient history.
- *Sinus arrhythmia*: a known phenomenon (condition) in younger people; heart rate increases as they breathe in and decreases as they breathe out.
- *Atrial fibrillation (AF)*: rapid chaotic depolarisation (contraction) of impulses through the atrial myocardium, replacing normal rhythmic activity by the SA node; can lead to palpitations as

the heart rate is increased (low risk rate below 100 bpm, medium risk heart rate 100–150 bpm, and high risk if rate over 150 bpm – Hand 2002).

- *Atrial flutter*: less common than AF; in contrast with AF the rate is regular and often the tracing is described as 'saw tooth' and rate is often 150, 100 or 75 bpm (Hand 2002).
- *Ventricular tachycardia*: a serious arrhythmia and requires urgent action
- *Ventricular fibrillation* (VF): the rhythm of cardiac arrest, fast irregular rate as the ventricles contract in a chaotic uncoordinated manner. In VF the heart ceases to pump and after about 10 s, the blood pressure falls and the patient loses consciousness. If left untreated, death follows in 3–5 min (Hand 2002).
- *Artefact*: muscular movement that can affect ECG reading/tracing
- *Electrical noise*: as above, but also occurs if leads or power cable are crossed, or the tracing picks up electrical energy from elsewhere, e.g. beds or infusion devices (NHS Lothian 2004).

Hampton (2006) also describes the difference of an ECG (with a 12-lead ECG) where the signal is detected by only five electrodes. One electrode is placed on each limb and the fifth is held on by a suction cup and is then manually (by hand) moved to different positions over the patient's chest.

Common problems and actions

Hand (2002) outlines several tracing problems and indicates they can usually be easily rectified (Table 17.2). Table 17.3 is a competency framework for recording a standard 12-lead ECG.

Table 17.2 ECG recording common problems

Problem	Action
Poor electrode technique often appears as irregular fluctuations (artefact) on the tracing	Improve skin contact, so remove any body sweat or hair, or change electrodes and ensure good skin preparation
Defective cables or a loss of contact with the electrodes produces sharp waveform fluctuations	Replace cable or insert further into machine
Muscular activity (artefact) appears as fast irregular fuzzy fluctuations	Ensure that patient is comfortable and relaxed or reposition electrodes
AC interference – fuzzy, thickened, regular pattern	Ensure that filter is on, check connections, make sure leads, etc. are not being pulled or crossing over. Do not touch during the procedure, and remind the patient to lie still
	If possible switch off other electrical source, e.g. bed; discuss with senior nurse first
Wandering baseline – up and down movement of ECG tracing	Ensure good skin contact, re-apply electrodes, make sure that the machine is close to the patient so that there is no pull on the leads or cable, etc.
Incorrect placement of limb leads – commonly right and left arm leads reversed	Check and swap right and left arm leads if incorrect
Misplacement of chest leads/electrodes	Check and confirm placement of electrode, e.g. V1 and V2 fourth rib space

Adapted from Hand (2002) and NHS Lothian (2004). (Reproduced with permission from NHS Lothian 2004.)

Summary

Recording an accurate 12-lead ECG is crucial. This is because the doctor (or registered nurse if a locally accepted role) will use this recording to make a diagnosis and plan appropriate treatment. Preparation and planning for the procedure and appropriate care throughout are therefore essential.

Case study 17.1

Fred Jones, aged 53 years, has been admitted for cardiac tests. He is anxious and has never been in hospital before. You have been asked to record a standard 12-lead ECG. Describe how you would prepare him for the procedure.

Case study 17.2

Betty Davis (aged 76 years) has been complaining of chest pain for 5 min and you have been asked to carry out a standard 12-lead ECG recording. Describe how you would position the electrodes and leads and carry out the procedure.

 ## Self-assessment

Assessment	Aspects	Achieved ✔
Patient	*Have you considered all aspects of this section?*	
	Patient assessment	
	Selection for lead and electrode placements	
	Communication and educational factors	
	Infection control and skin preparation aspects	
	Positioning patient and equipment	
Equipment	*Have you considered all aspects of this section?*	**Achieved ✔**
	Care of the equipment	
	Storage and maintenance of equipment	
Procedure	*Have you considered all aspects of this section?*	**Achieved ✔**
	Equipment and technique	
	Consent, communication and education	
	Problem solving	
	Recording	
	Reporting concerns and procedure completion	

Table 17.3 Competency framework competency: recording a standard 12-lead ECG

Steps	First assessment/Reassessment					Date/competent/signature
	Demonstration/supervised practice					
Recording a Standard 12-lead ECG	Date/sign	Date/sign	Date/sign	Date/sign	Date/sign	
	1	2	3	4	5	
1 Patient's identity confirmed as per local policy						
2 Procedure explained, verbal consent gained						
3 Assembled all equipment required, checked that ECG machine stocked						
4 Machine checked, cable/leads correctly in place, machine self test done, confirmed all settings set as standard						
5 Patient screened and prepared, undressed and jewellery removed						
6 Patient's comfort considered and positioning appropriate for safe practice						
7 Washed hands or used alcohol gel						
8 Skin sites on limbs and chest area selected correctly						

(Continued)

Table 17.3 (*Continued*)

Steps	First assessment/Reassessment					Date/competent/signature
Recording a Standard 12-lead ECG	Demonstration/supervised practice					
	Date/sign	Date/sign	Date/sign	Date/sign	Date/sign	
	1	2	3	4	5	
9 Selected sites correctly cleaned and prepared – sweat or hair removed						
10 Electrodes applied to designated sites, connections pointing in line with direction of cable and lead wires						
11 Confirmed all electrodes/leads connected to power cable correctly and positioned correctly						
12 Explained when procedure starts that patient must not move, talk or cough						
13 Waited 10 s for patient to settle and tracing to stabilise						
14 Pressed auto button and monitored tracing – ensure working correctly						
15 Confirmed ECG machine working and settings correct during procedure						
16 If problem with recording, checked and corrected problem						

17	Reassured patient during procedure								
18	Acted on concerns, if any, to appropriate person								
19	Checked final recording acceptable quality, then documented required information on paper recording								
20	Switched off machine								
21	Helped patient clean skin and dress, as necessary								
22	Explained next steps to patient								
23	Washed hands								
24	Machine removed and restocked, stored correctly								
25	Procedure reported to designated doctor or senior nurse – check local policy and document as required								

Supervisors/Assessor(s):

References

Dougherty L, Lister S, eds (2004) *The Royal Marsden Hospital Manual of Clinical Nursing Procedures*, 6th edn. Oxford: Blackwell Publishing.

Hampton JR (2003) *The ECG Made Easy*, 6th edn. Edinburgh: Churchill Livingstone.

Hampton JR (2006) *The ECG in Practice*, 4th edn. Edinburgh: Churchill Livingstone.

Hand H (2002) Common cardiac arrhythmias. *Nursing Standard* 16(28): 43–53.

Henderson H (1997) Electrocardiography. *Nursing Standard* 11(44): 45–56.

NHS Lothian (2004) *Recording a Standard 12-lead ECG NHS Lothian – university hospitals division*. Edinburgh: NHS Lothian.

Palatnik AM, Faran CK (2007) Get heart smart. *Nursing Critical Care* 2(3): 13–16.

Tortora GJ, Derrickson B (2006) *Principles of Anatomy and Physiology*, 11th edn. Hoboken, NJ: John Wiley & Sons Inc.

Tough J (2004) Assessment and treatment of chest pain. *Nursing Standard* 18(37): 45–55.

Index

Page numbers in *italic* type indicate figures; those in **bold** indicate tables or boxes. Please note that figures, tables and boxes are only indicated when separated from their text references.